Included **2 Video DVDs** *and* **3 Audio CDs**

The Magic of
Ilizarov

- **Techniques** • **Tips** • **Tricks**
- **Pitfalls** • **Methods**

L Prakash

MS (Orth), MCh (Orth) (Liverpool)
Institute for Special Orthopaedics
Chennai, Tamil Nadu

with contributions

Jishnu Baruah
MS (Orth), MCh (Orth) (Liverpool)
Dibrugarh, Assam

Sandeep Adke
MS (DNB) (Orth), FRSC (Kurgan, Russia)
Solapur, Maharashtra

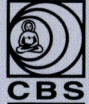

CBS

CBS Publishers & Distributors Pvt Ltd

New Delhi • Bengaluru • Chennai • Kochi • Kolkata • Mumbai
Hyderabad • Nagpur • Patna • Pune • Vijayawada

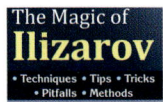

ISBN: 978-93-85915-93-2

Copyright © Authors and Publisher

CBS Edition: **2017**

Published by Satish Kumar Jain and Produced by Varun Jain for
CBS Publishers & Distributors Pvt Ltd
4819/XI Prahlad Street, 24 Ansari Road, Daryaganj, New Delhi 110 002, India.
Ph: 23289259, 23266861, 23266867   Website: www.cbspd.com
Fax: 011-23243014   e-mail: delhi@cbspd.com; cbspubs@airtelmail.in.
Corporate Office: 204 FIE, Industrial Area, Patparganj, Delhi 110 092
Ph: 4934 4934   Fax: 4934 4935   e-mail: publishing@cbspd.com; publicity@cbspd.com

Branches

- **Bengaluru:** Seema House 2975, 17th Cross, K.R. Road,
  Banasankari 2nd Stage, Bengaluru 560 070, Karnataka
  Ph: +91-80-26771678/79   Fax: +91-80-26771680   e-mail: bangalore@cbspd.com
- **Chennai:** 7, Subbaraya Street, Shenoy Nagar, Chennai 600 030, Tamil Nadu
  Ph: +91-44-42032115   Fax: +91-44-42032115   e-mail: chennai@cbspd.com
- **Kochi:** 36/14 Kalluvilakam, Lissie Hospital Road, Kochi 682 018, Kerala
  Ph: +91-484-4059061-65   Fax: +91-484-4059065   e-mail: kochi@cbspd.com
- **Kolkata:** 6/B, Ground Floor, Rameswar Shaw Road, Kolkata 700 014, West Bengal
  Ph: +91-33-2289-1126, 1127, 1128,   e-mail: Kolkata@cbspd.com
- **Mumbai:** 83-C, Dr E Moses Road, Worli, Mumbai-400018, Maharashtra
  Ph: +91-22-24902340/41   Fax: +91-22-24902342   e-mail: mumbai@cbspd.com

Representatives

• **Hyderabad**	0-9885175004	• **Nagpur**	0-9021734563	• **Patna**	0-9334159340
• **Pune**	0-9623451994	• **Vijayawada**	0-9000660880		

Printed at: Rashtriya Printers, Dilshad Garden, Delhi, India

Preface

Transosseus Osteosynthesis is a revolutionary concept in orthopaedics by which bone can be made to grow even after skeletal maturity. Not only bone, but nerves, vessels, tendons, muscles, ligaments, fascia and even skin can be made to grow. This is possible by a unique and revolutionary system introduced by GA Ilizarov of Kurgan, Siberia in 1951. The Ilizarov system produces miracles, which always cause awe, and elicits standing ovations in orthopaedic conferences, due to their apparently magical results.

This system gained popularity in 1990 and gradually rose to its peak until 2000, by when it had become popular all over the world, *with surgeons producing similar reproducible results worldwide*. Then came an era of wholesale modifications in the design of the apparatus, and an increasing tendency to replace the thin wires with thick Shanz pins. Around this time started a decline in the popularity of the system. Surprisingly, by 2015, the popularity of the system had declined to such an extent that it was infrequently used only in a few centres, and most younger generation orthopaedic surgeons were either unfamiliar with, or afraid of, this system.

When I resumed orthopaedic practice after a thirteen years break, I was surprised to find that Ilizarov had completely gone out of fashion, and both surgeons and patients were scared of the system. Having experienced the unique capabilities of this system, I understood that the problems were manifold. A few badly-applied frames and improperly done surgeries, wholesale design changes deviating from the Ilizarov principles, the heavy frame and rings, improper indications, lack of thorough understanding of the scientific principles, and a paucity of training facilities probably caused this decline in popularity.

The first five patients I saw after my return were all complications of internal fixations, and I applied the Ilizarov frame in four. The results (as I expected) were spectacular, and my internet posts and shares to various orthopaedic groups brought many comments and more questions. I suddenly realized that a large number of orthopaedic surgeons is unfamiliar with this magical system, and existing books are voluminous and too theoretical to allow a surgeon to actually operate after reading them.

This book attempts to fill that gap. If you are a young surgeon, with limited or no experience in Ilizarov system, this book will at least dispel all your apprehensions and allow you to begin applying basic frames, and experience the magic of osteosynthesis. If you are a practising Ilizarov surgeon or a specialist, you will find something to appreciate or criticize. I have shared my thirty years of experience with this system, and sincerely hope that my readers enjoy reading this as much as I enjoyed writing it in British English.

L Prakash

Foreword

I have the great pleasure of knowing Dr L Prakash for the last 30 years, and have seen him evolve from an aggressive surgeon to a mellowed, dedicated, observant, scientist, artist, genius, thinker and teacher. L Prakash, one of the earliest surgeons to perform Ilizarov surgery in Chennai, is one of the most experienced surgeons in this field. I have always admired his passion, both for his teachings and skilled surgical work.

In this book, he has reminded us of the forgotten Charnley's wisdom: "Orthopaedic surgeons should be more like gardeners than carpenters. And bones should not be viewed in isolation, but as a part of the limb."

It is thus both a pleasure and privilege to write the foreword of this wonderful book. This book is lucidly written and reads like a novel, yet it is as educative as a journal. The two significant scientific contributions of the book, which can be understood from a quick first reading, are a new classification of deformities, and a treatment-based classification of non-unions. Every aspect of this system is covered in a practical *how-to* manner, making it invaluable for any surgeon interested in, or using, this system.

Whether you are a resident junior surgeon, someone attempting to start this procedure, or even an experienced Ilizarov surgeon, there is certainly something that you can learn from this book. It is with great pleasure that I dedicate this book to the Art and Science of Orthopaedics.

Dr Mayilvahanan Natarajan
MS(Orth), MCh(Orth)(L'pool), PhD, DSc, FRCS, DSc(Hon)[3]

Acknowledgements

My father Mr TS Lakshmanan and mother Radha Lakshmanan, my friends, philosophers, guides, and gods.

My beloved sister Dr Pramila Ramaswamy, and Dr TS Ramaswamy, to whom I owe everything in my life.

My teachers in orthopaedics: Dr Ved Prakash Middha, Mr IW Young, Mr John Goodfellow, Mr MAR Freeman, Mr BM Wroblowski, Mr John Taylor, Mr CJ Monk, Mr Kieth Thompson, Mr William Boyle, Dr KH Sancheti, and Dr DP Bakshi who taught me all the orthopaedics I know.

Dr Mayilvahanan Natarajan, my best friend for always being there.

Dr Jishnu Baruah of Assam and Dr Sandeep Adke of Solapur for valuable contributions and inputs.

Dr RK Baruah, Dr Arvind Verma Jangid, Dr Nishant Ranjan, Dr H Das, and Dr Md. Arifuzzaman for clinical cases and examples.

Mr TG Seshadri, Mr M Babu and Mrs Tahira Begum, who helped me to stretch my day well beyond 24 hours.

My good friend and editor, Mr Ashok L Rajani, a wordsmith par excellence, for editorial suggestions and corrections.

All my patients who trust me with their life and limbs.

L Prakash

Contents

Introduction

Orthopaedic surgeons are generally a conservative lot. Most of us do not like to rush into doing anything new and untried. We wait for proven results before abandoning established methods. But once the method establishes its utility, we do not hesitate to jump on to the bandwagon. The field of Orthopaedics is full of turning points; each has heralded another era in patient care. And development of various new principles have relieved the sufferings of many. During the First World War, hundreds lost their extremities due to femoral fractures before Hugh Oven Thomas developed the **Thomas splint, s**aving countless limbs.

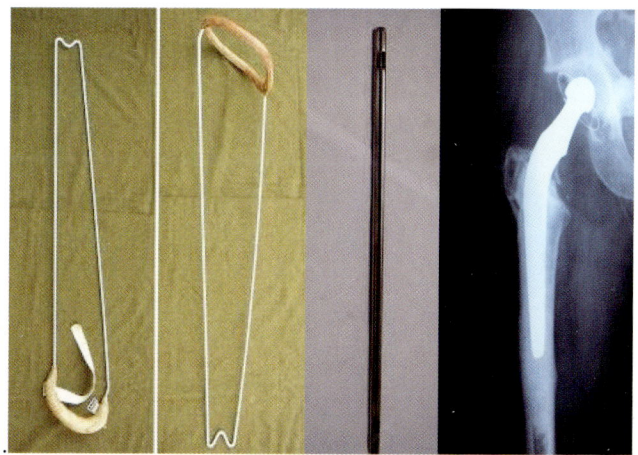

Picture 1: The Thomas splint, K-nail and Charnley hip have been turning points in orthopaedic surgery.

Operative treatment of femoral shaft fractures was revolutionized by **Kunchner** when he developed the intra medullary nail. **Charnley** came up with the principles of low friction arthroplasty, and this laid the foundation for joint replacements the world over. The Swiss **AO group** established the fundamental principles and biomechanical aspects of fracture healing and have achieved miracles in fracture fixation. All these great developments have initially been met with doubts and skepticism. But once their value was proven, surgeons came forward to accept the methods.

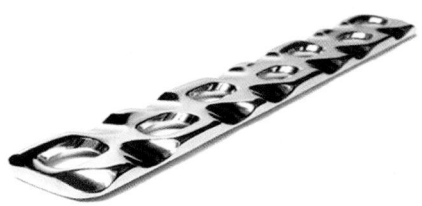

Picture 2: The AO group and its internal fixation methods have set standards for fracture treatment.

The development of Ilizarov fixations falls in the same category. Though invented as early as 1951 by Dr. Gavriil Abramobich Ilizarov, it caught the fancy of orthopaedic surgeons only in the recent past. Hundreds of difficult and complicated orthopaedic surgeries (performed in Russia, Italy, France, America and elsewhere) using Ilizarov's techniques bear testimony to the versatility of this system.

It is interesting to note that in the early nineties, when the ASAMI group was formed, there was a sudden increase in the use of this system. After a trail blazing season, where successful surgeons got miraculous results, while those not understanding the biomechanical aspects produced disasters, the system slowly faded away. A decade's overuse and misuse had made this system so unpopular that its use declined dramatically. By 2015, only a few and selected centres in the world regularly performed this complex and demanding procedure. However, in the recent past, the large number of diaphyseal non-unions caused by implant failures has again caused a resurgence of interest towards this system.

The so-called "improvements and developments" in the apparatus could probably be a cause for its declining popularity. K-wires are a little tricky to introduce; the fear of impaling vessels or nerves made many surgeons switch to thicker Shanz pins. However, the Ilizarov fixation is not just rings alone. The magic is principally in the thin wires. (I will reveal further details in the biomechanics part.) These so-called *improved fixators* and *hybrid fixators* were associated with numerous problems, which contributed further to its declining use.

At first glance, the Ilizarov system seems an extremely complicated and cumbersome system. But as one gets into the methodology of orthopaedic applications using the system, one realizes that this is indeed the beginning of a revolution. Amongst the therapeutic modalities in orthopaedic literature, this alone can be used in such diverse applications as fractures, non-unions, limb lengthening, deformity corrections, tumours, skin coverage, TIA, and even osteomyelitis.

In countries like India, this system has tremendous advantages. Bad results from improperly applied apparatus by surgeons unfamiliar with the biomechanics should not allow a revolutionary invention to be maligned.

1. Despite the numerous units of the apparatus, most components can easily be manufactured using locally available materials and manufacturing infrastructure.

2. The operation causes minimum trauma and blood loss to the patient; and unlike joint replacements, the operation theatre does not need to be very highly specialized.

3. The clinical material available in India in the form of a multitude of deformities lends itself wonderfully to this system.

4. The sudden increase of implant usage in fresh fractures, and the complications resulting from them, have produced an extremely large pool

of infected non-unions <u>with a properly done Ilizarov as the only alternative</u> <u>to amputation</u>.

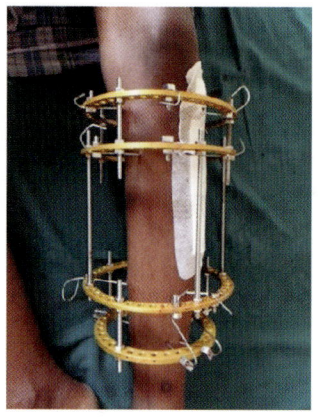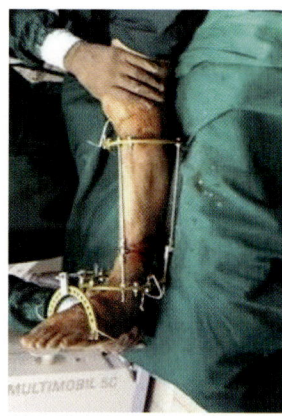

Picture 3: The Ilizarov apparatus has proved to be a revolution in orthopaedics.

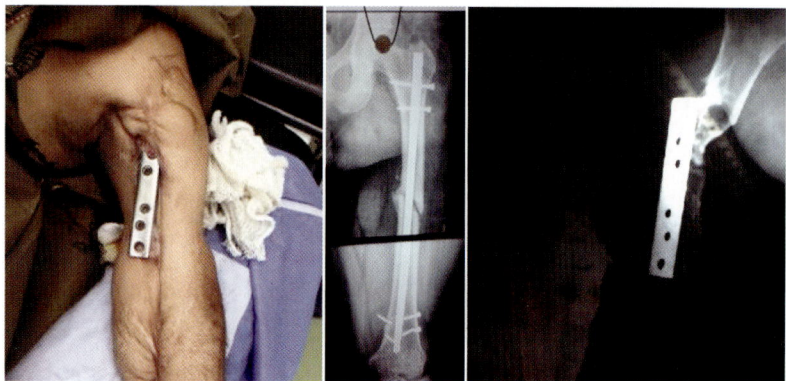

Picture 4: Complications from internal fixations are on the rise

My first introduction to this system was in 1987, when a group of Polish surgeons visited Madras. At that time, we had a patient with grade three compound fractures of both tibiae sustained due to a vehicular accident. The surgeons were willing to demonstrate their method; on one leg, an Ilizarov frame was used, which took over two hours for application. On the other side, our team applied a standard tubular external system in less than half the time. Though the patient recovered uneventfully and both fractures united well almost simultaneously, *the patient was a lot more comfortable with the tubular system than with the circumferential system.* I was personally not very impressed by the system then, and hence did not evince any further interest in using it.

It was only much later, somewhere around 1991, when there was a resurgence of interest in the methods of this system, that I realized I had thrown away a wonderful opportunity. What had gone wrong had been the **indication,** not the **system**. As with any other tool available to the orthopaedic surgeon, it is of paramount importance to have an indication right; then and only then will the patient and surgeon benefit from the procedure.

From 1991 to around 2001, I performed over 1000 surgeries, developed my own bangle paediatric fixator system, started a company manufacturing these instruments, and conducted over 70 courses and workshops in places as diverse as Colombo, Kuala Lumpur, Singapore, Dhaka, Indonesia, Thailand, Satna, Madras, Visakhapatnam, Davengere, Kollam, etc. which were attended by a large number of surgeons. During and after the courses, extensive feedback was received, and this helped me in a writing the first two versions of this book, keeping in mind the problems and doubts faced by most surgeons in using this system.

I was out of action from 2002 to 2015. After my return to active orthopaedic practice after 13 years, I was invited as guest faculty to a national Ilizarov conference with the original Kurgan team. Invited to give a few lectures, I struggled to locate old records and was preparing for my talk, when a sudden splurge of patients needing this system began coming to my clinic. In a month, I did about 11 cases, and each gave me different challenges. I had planned a career as a revision arthroplasty surgeon, but fate had decided something else for me! I was forced to research and re-learn about Ilizarov, which led to conferences, talks, publishers, and this book!

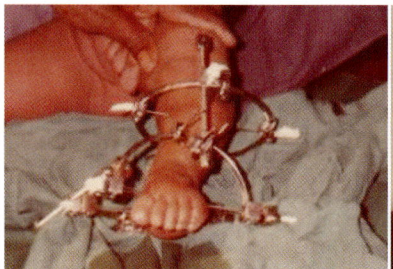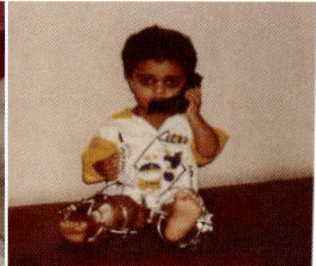

Picture 5: Ilizarov frame finds application in diverse situations

As a word of caution, I would like to add that this book on Ilizarov fixation systems is more of a hands-on manual than a text book. I have attempted to make you familiar with biomechanical principles, various instruments and the usage, different applications to the systems, and given a few examples of how system works. I have also given a *new classification of non-unions.* This is probably the first time that *deformities have been classified according to the therapeutic paradigms necessary for treating them.* The main idea is that if the reader is going to use the system occasionally, this comprehensive book should be a reasonably competent reference manual to help you to do the job well. In case you are embarking upon treating difficult and complicated problems, or you plan to concentrate solely on this system in your orthopaedic practice, it is advisable that standard text books on the subject be consulted or special training obtained at an institution where such procedures are being performed regularly. The three lessons which will be repeated throughout this book are:

1. Use the lightest and strongest ring that the patient can afford.

2. Try to use only K-wires as far as possible. Introduction of Shanz pins spoils the frame's biomechanics and leads to delay in bone formation.

3. Be prepared for a long haul, and motivate the patient accordingly. Patience is the most sought-after virtue during the use of this system. Unlike plates or nails, this is not a *fix and forget* surgery. Here constant tweaking, refining, adjustments and changes are needed. More like gardening and less like carpentry.

Ilizarov, the Man and the Machine

Gavriil Ilizarov was the sixth child of a poor Jewish peasant family in Białowieża, Polesie Vvodeship, Poland. Soon after his birth, the family moved back to Qusar, where he grew up. The family was poor and Gavriil was unable to attend primary school. However, he made up for it by passing the programme for missed school children when he was eleven years old.

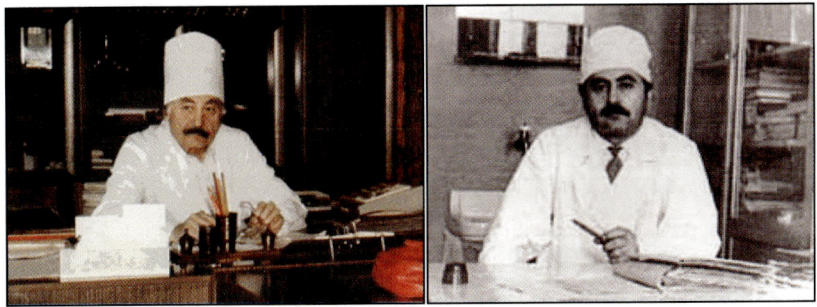

Picture 6: G.A.Ilizarov, the magician of Kurgan

As a child, when Gavril was seriously ill, he was cured by a medical assistant and was impressed by the profession of a doctor. This led to his enrolment in Buynaksk Medical Rabfac (an educational establishment set up to prepare workers and peasants for higher education). He then joined Crimea Medical School in Simferopol. After the outbreak of Communism in 1941, the school was evacuated to Kyzylorda, Kazakhstan. On completing his medical education in 1944, Ilizarov was posted to a rural hospital in Dolgovka, a village in Kurgan Oblast, Siberia, 2000 km east of Moscow. And it was here that the magic happened!

Ilizarov encountered a number of unstable fractures, splinted inappropriately. He was always of the opinion that the rigidity of a fracture immobilization was the cause of absence of discomfort. The splints were inadequate and external fixators were unavailable, because those were the Communist times. The best medical facilities only existed in Moscow, and Kurgan in Siberia was close to the so-called "rehabilitation camps", which were actually prisons probably harsher than today's Puzhal prison, a place where I had the good fortune of having spent a considerable time.

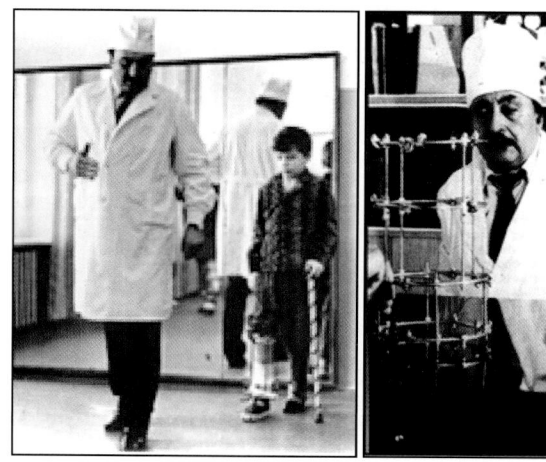
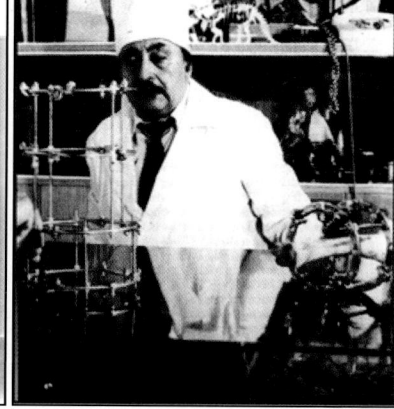

Picture 7: Archive photos of the master

At that time, the Politbureau of Moscow faced another problem: the **war-disabled**. Shells, bullets, grenades, blasts, compound fractures, segmental bone loss, discharging pus, popping out sequestrate, and hobbling anxious men were not too easy to handle in the top Moscow hospitals. Medicine in those times was highly politicized. And Communism meant equality for all except the Politbureau. I had the good fortune of personally meeting G. A. Ilizarov in 1991 and spent a considerable time with him. His translator was inadequate, but gestures conveyed his impressions. This is *my* translation of what he told me:

"In my country the bosses decide what is right and what is wrong. As a surgeon in War Veterans' hospital, I was earning 330 roubles, while the ward boy who pushed the stretcher to the operation theatre earned 360 roubles. In Moscow, they buy CT scans just as soon as they are invented. In Siberia, I had to beg for six years to get a portable X-ray machine."

It was under such dirty politics that two things happened simultaneously. The *powers that were* decided to start a hospital in frozen Siberia so that the war veterans could be shunted out of sight. And in 1955, they appointed Ilizarov as the Chief of the Department of Trauma and Orthopaedics in the Regional Hospital for War Veterans in Kurgan. By then, he had already tried out a bone stabilization system which produced such miraculous results that he was afraid to tell the world about it! It was spectacular enough to be considered black magic and could surely get him into trouble in communist Russia.

His out-of-the-box thinking was either an accident or sheer genius. Kurgan at that time had two major industries: a battle tank factory and bicycle factory! Using the engine bearing rings of the tanks, threaded rods (m6) from tank spares and spokes of bicycles, he created his own fixator: the ILIZAROV FIXATOR. Serendipity in action!

"I used wires because stainless steel threaded pins were unavailable. I discovered the process of tensioning by accident as I found that over tightened wires were painless with no pin track problems, as opposed to lax wires. Those spokes were not even stainless steel, just chrome plated iron. But still I got good results."

This stable fixator had quite a few inherent advantages, which even the inventor was not aware of! But that will come later. By 1954, he had accidentally discovered about corticotomy and regenerate. These were his own words in

Chennai shared during vodka and dinner. The translator was wholly inadequate, but Ilizarov had excellent body language and gestures. Here is what I understood of his talks:

"I got a segmental fracture tibia with bone loss. The upper fracture was closed an inch below the knee. The lower fracture was open two inches above the ankle. I put my fixator and wanted to compress the lower half. I did not want vessel kinking and planned for slow compression. I was willing to accept a two inch shortening. The patient was given a spanner, given instructions and sent home. I went away on a holiday. I saw him only after two months. He had misunderstood the instructions and distracted the proximal fracture while compressing the lower one."

I was not an Ilizarov expert when this talk happened in the lawns of a five star hotel in the early nineties over vodka. What I could not understand then suddenly came to me in hindsight. He would have advised a distal-to-proximal compression, but the confused patient would have done a proximal-to-distal, resulting in **a bone transport.**

"I was amazed!" Ilizarov gushed. "This was a little out of the ordinary," translated the sedate stone-faced translator. But the gestures said it all! And then was born a revolution in orthopaedics!

By accident he had discovered that by carefully severing a bone without severing the periosteum around it, one could separate two halves of a bone slightly, fix them in place, **and the bone would grow to fill the gap**. He also discovered that bone re-grows at a fairly uniform rate across people and circumstances.

These experiments led to the design of what is known as an Ilizarov apparatus, in which an osteotomy is gradually stretched by turning the nuts on a threaded rod, causing the dramatic appearance of new bone to fill the gap, provided the frame is precisely applied.

For a long time, Ilizarov faced disbelief, skepticism, resistance and political intrigues from the medical establishment in Moscow, which tried to defame him as a quack. However, the steadily increasing statistics of successful treatments of patients lead to a growing fame of Ilizarov throughout the country. He became known among patients as the **"magician from Kurgan"**.

*"So much politics in Russia in 1967! I had written my thesis **for Candidate of Sciences degree** and was all ready for submitting it, when a senior KGB officer's son had a gap non-union tibia, with nine failed operations in Moscow. I cured him, the grateful father pulled strings and got me a Doctor of Sciences for the same thesis!"*

And thus in 1968 he was a D.Sc. Another breakthrough came in 1968 when Ilizarov successfully operated on Valeriy Brumel (1964 Olympic champion and a long time world record holder in the men's high jump) who had injured his right leg in a motorcycle accident. Before coming to Ilizarov, Brumel had spent about three years for unsuccessful treatments in various clinics and had undergone seven major and 25 minor surgeries. After treatment at Kurgan in 1970, he could clear 213 cm in high jump.

But it was explorer and photojournalist Carlo Mauri, an Italian mountaineer with a tibial fracture from a skiing accident ten years ago, metal fixation, infected non-union and oozing pus, who became his celebrity patient. On the urgings of his Russian colleague Yuri Senkevich, Carlo Mauri travelled to Kurgan in the Soviet Union, where Ilizarov treated this tibial fracture. Italian doctors had long given up hope of any surgical improvement to the leg. Ilizarov distracted the stiff non-union in the tibia by 2 cm, healing the pseudoarthrosis, corrected an equinus deformity by distraction and lengthened his leg. Mauri dubbed Ilizarov "the Michelangelo of Orthopaedics".

On Mauri's return to Italy, the healing of his leg amazed local orthopaedic surgeons. Subsequently, Ilizarov was invited by Antonio Bianchi-Maiocchi and Roberto Cattaneo to be a guest speaker at the AO Italy conference in 1981 in Bellagio. Ilizarov gave three lectures at the conferences to more than 200 delegates from Italy, France, Switzerland, Austria, and Germany. At the end of the lectures, Ilizarov earned a ten minute standing ovation. This was the first time Ilizarov spoke outside the Iron Curtain.

In 1986–1987, the technique was brought to North America by Victor Frankel, president of Hospital for Joint Diseases, and Dror Paley and Stuart Green, who edited the first English translation of Ilizarov's book in 1992. Over 300 American orthopaedic surgeons attended an international symposium in 1987 in New York by the Hospital for Joint Diseases and M/s Smith & Nephew to hear Ilizarov's lectures. Smith & Nephew started the distribution of the Ilizarov external fixator in the USA and worldwide. And then of course commercialism took over!

I met Ilizarov in 1991 a few months before his death. This is my translation of what I could understand:

"I'm waiting to be made a member of the Academy, Russian and USSR."

By now however he had accumulated dozens of international awards and enough column centimetres (nay, metres) in newspapers to make him an unforgettable part of orthopaedics.

The opposition by the Moscow medical establishment continued until the last years of Ilizarov's life. Only in 1991, just one year before his death, Ilizarov was elected a full member of the Russian Academy of Sciences. Despite numerous awards and world-wide recognition, he was not elected to the USSR Academy of Medical Sciences.

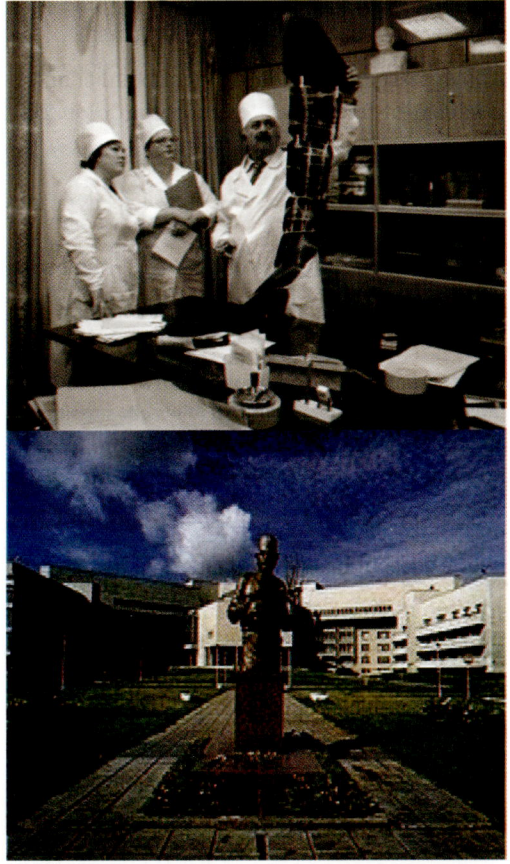

Picture 8: The Kurgan hospital has honoured the master with this bronze statue

I had a chance to spend quality time with his long time assistant Shevetsov in 2015 during the Solapur conference; this time, the interpreter was better. And I end this chapter with Shevetsov's opinion of Ilizarov:

21

"Ilizarov was a meticulous scientist, a little stubborn, and difficult to change. Once he had found the formula, and after meeting with Kritchner, he was of the opinion that frame dynamism is only wires. Exchange a single wire with a pin and you mess up everything. вы испортить." (You spoil everything!)

Micromotion, callus formation, and post fracture bone behaviour

Fractures seem to have minds of their own insofar as their healing time is concerned. Of course, there are certain norms and principles that the fracture healing adheres to. All of us have experiences of similar fractures taking very different courses in spite of identical methods of management. If we pause to think, similar transverse tibial fractures in young adults, all treated by a locked tibial nail, take different times to heal. Similar results have been reported with treating closed tibial fractures with a long leg cast followed by PTB casts. Few of them throw abundant callus and consolidate in under three months, while a number of them remain mobile at the end of a year. Further, some throw an abundant callus but no evidence of a bony bridge. On the contrary,

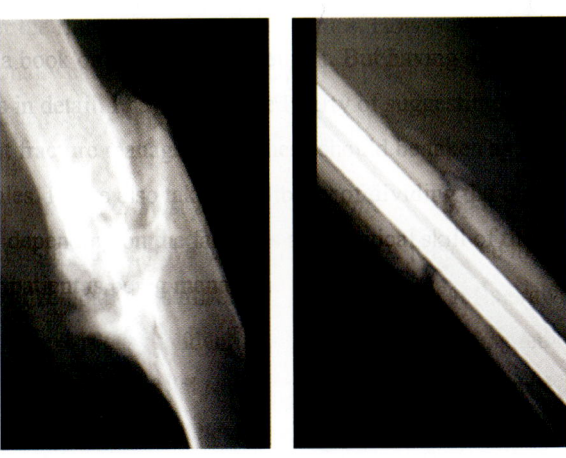

Picture 9: Whether treated with a plaster or internally fixed, non-unions do happen

23

others show little evidence of external callus, but go on to a sound union relatively fast.

Should this not make us pause and think? Do we know enough about the processes of fracture healing? Is it not essential to have a more detailed knowledge of the fracture healing process to enable us to plan a more scientific manner of fracture management towards the ultimate goal of speedy return to function?

If we examine orthopaedic literature, we find a lot of established factors which have a very significant bearing on fracture healing and the time taken to achieve the same. Children, of course, heal faster than adults, and upper limb fractures heal a lot faster than lower limb fractures. Bones that have a precarious blood supply or fragments that are starved of blood (either due to their anatomical situation or due to surgical manhandling) will logically suffer from a delay in callus formation. The questions that arise at this moment are:

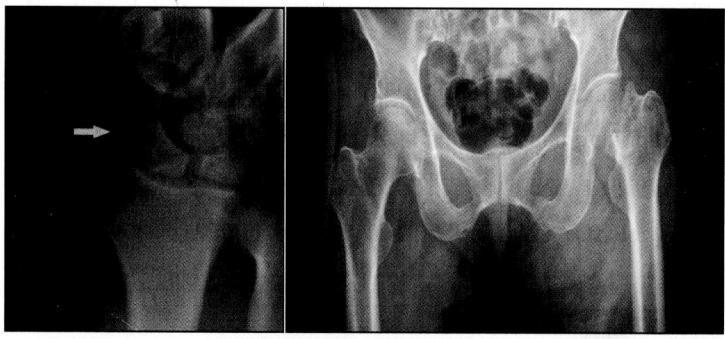

Picture 10: Scaphoids and neck of femurs were identified as non-union sites by anatomists long ago.

Whether callus alone is all that important?

Do we desire callus, or do we want bone bonding?

If we analyze published literature, it would emerge that the anatomist has done more research into fracture healing than the surgeon. Scaphoid fractures, neck of femur, lower tibia and ulna have all merited extensive study by our anatomist colleagues.

Children, having a faster metabolism, are obviously endowed with a much better perfusion. Upper limbs, being closer to the heart, are not gravitationally dependant and get a better blood supply. Naturally fractures in these will heal faster and better, or at least better callus will form. But unfortunately, not much effort has been made in identifying the factors that aid bone bonding.

It has been realized from ancient times that man does not heal bones; Nature does. From Egyptian times to our own Sushruta, Hippocrates to Bohler, or Hugh Owen Thomas to Sarmiento, the general consensus was that bones retained immobile in anatomical position would heal, if given time! Against much opposition, it was **Augusto Sarmiento** who advocated return to weight bearing while still in a cast.

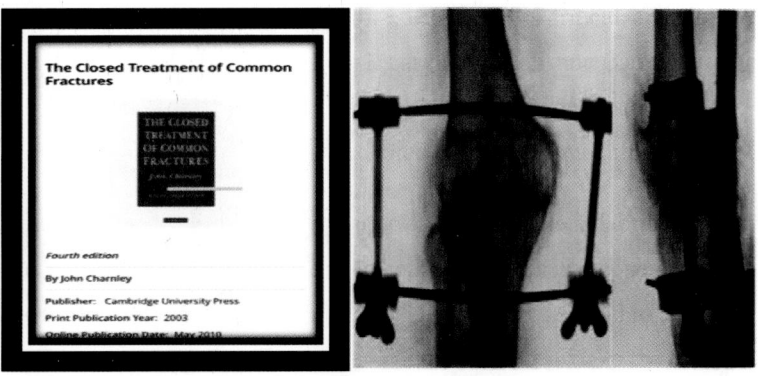

Picture 11: Sir John Charnley understood that compression causes bone bonding.

He reported that compression makes fractures heal faster!! This thought was expanded upon by Charnley.

Sir John Charnley was a genius. His book on closed treatment of common fractures is still a classic. He realized early that compression of bone ends speeds up bone healing. His compression clamps revolutionized knee arthrodesis which was previously an uncertain procedure.

His work was expanded in a linear fashion by the AO group of Switzerland, who can be credited with extensive biomechanical, animal experimental and clinical research, leading to pioneering and extensive developments in the knowledge of fracture healing and newer treatment modalities. Their initial studies were concentrated exclusively on compression, leading to union without visible callus. "Primary Bone Healing" was the key phrase. Their rule book said thus:

1, Hypertrophic non-unions did not require any grafting.

2, Atrophic non-unions would join if resected and compressed, provided a little shortening was acceptable.

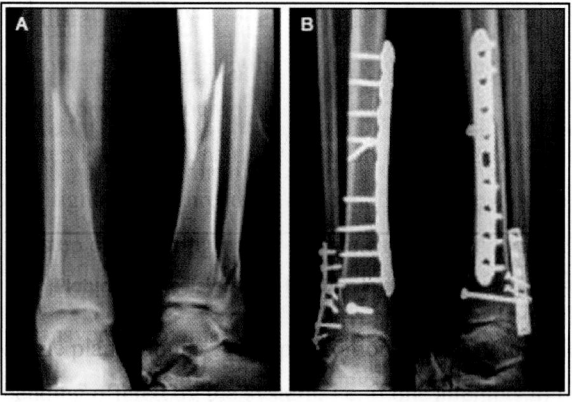

Picture 12: Primary bone healing is not always a good thing.

3, Fresh fractures had to be rigidly fixed and primarily compressed if one had to get them to unite.

Even fracture healing was defined either as primary or secondary. Fractures were not accepted as properly fixed if there was evidence of callus. A proper rigid and compressive fixation was invariably associated with apparent healing without a callus formation. But AO methods did not stand the test of time.

Trouble started with troublesome implants associated with full function and radiological *Primary Union*. This was the group of patients who were back to work; X-rays looked perfect, but patients had minor implant irritation due to protruding screws, or fibrosis around metal (one to three years post surgery). However, in a few of them, the fracture just fell apart when the implants were removed, proving that it was the implants which were bearing weight and functioning. Bones were still not inclined to get united! This made the AO hastily announce their implant removal guidelines in 1987, in which they urged caution.

By now, the AO group realized that callus is not a bad thing after all. They came to understand that though callus formation and bone bridging were different yet interrelated factors, it did not necessarily mean that bones have to always unite without callus. *Primary bone healing* was not always the desired thing! Instances of fractures falling apart two years later when the plate was removed, situations of a radiological trabecular continuation after three years was proved false after implant removal, cases when the surgeon was in a dilemma whether to remove the implant or not all contributed to the newer development of *dynamization*.

Once the fracture become sticky and was on its way to mending, would it not be appropriate to allow nature to take charge? Was there not enough truth and evidence to back Sarmiento's teachings? Was callus detrimental?

As the Swiss group was developing and researching the other parameters of bone healing, they too realized what Charnley had propounded earlier. The findings were strikingly clear: *There was no rigidity about rigidity of fixation.* Micromotion was in fact beneficial, provided it was applied in the correct manner and direction. Callus formed due to micromotion could indeed be beneficial if it was conducive to bone healing and a bone would heal much faster, more rapidly and better if assisted by callus, rather than on its own. The interlocking nails that gave an extremely rigid fixation were dynamized by removal of distal or proximal screws to allow motion at the fracture site, thus aiding and assisting the healing of fractures.

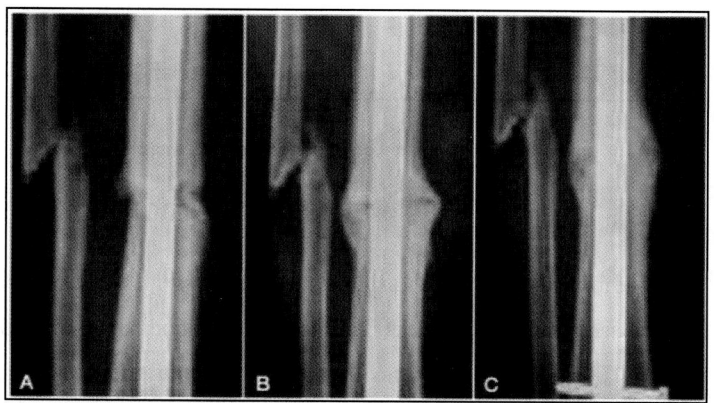

Picture 13: Linear telescoping or dynamization throws up a lot of callus

Mention should be made here of the work of De Bastiani of the University of Verona in Italy and his Orthofix fixators. He too realized that after the fracture had become sticky enough to make sure that displacement would not occur, if the rods or even the pins were loosened, the micromotion resulting from this loosening would definitely speed up callus formation and fracture healing. Orthofix International stemmed from his work. During the end of the 1970s, Bastiani proposed the concept of *"Dynamization"* based on the natural ability of

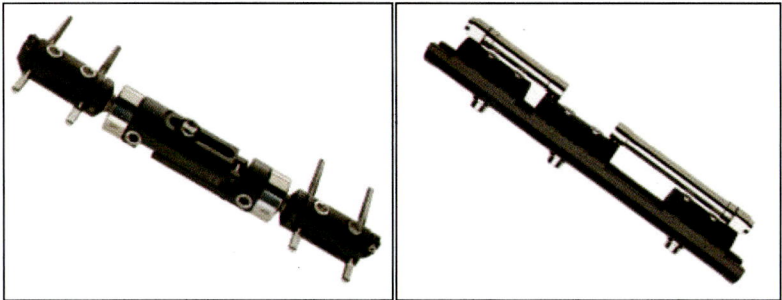

Picture 14: The Debastiani Orthofix fixator

bone to repair itself. He developed a modular system of external axial frame devices that could be fitted to a bone, allowing micromotion at the fracture site to stimulate bone healing. De Bastiani founded Orthofix Srl in 1980 in order to continue the development of the device and launch it as a commercially available product.

Sarmiento, in his monumental work on cast bracing, had earlier propounded the same theory! Beneficial micromotion after the fracture has become sticky enough to resist displacement will surely lead to a much faster fracture healing and bone bonding.

A very interesting factor emerges at this juncture. The AO dynamic compression plates with their very rigid fixation and extremely mechanical primary compressive action lead to a perfect primary fracture healing in most cases. But there have been a large number of patients where this has gone wrong despite a strict adherence to AO principles. This is what forced the ASIF group in Switzerland to revise their theories. Surprisingly, the problems after the usage of AO type DCP plates in India have been relatively infrequent. An observation in this context has been made by Dr. G. A. George of Kollam, Kerala:

"India being a poor country. most patients cannot afford costly imported plates and screws. Most DCPs that are being used are not AO DC plates but AO type DCPs made locally. If one takes the trouble of studying the profile of the locally available plates, one finds that the holes in the plate do not have a compressive profile at all. Plates look like the Swiss ones, but actually have just oval holes instead of compressive profile holes. These oval holes cannot be used with a loaded drill guide and do not give any compression at the fracture site whatsoever. However, their ovality permits micromotion in the linear direction while rigidly preventing angular, rotatory and distraction forces. Thus all the DCP plates made locally seem to make fractures heal rapidly with some amount of callus and our surgeons are not troubled with the handicap of rigid fixation. " This observation by a keen surgeon throws a lot of light over the problem of union versus callus.

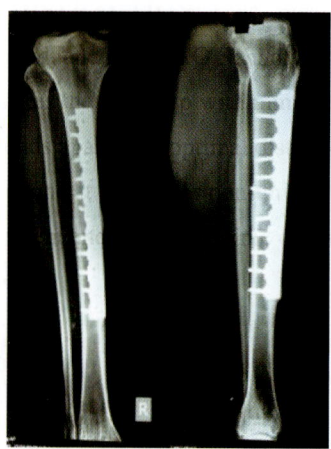

Picture 15: Oval hole DCPs unite with visible callus due to linear motion.

With the above factors in mind, I was forced to get my mental ball bearings rolling and set the gears clicking to understand if some fundamental principles about healing of fractures could be laid down. I do not claim to have made any earth shattering discovery! I would just like to share with you, my dear reader, my experiences and thoughts. My observations and theories! My knowledge from the published literature and my observations from my clinical experience! All I request is that you indulge me! And pardon me if I am erratic or dogmatic.

I am placing before you my theories regarding fracture healing and its relevance independent of established factors like age, site, type, communition, communication to the exterior and infection. *Fracture healing has a lot to do with micromotion.* After a bone breaks, nature makes a war front effort to bond the bone. The torn micro vascular structures bleed. A hematoma forms. The calcium metabolism is stimulated and hydroxyapatite crystals jump to the site of bone breakage. Then start nature's efforts to glue the break; the subsequent steps taken by the body are entirely dependent upon the factors prevailing at that time. Capillaries that supply the callus will obviously keep supplying if not disturbed.

If a fracture is distracted, it will obviously have no surfaces to bond. Thus all femoral shaft fractures treated by indiscriminate over traction will definitely have to go into a non-union. Humerus fractures treated by hanging casts suffer the same fate. Straightforward moral: No callus, no union!

Examples of hanging casts for the fractures of the shaft of the humorous, tibia fractures treated by calcaneal pin traction and mid shaft femoral fractures treated by heavy skeletal traction are all too well known to senior surgeons familiar with conservative management.

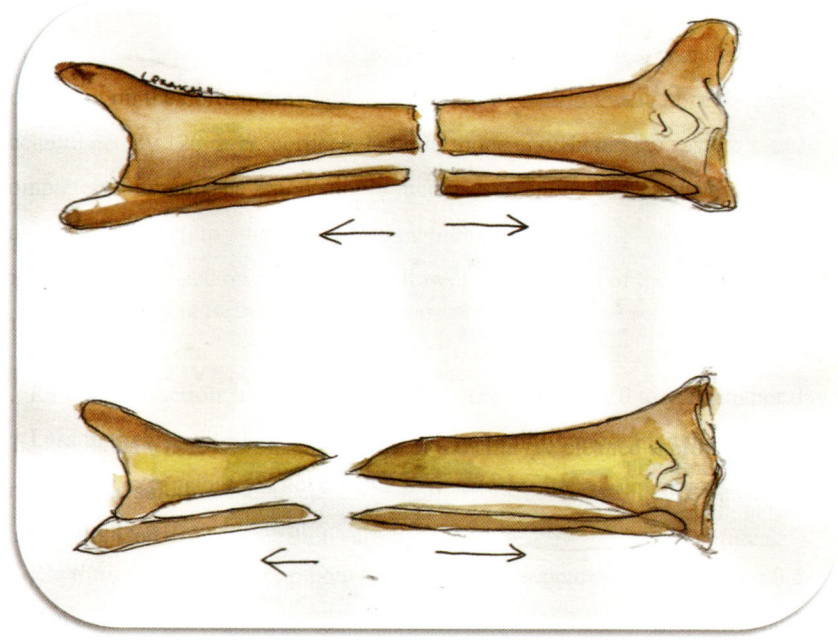

Picture 16: Distraction causes atrophic non-union

Thus we can infer that distraction produces a non-union. With no stimulus for callus formation, an atrophic or hypotrophic non-union occurs.

On the other hand, if a fracture is rigidly immobilized, there is enough stimulus for bone bonding, but not enough for callus. The greater the compression, and greater the degree of rigidity of immobilization preventing micromotion, greater is the lack of callus formation. Visible callus seen on radiographs, fancifully termed as external callus, is never in evidence. Obviously, bone bonding or the rate of healing cannot be evaluated clinically. This causes enough hardships to the clinician to make him confused about the processes of bone bonding.

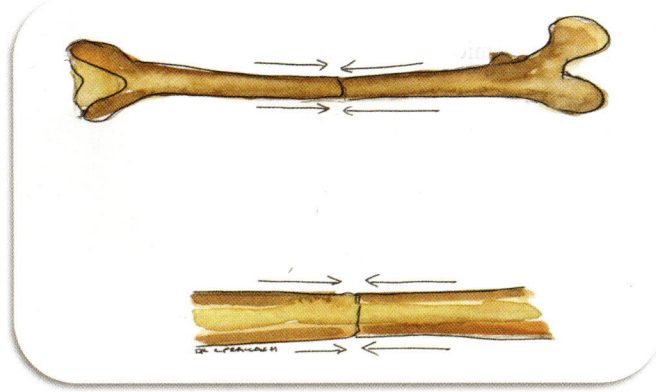

Picture 17: Primary compression causes union without much callus.

On the contrary, if the fixation is not rigid, the micromotion that occurs will show new bone formation. The callus seen after *inadequate fixation* (with due apologies to the AO group), is considered as secondary healing. On the other hand, if the fixation is extremely rigid, it is difficult to distinguish the state of the fracture from Day 1 to Day 100. No external callus is in evidence and it is quite possible to err on the side of fanciful imagination of trabecular continuities. We all have experiences of plates removed after 18 months and the fracture still falling apart!

Thus, the second conclusion that emerges is: *Massive compression does not allow satisfactory bone bonding*. Too rigid an immobilization produces no callus and the bonding of a fracture that occurs cannot be termed strong.

If micromotion occurs at the fracture site, it stimulates callus formation. By this, it must by no means be inferred that callus formation and bone bonding are the same! The type of callus formation directly depends on the degree of micromotion. Woolf's' law explains the piezo-electric influences and the deposition of calcium hydroxyapatite $(Ca_5(PO_4)_3(OH))$ at the site of bone breach, as a result of movements at the fracture site. Each day, nature sends in its influences. Mini capillaries will flood the fracture site. Callus will be deposited. Nurtured with an atmosphere of immobilization, this immature callus will heal and solidify. If micromotion continues, then additional callus will be thrown up. Many times, the callus formed is more than needed to join the bones and produce bonding. But it still continues to form as long as the stimulus continues.

Based on the above, it can be only logically inferred that if the fracture situation is subject to angular micromotion, the hinge of the angle will have compression. The pylon of the angular motion will be subject to distractive and compressive forces, and this will lead to a one sided hypertrophy and no bone bonding. Thus we are likely to have a situation where *angular micromotion produces a one sided hypertrophy.*

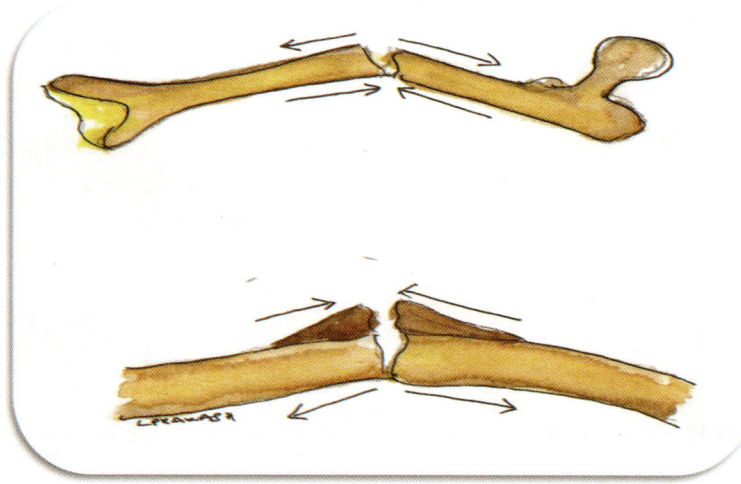

Picture 18: Angular micromotion causes hypertrophy at compression axis but atrophy on the distraction point and produces a horse hoof non-union.

Let us now look at the scenario that allows a rotatory motion at the fracture site. Each day, at a specified speed and rate, callus formation occurs. Even rotatory compressive micromotion is conducive to this callus formation. But even before the two ends have a chance of joining, the next bout of rotation occurs and breaks the bondage. Callus formation however continues unrelented and thus forms a hypertrophic non-union. Horse hoof or elephant foot? Whatever you call it, the fact remains that this pattern of motion (which stimulates bone formation but does not allow bone bondage) will cause a hypertrophic non-union. The third conclusion: *Rotatory micromotion thus causes a hypertrophic non-union.*

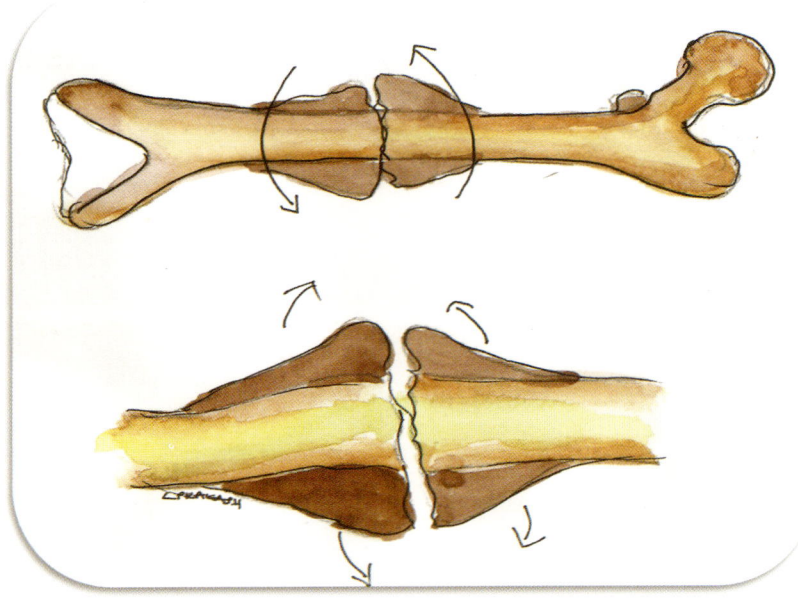

Picture 19: A rotatory micromotion causes hypertrophic callus without union. Elephant foot type.

The other end of the scale is a side-to-side shift. Here, there is no contact between the broken ends, thus no stimulus is possible. Irrespective of the amount of motion, even if it is a macro or mega motion, as there is no stimulus, obviously no bone will form. Thus happens the atrophic non-union, bringing us to our fourth conclusion: *Side-to-side shift without regular bone contact causes an atrophic non-union.*

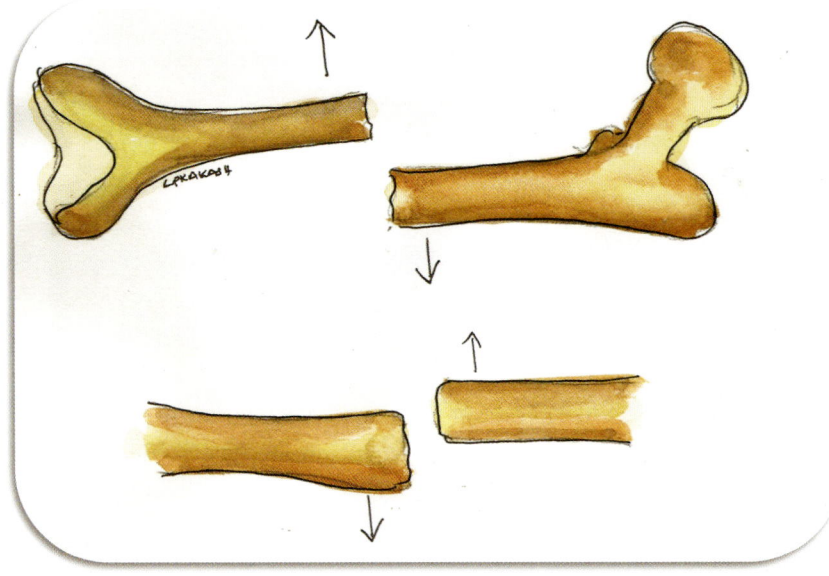

Picture 20: Side-to-side shift causes atrophic non-union.

At this stage, it can be safely inferred that a *micromotion which is minimal but in the axis of linear push pull, delivers the optimal compression and distraction to stimulate the formation of healthy callus,* and the callus will eventually be of the type that will ensure bone bonding. Having understood this in the last few decades, even the AO School has revised its opinion about rigidity of compression and they too are talking about micromotion. These observations assume greater credibility when we realize that if a tibial fracture on a uniaxial frame is slow to throw callus, we are advised to dynamize it by loosening the clamps at one end. Likewise with interlocking nails, after the fracture has become sticky, it is advised to remove the distal locking screws to permit dynamization allowing for a quicker fracture bonding.

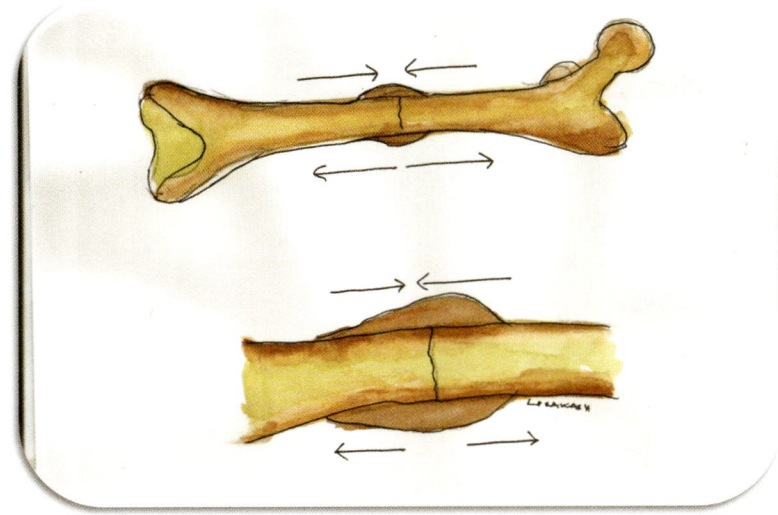

Picture 21: Telescopic micromotion with rotational stability causes union with healthy callus

Many examples abound in our clinical practice to prove this contention. When a fracture is on external fixator for quite some time and there is no evidence of callus, an occasional patient attempts to walk and loosens a few pins. Micromotion happens in the linear direction and a rapid production of callus results. Likewise, if fractures are treated by plaster immobilization of a joint above and below until the fracture is sticky, and then when cast braced, the mere fact that mobility is stimulated results in a rapid growth of callus at the fracture site.

THE ACCIDENTAL DISCOVERY

Gavril Ilizarov made a revolutionary discovery purely because of a concatenation of three accidents: Battle tanks, bicycle factory and war veterans' hospital. If we understand the biomechanical principles of the ring fixation system, we can appreciate how this handles fracture healing. The rigid fixation of the threaded rods to the ring assembly resists rotatory and angular stresses and thus favourably eliminates the harmful micromotion. Pure massive compression and distraction can be clearly avoided at all times by simple screw turnings, keeping the surgeon in control at all times. And of course, the icing on the cake is K-wires, which are used for bone-to-ring anchorage.

Unlike uniaxial pins acting as cantilevers and allowing extreme rigidity in one axis and inadequate stability in the opposite axis, tensioned pins not only allow for a uniform distribution of forces along the entire length of the wire, but a tensioned wire is never completely stiff! Thus the wire will buckle, but only in one axis and that too under load. Once the load is removed, it will immediately return to its pre-deformation state. This lurchiness at the pin bone site is capable of delivering the telescopic compressive dynamic forces at the fracture site, in spite of the rigid anchorage between the frame assembly and the rods.

Thus, with Ilizarov frames, we are able to retain beneficial micromotion at the fracture site, and at the same time avoid harmful micromotion. Likewise, the immense rigidity in all other planes makes it unnecessary to wait until the fracture becomes sticky before subjecting the fracture to dynamic stresses. Rather, the frame itself allows controlled dynamization from the day one!

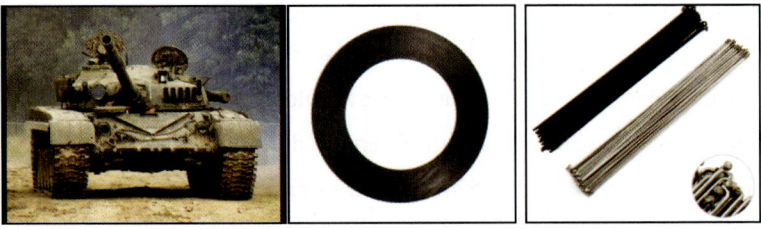

Picture 22: Battle tank steel gaskets and bicycle spokes made the first Ilizarov frame.

With the above preamble to the movements at the fracture site, and in line with the present opinions about fracture healing, the present generation surgeon may no doubt be faced with various methods of fracture management. From the primitive wooden splints to rigid internal fixation, from uniaxial to Ilizarov external fixation, fracture management has seen innumerable methods. There can of course be no hard and fast rules regarding how to treat a fracture. Each system of approach has its own prejudices and shortcomings. Dogmatism about one system always causes surgical embarrassment.

SO WHAT CAN WE INFER FROM THE ABOVE IS;

1. An implant which attempts to functionally bypass biology has a good chance of failure.

2. Bones heals despite internal fixation, *certainly not due to them*!

3. Nailing buggers up the medullary blood supply, while plating screws up the periosteal and nutrient supplies. Screw holes cause thermal necrosis.

So internal fixations are not biological, but only tools for early return of patient's functions. If a patient is patient, and can afford a few weeks or months of compliance with treatment away from his work and responsibilities, almost all diaphyseal fractures can be treated conservatively with excellent results.

This is NOT a book on fracture management. But having discussed fracture biomechanics in detail, I have taken the liberty of suggesting some norms and theories about fracture management. These should be taken as suggestions rather than rules. I have also taken the liberty of dividing the management into three groups, depending on the facilities and surgical skill of the centre where the particular patient is being managed.

FRACTURES IN CHILDREN:

1. Almost all fractures have to be managed conservatively, except intraarticular fractures (where an open reduction and stabilization with K-wires may be preffered).
2. If a C-Arm is available, a percutaneous pinning after closed reduction is acceptable. Never plate children!
3. Except in femoral fractures in children around 14 years or above, internal fixation should be avoided in children as far as possible. Where prolonged traction is not desired by parents, femoral fractures can be nailed.

FRACTURES IN THE ADULT:

1. Intraarticular fractures have to be managed by accurate reduction and proper fixation, but only if facilities are adequate. An infected implant is an irritation to the surgeon and a lifelong misery to the patient.
2. Fractures that will not unite conservatively, e.g. femoral neck, should be routinely operated.
3. Undisplaced or reducible comminuted fractures, unless intraarticular, should be managed conservatively by an accurate reduction and immobilization followed by rapid cast bracing. The only reason for operations in this group will be unacceptability of plaster by the patient.

FRACTURES IN THE POOR OR UNDERPRIVILEGED:

1. Please ensure that economic burden of treatment does not spoil the life of a whole family!
2. A mal-union in a functional position or a functional pseudoarthrosis is better than pouring pus or an infected implant!
3. Please remember that functional results are always more important than radiological or anatomical results!

Bio-mechanics and pathophysiology of the Ilizarov system

Here, we shall briefly discuss the bio-mechanical principles involved, specially focusing on the differences between the standard uniplanar and biplanar fixators *vis a vis* the triplanar ring fixation system.

Linear stiffness

Ring fixation system is less stiff in the linear axis than conventional single plane systems. But there is an increased elasticity characterized by an instant return to its pre deformation state after removal of the deforming forces. This means that

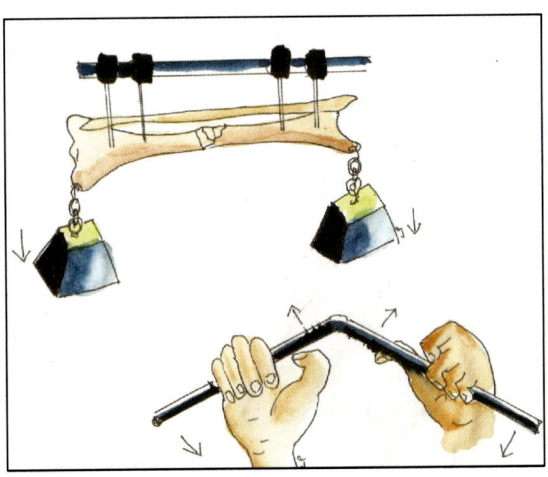

Picture 23: Resistance to bending is called linear stiffness.

though the Ilizarov frames are less rigid than conventional frames, they are inherently dynamic. Ilizarov fixation systems are more elastic and therefore, more biological than conventional systems.

Shear stiffness

This refers to the resistance of the fixator to rotatory stresses. In case of conventional fixators, this stiffness is very high in the plane of the pins and low in the plane without the pins. If we try to imagine a rigid uniplanar system like

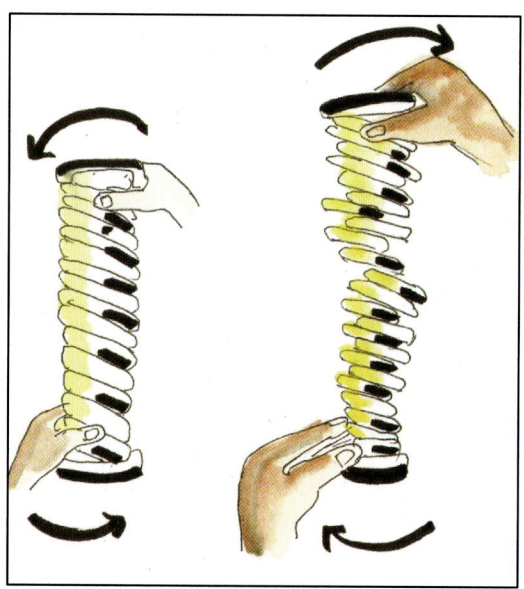

Picture 24: Resistance to twisting is shear stiffness.

orthofix or a single plane tubular AO type fixation, it is easy to understand the resistance to bending offered by the system, i.e. if one attempts to bend the system in the axis of the pins and fixator, a tremendous amount of resistance is encountered. But if the same forces are applied in an axis at right angles to the plane of the pins and fixator, much less resistance is encountered. Conversely, with the ring fixation system, shear stiffness is more uniformly distributed in the circumferential plane depending on the placement of the connection rods.

Axial stiffness

This is the ability of the fixator to resist compression distraction. In other words, if the fixator is applied with a gap between bone ends, the high axial stiffness will lead to greater resistance to gap closure. Conventional fixators have high stiffness to axial loading, but low stiffness to bending loading. On the contrary, Ilizarov fixators have low stiffness to axial loading and high stiffness to bending and loading. Thus, we find that conventional fixators are not inherently dynamic but need to be dynamized. Dynamization of conventional fixators is achieved by the telescopic facility and is not always physiological, because mechanical problems like jamming of the telescopic rods can frequently occur. On the other hand, the tensioned wires inherently allow for elastic micromotion in the linear axis, and hence afford the opportunity for physiological dynamization.

On studying the literature regarding the relation between micro movement and fracture healing, it is evident that cyclical axial micromotion is beneficial, whereas transitional and rotatory shear at the fracture site are detrimental to union/ healing. With compressive immobilization, no callus forms and healing occurs by what was termed as "primary bone healing". Later studies with the use of semi-rigid devices showed that the micro movement actually produces an increased amount of callus. Uncontrolled movement will not only produce excess callus, but will also lead to a situation by which the fracture will fail to unite by a bridging callus, leading to a hypertrophic non-union. Hence, it appears that the ring fixation system possesses some of the most optimal biomechanical characteristics for fracture healing by permitting the desired movement and resisting the detrimental movements in an assembly

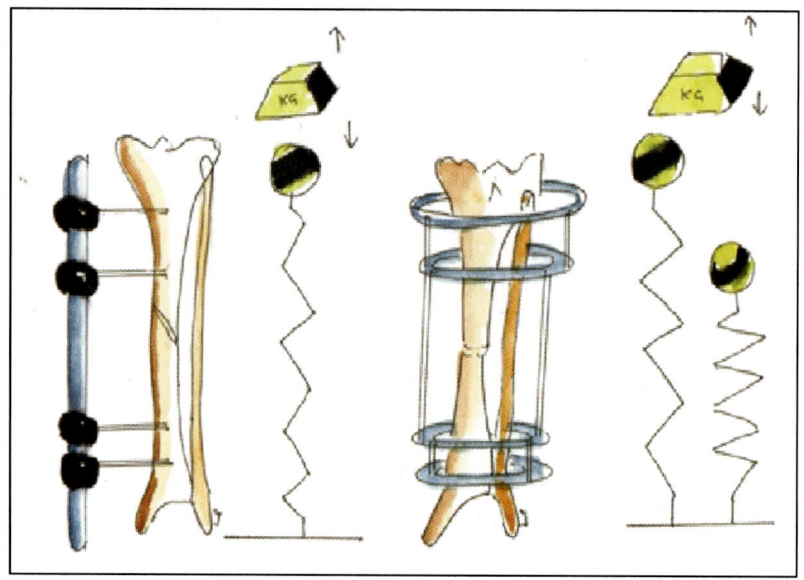

Picture 25: Resistance to collapsing is axial stiffness.

PATHOPHYSIOIOGICAL ASPECTS

Over the years during which this system has been in use, an entirely new dimension to the pathophysiology of the bone and soft tissues has emerged. These phrases were first introduced by Ilizarov.

CORTICOTOMY: We all perform *osteotomy*. So what is *corticotomy*? It is no different, except for the manner in which it is performed. Through a very small incision, the bone is exposed. *The periosteum is cut longitudinally*. A specially designed chisel is introduced inside the *periosteum* and cuts the cortex alone without theoretically disturbing either the *periosteum* or the medullary blood supply. (Whether this is always practically possible is a matter of conjuncture.) The posterior aspect of the cortex, unapproachable by the chisel, is broken by gentle external manipulation.

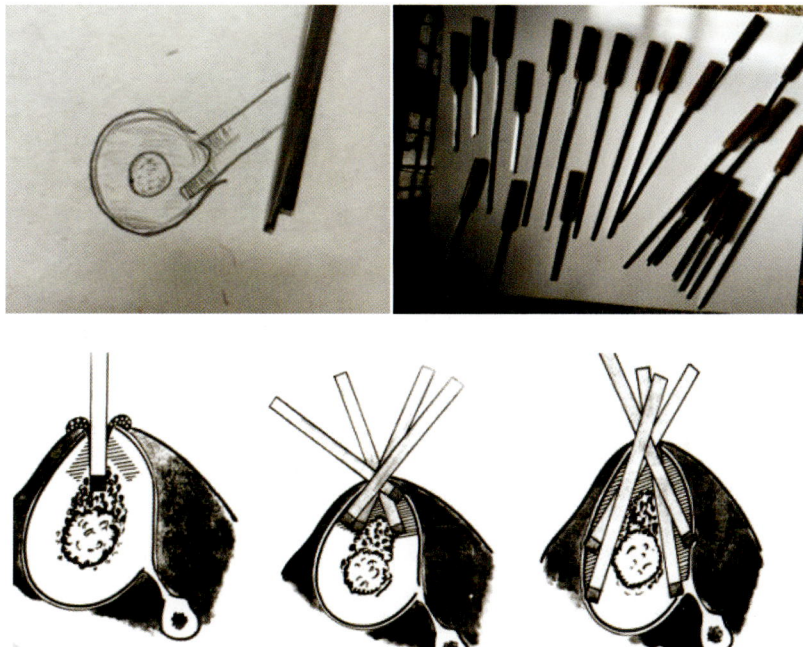

Picture 26: The special chisels used for corticotomy and the method of cutting cortex alone without damaging periosteum and medulla.

REGENERATE: An English translation of a Russian word used to describe the new tissue generated as a result of lengthening operation. This tissue forms at the corticotomy site after the elongation procedure is started. Though this initially referred only to the callus and bone that developed due to distraction, "regenerate" now also refers to skin, sub cutaneous tissue, fat, tendons, muscles and neurovascular structures in that area, which all expand simultaneously.

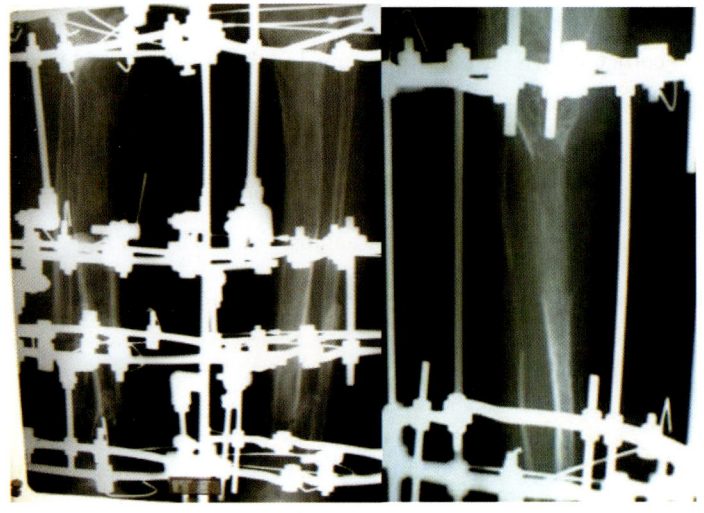

Picture 27: Gradual distraction produces new bone, called regenerate.

COMPRESSION AND DISTRACTION: These mean the same as they sound. As John Charnley reaffirmed, and as the AO School has stated, compression of the bone ends together makes them join up with minimum callus. Distraction means keeping the bone ends apart with optimal distance. Distracting the bone ends either produces new bone at the site or non-union and cyst formation, depending on the environment and the speed/ time of distraction. More details are given later in this chapter.

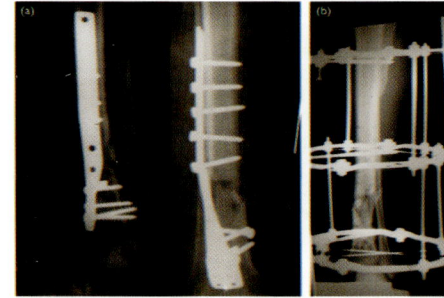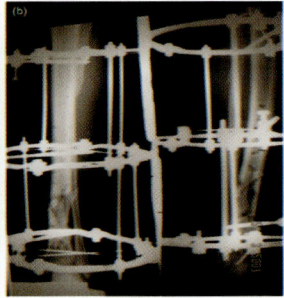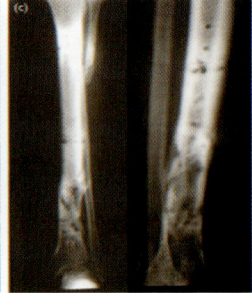

Picture 28: Bone transport is a unique concept of this system

BONE TRANSPORT: This is a fantastic concept where one treats a gap non-union. A corticotomy is performed proximal to the gap and the middle fragment is pulled away from the upper fragment as in bone elongation. As a consequence, this narrows the bone gap, and the middle and lower fragments are compressed together to produce union. This technique is of great value in pseudoarthrosis, and infected gap non-unions.

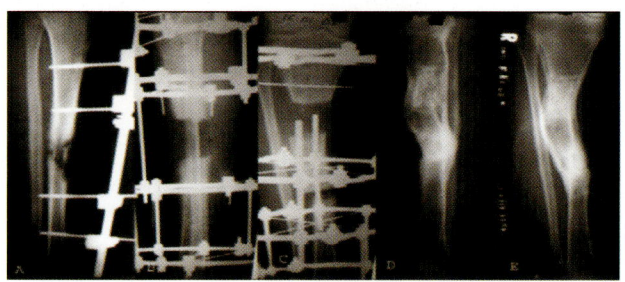

Picture 29: Bone transport is a unique concept of this system.

DISTRACTION OSTEOGENESIS: This is defined as a mechanical induction of new bone between bony surfaces, generated when they are gradually pulled apart. Based on numerous clinical, histopathological and experimental studies conducted the world over, it can be summarized that the bone formed as a result of distraction osteogenesis has the following characteristics:

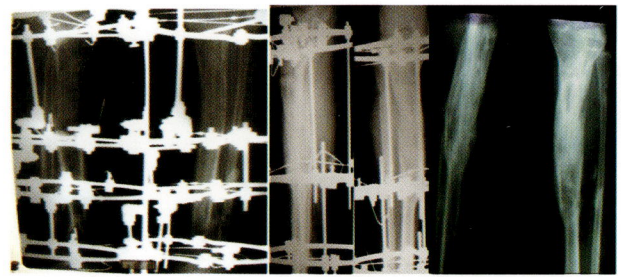

Picture 30: Distraction osteogenesis and regenerate formation

For the first two weeks, the gap is filled with a fibro vascular network; in about two weeks, mineralization first starts. From then on up to three months depending on the corticotomy and the mode of distraction, new bone tends to accumulate. By 120 days, cortices, lamellar bone and Haversian system are all completely formed. The blood supply increases in spurts and grows over vascularization; up to 300 times occurs which seems to bring about most of these changes. Based on studies, the following parameters of the protocol are important:

1. Rate of distraction: This should be within the range of 1.0 to 1.5 mm per day. Less than this will cause the bone to bridge rapidly; more than this, the vascular expansion will not be able to match the rate of elongation, leading to inhibition of mineralization.
2. Rhythm: 0.25 mm every 6 hours produces adequate osteogenesis. Two 0.5 mm expansions (12 hours apart) showed a decrease in osteogenesis. One 1 mm expansion (every 24 hours) slows down osteogenesis significantly.
3. Gap: The initial gap at corticotomy should not exceed two mm.

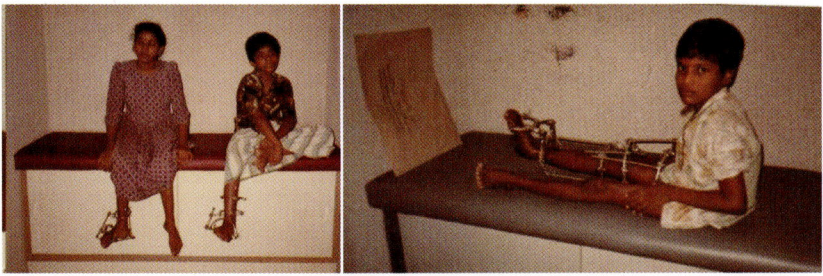

Picture 31: Ilizarov is versatile and highly efficient system with excellent patient compliance. It works in all age groups and both sexes equally well.

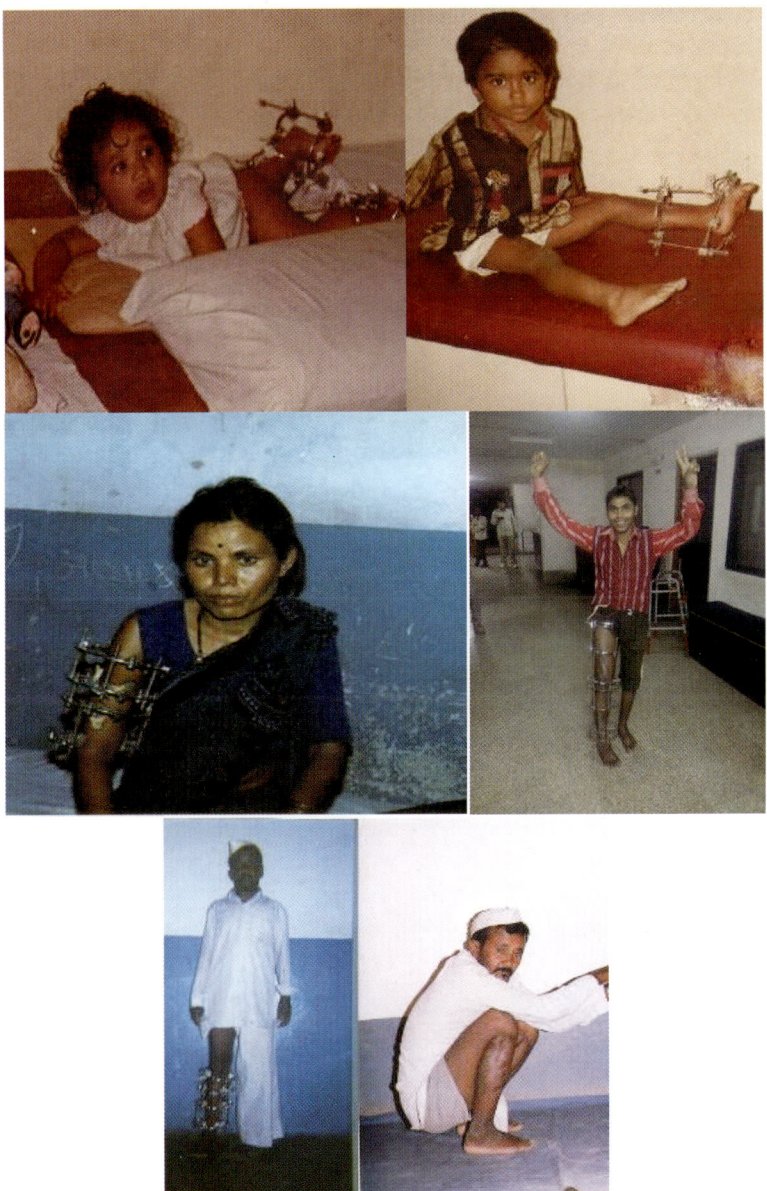

Picture 32: Ilizarov is a system independent of age, sex, race, region, and fracture with universal applications.

4. Latency: This is the time interval between the operation and start of distraction process. A latency of over three weeks will cause a rigid bridge at the corticotomy site. If the damage to medulla is minimal, distraction can be started on day one. If there is some damage, one can wait up to ten days before beginning distractions.

In any case, the most important advantage of this system is that the patient is allowed and encouraged to begin full weight bearing from day one and return to function, the bulky apparatus notwithstanding, and he himself controls the distractions and compressions under supervision.

Components of the Ilizarov System

Most mechanical devices contain various components. Each component is incomplete on its own, but put together, the machine comes to life. Similarly, the Ilizarov fixator has different components; joined together, they make a frame which works wonders.

These components can be divided into primary, secondary and tertiary components. The primary components join the bone to the first level component systems. The secondary components join the primary components. Tertiary components are not parts of the frame, but include the special instruments needed to put the frame together. Primary components include the K wire, the rings and the wire fixation bolts. Secondary components are additional supports which make up the frame; these include threaded rods, partially threaded rods, telescopic rods, graduated telescopic rods, slotted threaded rods, supports and posts, hinges, plates, simple bolts and nuts, threaded sockets and bushings, washers and wire fixation buckles. The tertiary components include spanners and different types of wire tensioners.

I will take up each of these separately for *I find it essential that one should have a fairly good knowledge of these components as regards their characteristics, functions and applications before actually proceeding to start operating.* The Ilizarov frame system is neither standard nor are the components specific. Each component can perform more than one function. In addition, one can use the frame without using many of these components. However, in the interest of precise mechanical force applications, a compromise by lack of specific appendages will cause problems.

The original Ilizarov system had some specific components. These later underwent additions from the ASAMI and the French group. Later American and Canadian surgeons introduced wholesale modification to the components. Thus, if one looks into the array of components available today, one is sure to find a lot of differences in the variety as well as dimensions of components offered by various manufacturers. In addition, there is a constant endeavour by different people to modify and improve on the design and materials of the components, preventing the possibility of standardization.

My 25 years of experience with this system has convinced me that the original Ilizarov is still the best and produces reproducible and miraculous results. I now believe in using an all-wire construct and am strongly against use of Shanz pins, except probably in proximal femur. The only improvements in the system, in my opinion, are in the fields of material research to produce a lighter and stronger system. Thus I will be describing only the components of the original Ilizarov system.

PRIMARY COMPONENTS

K-WIRES

This is the most important component while erecting a frame. When Ilizarov started his work, he used bicycle spokes ground to pointed ends. Later, after meeting Krichner, he switched over to stainless steel wires, which, though not as elastic as bicycle spokes, were totally corrosion-resistant and biocompatible.

The modern day wires are very different from the standard K-wires used in bone surgery. Cold drawing and special manufacturing processes produce wires of stainless steel with proper hardness and elasticity. They are available in many diameters and different lengths. The most common wire is 1.8 mm in diameter and at least 250 mm long. There are two types of tips: Bayonet shaped is specially designed for use in diaphysial cortical bone as it does not overheat the bone; Trocar point is for metaphyseal cancellous bone, and enables one to have better control over the direction of the wire.

It is very important to use the correct type of wire because this will, to a very large extent, decide the course of operation and the post-operative comforts of the patient. The original Ilizarov wire is stiff and can be drilled straight through the bone without buckling or twisting. It is extremely elastic and has an inbuilt springiness. It is capable of being tensioned, and has a very low malleability and elongation index. It has a reasonable breaking point and should, under ordinary circumstances, withstand a load of over 175 Kg before it breaks. The dimension of the wire depends on the application. In the ordinary course of events, one uses a 1.8 mm wire. This is the thickest possible wire that will withstand the stresses of tensioning. In younger patients and those with softer bones, a 1.6 mm wire should be used. Wires thicker than 2 mm will approximate S*chanz* pins in their characteristics and are hence not very suitable. Wires thinner than 1.2 mm have a very low breaking point and are hence incapable of being tensioned enough to bear the tremendous forces that an Ilizarov frame requires.

OLIVE WIRES

This is an original concept of Ilizarov, where a stopper is incorporated onto the wire and provides many special functions such as interfragmentary compression, axial loading or translation of bone fragments. In case an olive wire is not available, one may construct a wire on the table by producing a kink or twist in an ordinary wire. The original olive was indeed olive shaped with a pointed tip. This, on occasions, would be incorporated into the bone because of its tapered shape. Subsequent designs have more spherical olive wires which provide adequate stopper activity and at the same time do not get stuck in the bone.

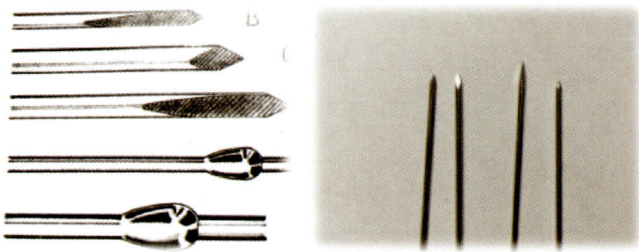

Picture 33: Trocar tip, Bayonet tip and olive wires

The following are the uses of olive wires:

1. The principal use of an olive wire is to apply an interfragmentary compression. This is especially useful when one is dealing with small and butterfly fragments
2. If there is a shift or angulation of the fragments during the operative procedure, then the olive wire can be employed to statically or dynamically correct the deformity during the course of treatment.
3. In osteotomies and deformity corrections, intra-operative and inter-treatment shifts in the direction of force applications produce a desired bone alignment.
4. In bone transports where the fragment is too small to allow for a ring application, two crossed olive wires give a sufficient grip and pull, while occupying hardly any space.

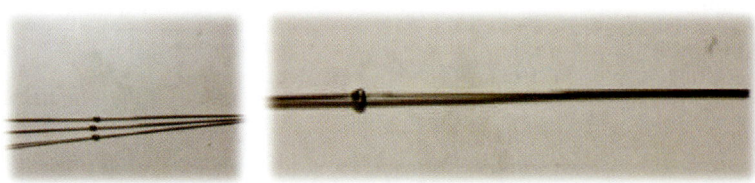

Picture 34: Olive wires have many uses

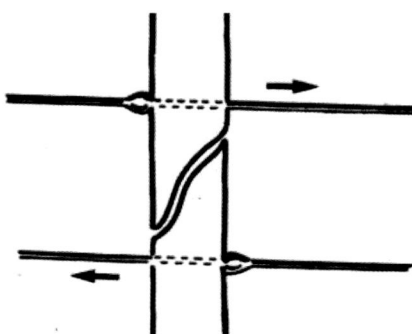

Picture 35: Olive wires can be used to produce interfragmentary compression

5. In operations where one desires to augment the diameter of the bone transversely, and those where a lateral shift is desired (as in the case of TAO), olive wires are essential.

6. In frame applications for deformity corrections, especially in the foot, where it may be possible to use two crossed wires, a single olive wire with the olive placed in the direction opposite to the shift axis will prevent the side-to-side translation of the half ring.

RINGS

Rings are available in different sizes and the number of holes varies according to the size. The original Ilizarov fixator has 12 sizes of rings with internal diameter ranging from 80 mm to 240 mm and number of holes from 8 to 24. In normal practice, the size of the ring used will depend upon the girth of the extremity. One must attempt to leave at least 2 cm gap between the skin and the ring to accommodate soft tissue swelling. Mechanically speaking, the smaller the ring, the greater is a possible tension. Thus the smallest possible ring that can be comfortably accommodated should be used.

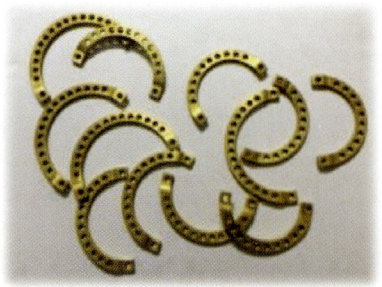 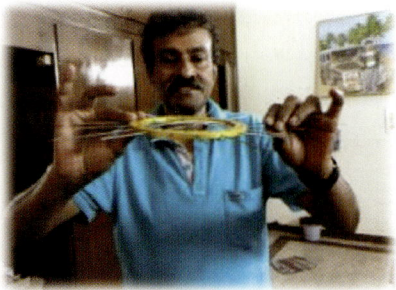

Picture 36: Rings come in various sizes and materials.

The rings in the original Ilizarov sets were made of A818 420 stainless steel. This is magnetic steel with inherent heat treatability and elasticity. This property is essential to avoid deformation of the rings when extreme tension is applied on the wires. In addition, the weight-bearing stresses may cause minor deformations of the rings during the process of loading. Ideally, the rings should return to the pre-deformation state as soon as the deforming forces are neutralized. The disadvantage of using this material is primarily its weight and radio opacity.

A lot of research is in progress to explore the possibility of producing these rings with lighter materials like aluminum, fibre glass, carbon reinforced plastics and lighter alloys of titanium and vanadium. The newer alloys are no doubt much more expensive than steel, but offer patients the comfort of a very light frame and a more precise distribution of forces across the various frame components. In addition, plastic, fibre and carbon based non metallic materials have the advantage of being transparent to X-rays and hence a much better visualization of the bone quality can be made. But the fact remains that these materials are very expensive and may be out of the reach of the average patient coming for treatment in our clinics.

I have recently developed an extremely light weight ring system from special alloys used in the aircraft industry. These have been tested both in the laboratory and on patients and should be launched commercially soon. As the only factor that interferes with the patient compliance is the bulk and weight of the system, lighter rings are the way to go and would probably replace all the heavier versions in due course.

FULL RINGS

These are complete circles and have two advantages. Firstly a complete circle is decidedly more rigid than two half rings bolted together. Secondly, two extra holes are available for rods and wires. Newer design edge-drilled full rings give additional wire holes for a more exact frame application.

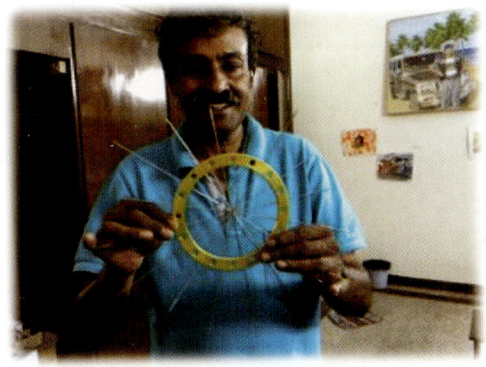

Picture 37: An edge drilled light weight ring invented by the author

The disadvantages are:

1. It must be passed over the extremity before wire insertion (as it would be impossible to place the full ring at the desired place, passing it over the wires and existing rings).

2. Any condition that necessitates ring removal during the course of treatment (for example edema) will make it impossible to remove it unless you dismantle the entire frame or cut the ring.

3. During the course of treatment it is impossible to change the diameter of the ring, which is possible with two half rings bolted together. In the latter case, one would have to just remove the connection bolts and add a straight plate between the two halves of the ring, and this would increase the effective internal diameter of the ring.

Therefore, if at all used, a full ring should he used as the distal most ring, which would make its application and removal easy. The photo below shows as a full ring as the last ring.

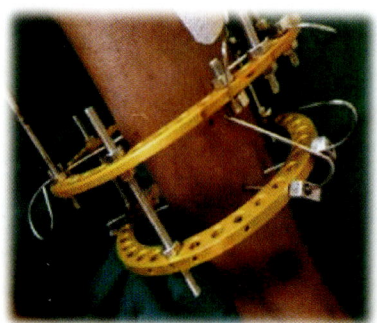 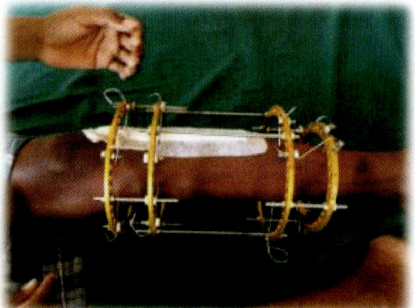

Picture 38: Full rings used as distal most ones give a couple of additional holes.

HALF RINGS

Two half rings bolted together making a full ring. This normally constitutes the most common form of ring. These half rings can also be used alone in various locations like proximal humerus and proximal femur. A half ring on its own is not a very rigid structure. Thus too much tension across the ends of the half ring will cause it to buckle. Fortunately one can overlap two half rings in any manner to construct either full rings, 5/8 (five eights) rings, 2/3 (two third) rings or anything in between. The following photos show a few combinations.

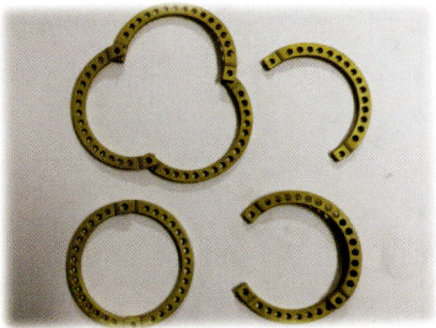

Picture 39: Half rings can be joined into different shapes

5/8TH RINGS, HALF RINGS WITH CURVED ENDS AND ARCHES

5/8th rings are five-eighth of a circle and when placed near a joint, allow freer movements than full rings, without restriction. They are also useful for areas with soft tissue damage, skin loss or places where a daily dressing is required. Arches are curved in shape and have larger width and thickness than rings. The holes are arranged in two rows. In the original Ilizarov system, they were meant especially for fixation around the proximal end of femur and humerus.

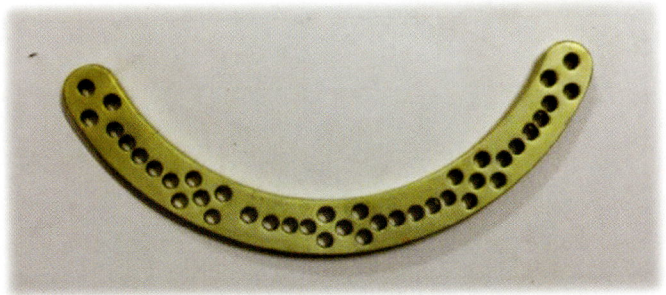

Picture 40: Ilizarov and Italian arches find use in proximal humerus and tibia

WIRE FIXATION BOLTS:

Wire fixation bolts, used to fix the wires to the ring, are of two types according to the relation of the wire to the hole on the ring over or beneath which they pass.

1. CANNULATED WIRE FIXATION BOLT

This has a central hole beneath the head of the bolt. After insertion of the wire and placement of the ring across the wire, the bolt is used for the *wire-to-ring* anchorage if the wire lies exactly in the centre of the hole. This gives a very firm grip, resists loosening, and is very versatile in one aspect. If the wire gets loosened during the course of treatment, one needs to just twist the nut, thereby attempting to wind the wire around the shaft of the nut, and achieving adequate tension in the wire.

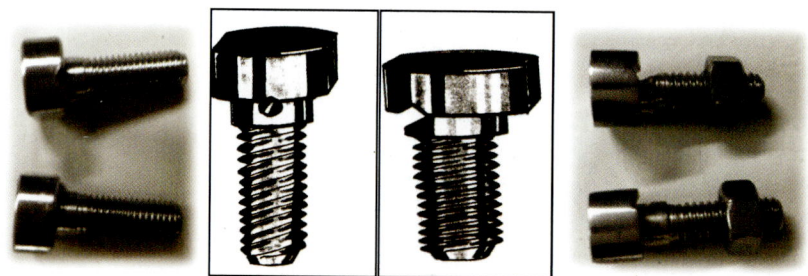

Picture 41: Cannulated and slotted wire fixation bolts

2. SLOTTED WIRE FIXATION BOLT

The slotted wire fixation bolt has a slot offset to one side on the under surface of its head. This bolt is used when the wire is off-centre in relation to the diameter of the hole.

Some wire fixation bolts have a vertical threaded socket in the head to permit the fixing of an extra rod compensating for an additional hole if the same is needed.

3. WASHERS

Use of washers along with nuts and bolts ensures rigid fixation. These are of the following types:

Simple washers have two flat surfaces with a central hole with a diameter slightly larger than the thread of the bolt. They are used when the wire emerges slightly above the linear axis of the ring and the anchorage of the wire could cause a pressure to the skin/pin junction.

Side slots have an eccentric slot on one surface while the other surface is flat. This serves the same purpose as a slotted wire fixation bolt. An off-centre wire can be passed through the slot and is fixed with the help of a common bolt and nut to the ring.

Conical washers have two components, one convex and the other concave. The hole in the two components is slightly larger than the thread diameter of the bolt and by a swiveling action, an angulation of up to 15 degrees between the ring and the wire can be achieved. This is particularly useful when the wire emerges a few mm away from the ring either above or below it.

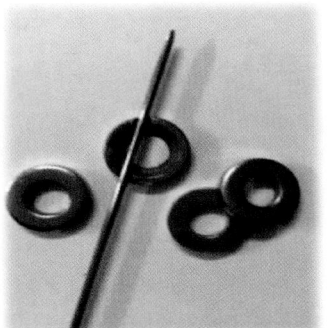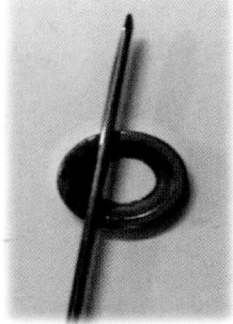

Picture 42: Washers are available in many types.

Wire fixation buckles are of two types and are used to fix K-wires to the rings. Their advantage is that they do not require holes for their own fixation to the rings and are hence useful in situations where the number of holes is at a premium because of crowding of other components on the ring.

SECONDARY COMPONENTS

THREADED RODS

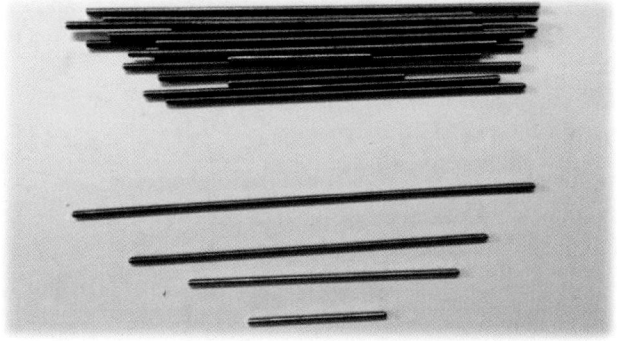

Picture 43: Threaded rods

Threaded rods, the most important secondary components in a set, are available in a large number of sizes and are used to anchor various ring assemblies to one another; by moving the units over the threaded rods, the rings can be compressed or separated uniformly while maintaining a proper alignment in both planes. Shifting of the threaded rods from one hole to another can also rotate the ring, allowing control in all three planes.

The original Ilizarov system had threaded rods varying in size from 60 mm to 400 mm. These were M6, i.e. rod diameter 6 mm. The *pitch* (distance between 2 consecutive threads) was 1 mm, meaning that one full turn of the nut would give a 1 mm distraction or compression in linear axis. This is the commonest threaded rod in use today, but rods of smaller diameter (M4 for paediatric use) and larger diameter (M8 for femurs and bulky patients) are also used. It is essential to know the pitch and plan the screw turnings appropriately, so as to obtain all corrections in the precise plane to the exact mm.

PARTIALLY THREADED RODS

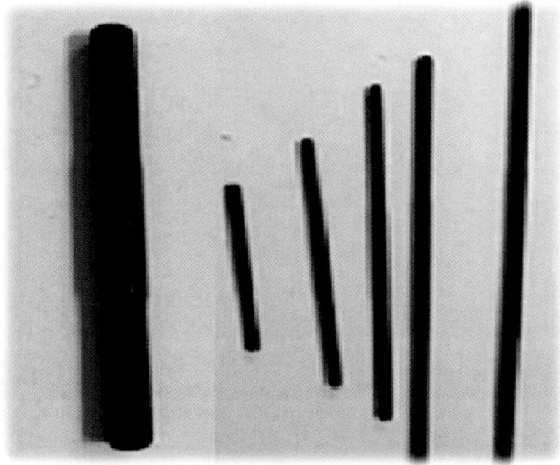

Picture 44: Partly threaded rods

Partially threaded rods are threaded at both ends but not in the middle. Naturally, they are stronger than fully threaded rods and resist bending and deformation. As compression and distraction are required only close to the rings, these have found favour in specific situations. Partially threaded rods are available in sizes from 60 mm to 400 mm.

TELESCOPIC RODS

Telescopic rods are hollow tubes with one end bearing threads that can be screwed or bolted on to rings. The normal threaded rods slide easily into the telescopic rods and with nuts can be made to expand or distract in a more controlled fashion. Modern threaded rods with graduations, markings or square nuts with numbers on each side, allow for precise measurement of the distraction achieved. In distractions and elongations, a telescopic rod is more advantageous than conventional threaded rods, because it precisely measures the amount of distraction and is more patient-friendly. These advantages are countered by the slightly increased weight and a much higher cost. If the patient is intelligent, and understands the principles of surgery, a simple threaded rod is sufficient.

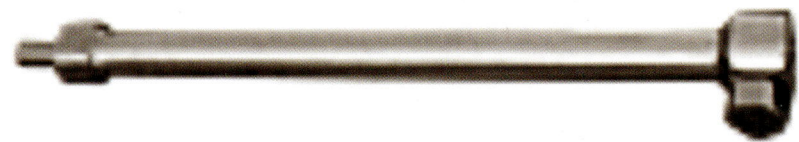

Picture 45: A telescopic rod with nut markings.

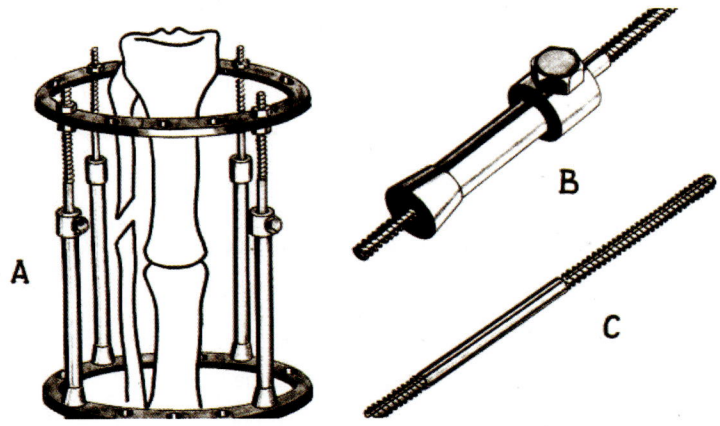

Picture 46: Telescopic rods

SLOTTED THREADED ROD

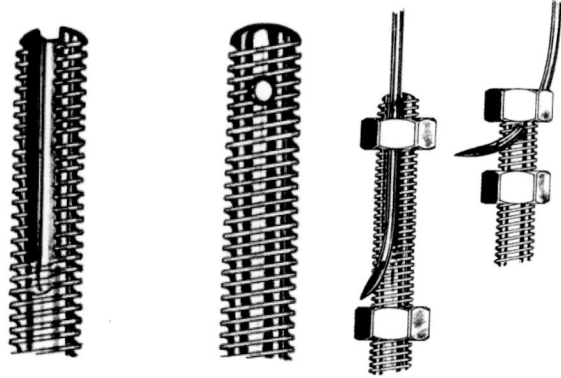

Picture 47: Slotted threaded rods

This is one of the Ilizarov concepts that adds to its magic. The purpose of slotted threaded rods is to achieve a pull in a direction at right angles or other angles to the main frame. These rods have a groove or slot longitudinally along their axes. Once a wire is placed into the slot and a nut tightened, the threaded rod becomes an extension of the K-wire. Now distracting the rod pulls the wire in the desired direction. This is not only invaluable in three dimensional deformity corrections, but of great use in TAO, transverse expansions and similar conditions.

This rod is also used to produce interfragmentary compression by pulling the fragment while treating comminuted fractures with a large butterfly fragment and oblique tibial fractures with displacement. This is accomplished in the following way: An olive wire is drilled through the bone fragment to be pulled. The opposite end is threaded through the slot of the rod being mounted on the frame with its long axis parallel to the olive wire. Tightening a nut pulls the wire and the bone fragment achieving a compression in the desired direction.

SUPPORTS AND POSTS

These are solid bars with flat rounded heads. They are available in four sizes and have one to four holes. Posts are of two types. The male post has a threaded end while the female post has a threaded hole. The male post accommodates standard nuts and the female post has threading corresponding to either nuts or threaded rods.

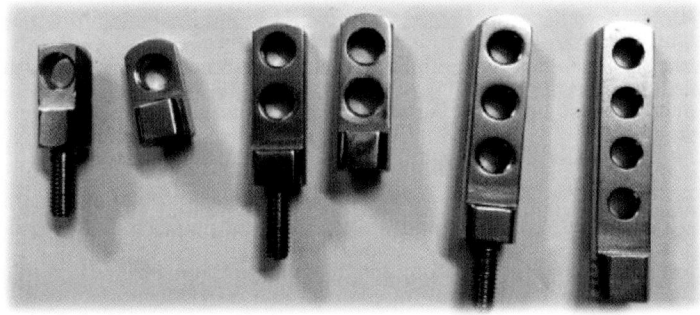

Picture 48: Single and multiple holed posts.

Posts have four uses:

1. Additional wires can be passed in close proximity to rings without the use of additional rings.
2. If wires are accidently or deliberately drilled obliquely (to avoid vital structures) with an offset of more than 15 degrees, posts can be used to fix this wire and avoids undue tension on soft tissues.
3. Two posts can be joined using a nut and a bolt and will act as a hinge. This hinge is then connected to the system with threaded rods; by gradual change in the angle of the hinge, deformities can be corrected.

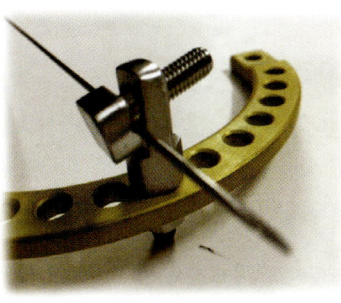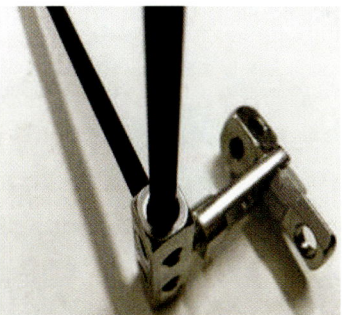

Picture 49: A combination of posts produces hinges

4. Male and female posts can be mounted through a single hole on either side of the ring to stabilize and improve fixation in two or more planes.

HINGES

Hinges are similar to posts both in form and function, the only difference being the thickness and number of holes. As opposed to posts, a hinge has only one hole.

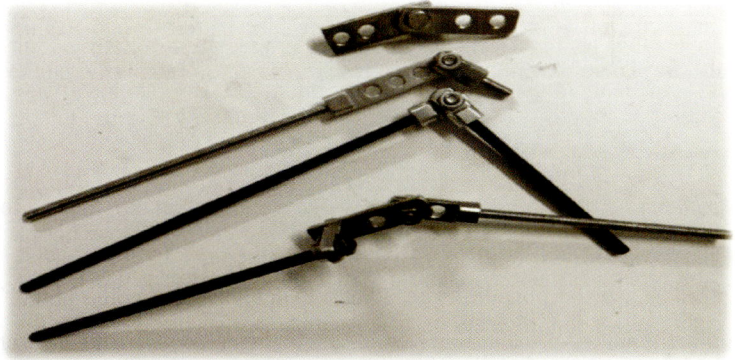

Picture 50: Different hinge possibilities

PLATES

Plates are static fixation devices to anchor various components of the frame. During the operation if it is felt that a particular configuration is full and final and would not warrant any change during the further course of management, then one employs plates. Either straight or twisted, plates come with different hole sizes.

Straight plates are of varying lengths with uniform holes. The shorter plates have just two holes and are useful for connecting rings of different diameters.

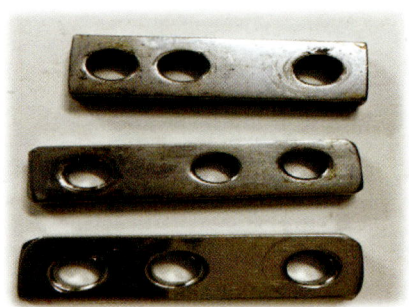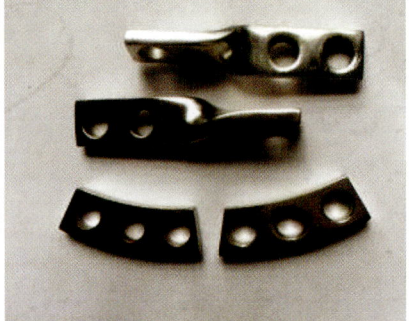

Picture 51: Straight, curved and twisted plates

Longer connecting plates can be used instead of threaded rods in a static assembly where one does not require compression or distraction.

Curved plates are used to increase the circumference of a ring so that an obliquely drilled wire going beyond the ring can be accommodated within the frame.

Twisted plates, as their name indicates, are twisted in the middle by 90 degrees so that the two halves are at right angles to each other (like a propeller). Thus one component can be connected to the horizontal plane while the other to the vertical plane. These are extremely useful in combination with hinges for a three dimensional deformity correction.

BOLTS AND NUTS

Bolts and nuts are used to fix half rings together or to join different components of the system with each other or with the ring while erecting a frame. The nuts are hexagonal and the bolt heads are either oblong or hexagonal. Each set or system has uniformity in the hexagonal span of the nuts, and bolts and this span usually corresponds to that of other components like threaded sockets, posts, hinges, etc. to allow for the use of the same set of spanners for all the components.

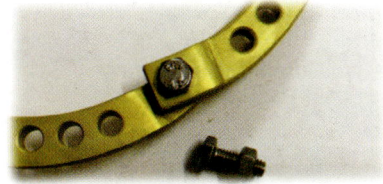 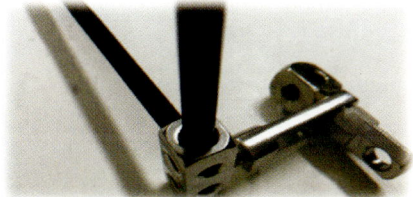

Picture 52: Nuts and bolts anchor various components to one another

THREADED SOCKETS AND BUSHINGS

Both these components serve as additional connecting devices and aid the stability and length of the rods. Sockets are hexagonal and threaded at both ends. Each has a threaded hole at the centre perpendicular to the long axis. The most common use of a threaded socket is to increase rod length. On many occasions one may need to use a rod longer than what is available. In these circumstances, it is an easy matter to thread the socket to one end of the threaded rod. An additional threaded rod is now screwed on to this socket, which increases the length of the threaded rod. The central thread is at right angles to the long axis of the socket. This is employed when one wishes to connect two threaded rods at right angles to one another.

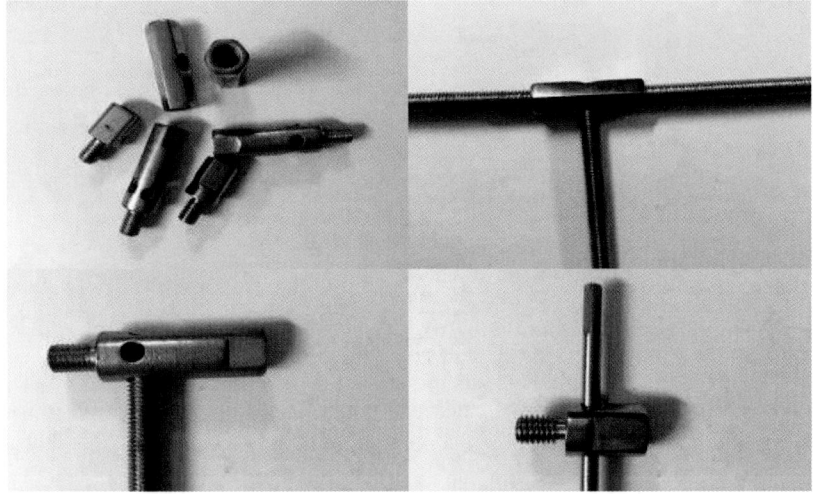

Picture 53: Threaded sockets and bushings can be used in various combinations

Bushings are cylindrical; each has a threaded perpendicular hole at the centre. What makes them different from sockets is that the lumen running along the long axis is not threaded. These components come in handy for attaching various components to rings and to each other.

TERTIARY COMPONENTS

SPANNERS

Spanners are used to tighten nuts and bolts. Normally spanners are open at one end and ring type at the other end. The open end can be slid into closed spaces, while the ring spanner gives greater ease of operation. On occasions, it is desirable to use a box spanner or a swivel spanner for linear applications. Each set employs spanners that uniformly fit all components.

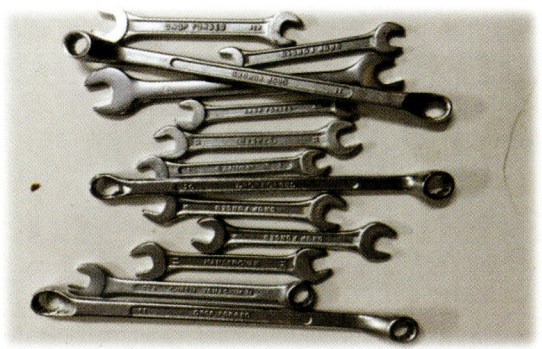

Picture 54: Spanners open and closed

Spanners have a tendency to slip and fall on the floor during surgery. A good set will have at least half a dozen spanners, open at one end and closed at the other. In addition, thin spanners, Allen keys and box spanners should be a part of the set.

WIRE TENSIONER

Unlike uni- or bi-axial fixators (where thick Shanz pins act as inelastic cantilevers), Ilizarov assemblies depend on stretched wires to give them strength while retaining elasticity, just like stretched veena or piano wires. To make the K-wires and in turn the assembly fairly rigid (so that it withstands the enormous stresses of weight bearing and loading), adequate tension is essential in all the wires. In simple language, tensioning is anchorage of the wire to the ring assembly after it has been tightly pulled apart at both ends. The required tension to be applied ranges from 50 Kg to 130 Kg and differs according to the usage and number of wires. According to Ilizarov, the tension levels for different applications are as follows:

1. For a single wire on a half ring, 50-70 Kg is adequate. Any more will cause ring deformation or twist.

2. Drop wires need 50-70 Kg, wires in children about 110 Kg, and wires in adults on full rings around 120-130 Kg of tension. This is the maximum acceptable mechanically and physiologically.

3. Olive wires need 100-110 Kg tension when used for strategic placement, but 50 to 60 Kg tension is adequate for inter-fragmentary compression.

4. For 1.6 mm wire, 100 Kg and for 1.8 Inn-T wire, 120 Kg tension are optimum.

5. With more than 2 wires on a ring, tension up to 140 Kg is acceptable.

Various methods are employed for tensioning the wires.

1. Direct mechanical pull

After transfixing one end of the wire to the ring, the other end is grasped by pliers and pulled, after which it is fixed. This method does not measure the tension imparted to the wire, and unless the surgeon is a superman, does not give an adequate amount of tension. *This is not recommended for general use and is mentioned only to be condemned.*

2. Conventional manual tensioner

This was devised by Ilizarov and consists of a two pronged instrument with a right angled threaded bolt. The bolt has a central cannulation through which the protruding end of wire is passed. One end of the wire is anchored to the ring using a wire fixation bolt or washer. The arm of the tensioner is now rotated, which exerts a linear pull on the wire. The wire is periodically tapped with a spanner after each turn; when a tinny piano-like sound is heard, the other end of the wire is anchored to the ring. This is an excellent method and should be used when a dynamometric tensioner is not available.

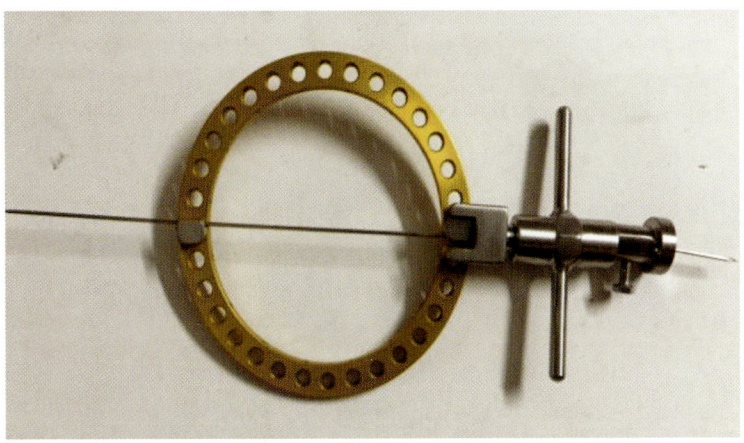

Picture 55: Manual tensioner

3. Manual tensioning bolt

In the screw nut assembly used here, one end of the wire is fixed to the ring and the other end is passed through the screw nut assembly; the screw is opened using wrenches. After each thread is opened, a certain amount of tension is achieved and this process is continued until the desired tension is achieved.

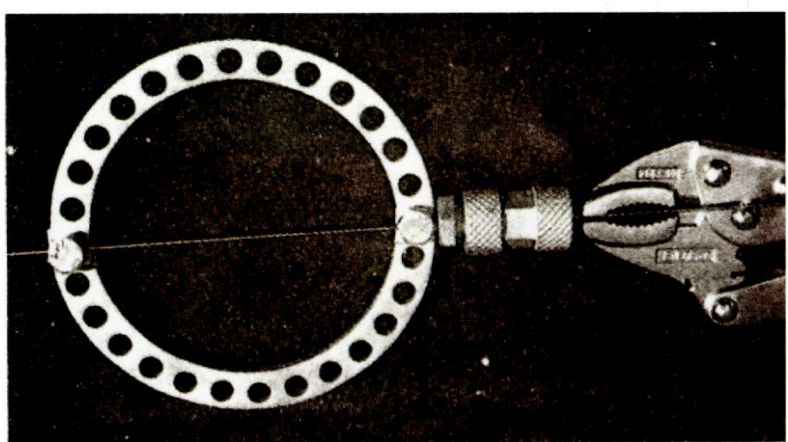

Picture 56: Hollow bolt tensioner

The Prakash nut Tensioner is a very simple device based on this principle. A large bolt with a hole through it in the linear axis and a wide nut are used. Each full turn of the nut gives 15-20 pounds of tension. 5 or 6 full turns give the required tension to the ring. This is an excellent system but needs some experience, because over-tightening can break the wire and prolong the surgery. Experimental studies have shown that the relation between turning the nut and tension generated is not proportional. In the initial stages, only 8 to 10 Kg are generated per full turn. As the tightening progresses, 15 to 20 Kg tension is generated per turn; this continues until the fifth or sixth turn. At this stage, when the nut is further turned, as much as 30 Kg tension is exerted per turn. Thus, one needs experience with the Prakash nut type Tensioner to achieve adequate tension, and know when to stop. Constant tapping with the spanner to locate a tinny sound will most often do the trick.

4. Turning the wire fixation bolt

This wonderfully simple technique was originally described by the master himself. This is done by first fixing one end tightly and then turning the wire fixation bolt on the opposite side by one half-turn attempting to wind the nut around the bolt and tightening the nut. Here again, the amount of tension imparted cannot be measured in terms of quantity. An original reading of this description hardly conveys how turning the nut could increase the tension. Actually, after anchorage of the wire to the nut, twisting the nut will attempt to wind the wire around the nut, which will pull the wire and impart tension.

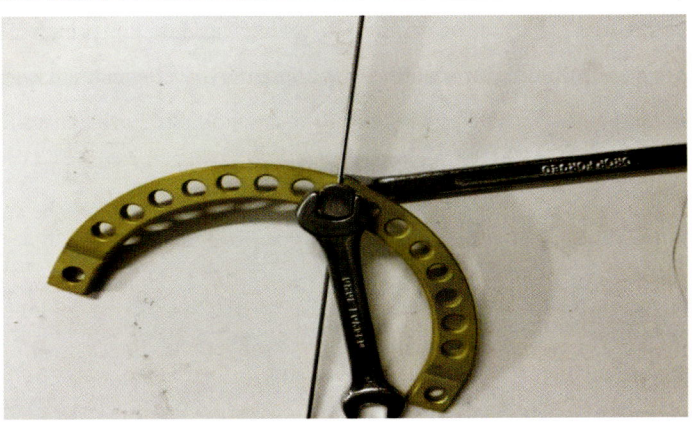

Picture 57: Wire tensioning by bolt twisting

5. Dynamometric wire tensioner

This is a spring loaded device with the tension measurement marked for imparting precise measurable tension to the wire. The principle is very simple. One end of the wire is anchored to the ring. The other end is threaded to the dynamometer. The handle is twisted. The inbuilt spring pulls the wire to a predetermined extent. This is quantifiable and measurable. The external scale displays the exact tension that is being administered. Once a satisfactory level of tension is achieved, the other end is tightened to retain the tension. It is desirable to use this type of tensioner wherever possible. But unfortunately because of the very high cost this may not be always available. The other disadvantage is that springs of good quality and consistent performance seldom withstand steam sterilization. Consequently this instrument needs very special care while handling and sterilization and is subject to repeated breakdowns. Even when the surgeon prefers to use the dynamometer routinely, it is essential to have an ordinary manual device as a standby.

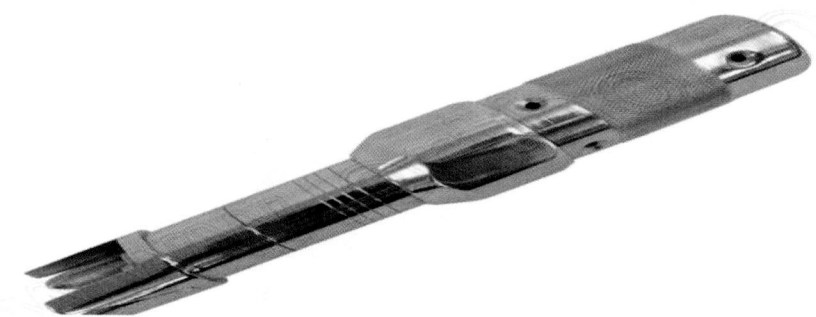

Picture 58: Dynamometric tensioner.

While using any of the other above mentioned methods when dynamometric wire Tensioner is not available, the best way to ascertain that the wire is sufficiently tensioned is to lightly tap the wire with a spanner after each turn. An untensioned wire gives a dull note, but the note changes with each successive turn and a properly tensioned wire gives a high pitched musical note like a tight piano string.

Care of instruments

Most of the components are reusable, except for the K-wires and rods that have either become bent or where the thread is cut or slipped. Most secondary components are made of non-corrosive stainless steel alloys and their cleaning and sterilizing procedures are the same as for other orthopaedic instruments and implants. It is important that prior to starting surgery, one has a complete range of instruments and implants available and that different sizes of rings, full range of lengths of wires, and all additional paraphernalia are kept on hand. Further details on this aspect are covered in the chapter on preoperative planning.

Indications and contraindications of the Ilizarov system

Unlike other systems, it is not possible to clearly spell out the absolute and relative indications and contraindications of the procedure. Russian literature describes indications for conditions such diverse as fractures, non-unions, osteotomies, Ollier's disease, Burger's disease, and even osteomyelitis and fibrous dysplasia. The extent of indications is so large that Russian literature comments that *"Western orthopaedic surgeons not familiar with this method will not comprehend the vast potential of this system."*

In my opinion, when two or more methods achieve the same function, the simpler method should be chosen. Thus, simple fractures which would heal well with a plaster application are best treated conservatively rather than undertaking all this trouble both for surgeon and patient. Similarly, simple diaphyseal fractures that can be internally fixed should be simply fixed. As with indications, one must more importantly knows the contraindications, because the balance of practice is achieved only when one knows *when not to do*. Thus I have divided the indications into four groups:

1. Conditions where Ilizarov frames *are more useful* than conventional methods and *should* be used

2. Conditions where Ilizarov frame *may* be used

3. Conditions where Ilizarov frame *should not* to be used.

4. *Questionable* indications

It is to be understood that this classification of the indications is entirely based on my personal experiences and available publications in English literature. It is however possible that an expert Ilizarovian may be able to achieve miracles even in conditions listed above as relative or questionable. What is important is that we must not forget our primary aim: *To treat the patient and to treat him or her well!*

It is very simple to understand that the patient on an Ilizarov frame for prolonged periods undergoes a certain amount of physical and psychological trauma. In addition, the frame application demands a fair amount of mechanical understanding and surgical skill. Furthermore, the system has a definite learning curve for the surgeon. With all these in mind, it is better to evolve a system of protocols whereby we restrict the use of this system for conditions where other conventional methods have not worked or will not work.

Conditions where Ilizarov frames are more useful than conventional methods

1. Congenital pseudoarthrosis of tibia

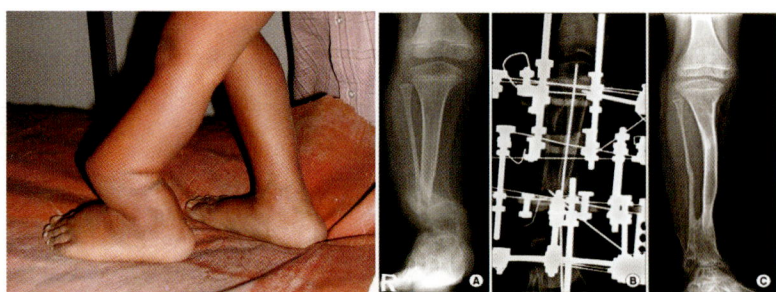

Picture 59: Congenitial Pseudoarthrosis

2. Refractory non-unions and pseudoarthrosis of all long bones.

78

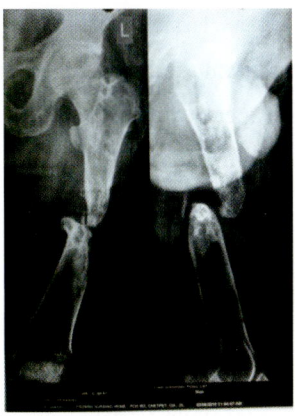

Picture 60: Refractory gap non-unions

3. Limb length elongation in appropriate situations, especially inequality. Cosmetic lengthenings are being done, but I neither do them nor recommend them. You can't treat lack of confidence by making someone taller!

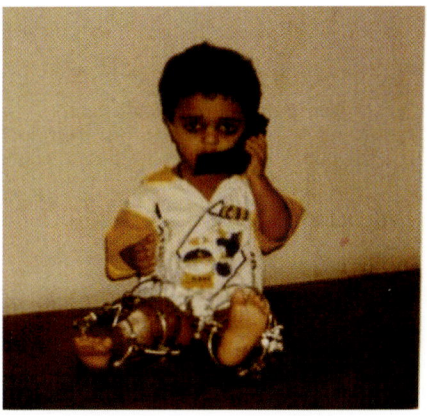

Picture 61: Limb lengthening

4. Intra-articular fractures with multiplanar deformities. Here a ligamentotaxis is used.

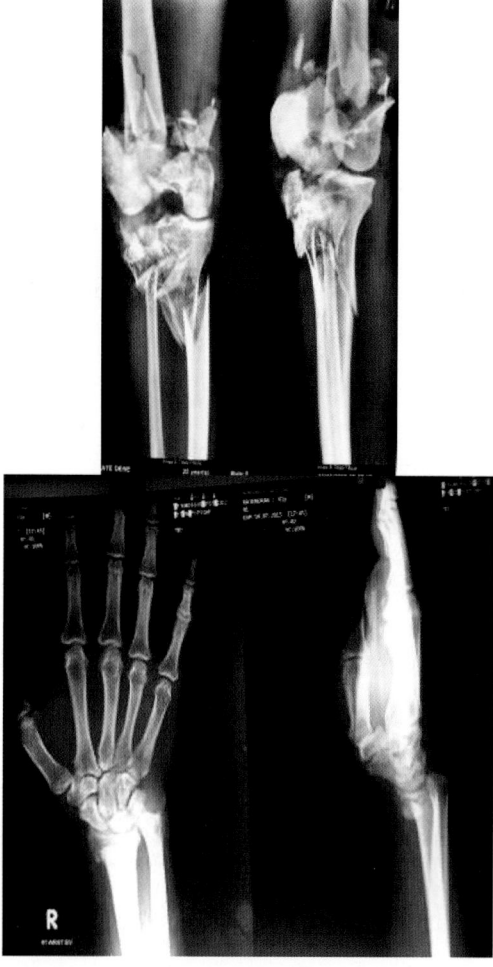

Picture 62: Complex intra-articular fractures.

5. Massive intercalary bone loss

6. Lengthening or shaping of amputations stumps

7. Complex multi-planar deformities where soft tissue releases have failed or will not work

8. As a salvage procedure in methods where conventional fracture management has failed to achieve the desired effect

Conditions where Ilizarov frame may be used

1. As an external fixator like any other external fixator
2. Correction of joint deformities not possible by soft tissue releases
3. In simple non-unions where bone grafting is not desired either by the patient or the surgeon
4. Arthrodesis and joint fusions

Conditions where Ilizarov frame should not to be used

1. Open fractures when soft tissue loss is best treated by single plane fixator for freer access to secondary procedures
2. Intra-articular fractures, which are best treated by accurate open reduction and internal fixation. However, a skilled Ilizarov surgeon can get better results than plates in intra-articular fractures by a judicious combination of olive wires and hinges!
3. Simple long bone shaft fractures which can be properly treated by nailing, plating or plasters. The tendency to use Ilizarov frames in these conditions should be strongly discouraged.
4. Fresh fractures in children
5. Minor limb length discrepancy which can be easily equalized by standard Epiphysiodesis, shoe raise or even reassurance

Questionable Indications

1. Chronic and acute Osteomyelitis
2. Burger's disease

3. Primary treatment in deformities like polio and club foot, without trying conventional means of correction

If one reads the literature propounded by Russians and by their followers like the ASAMI group, with regard to their experience with Ilizarov frames, it would appear that almost all the pathology of the locomotor apparatus can be successfully treated using Ilizarov frames. But as the practising surgeon, it is recommended that one uses this as the invaluable tool for selecting specific conditions which are not manageable by other methods, until one gains adequate experience to be able to tackle difficult problems (which were earlier considered insurmountable).

Surgical Technique for the Ilizarov System

Original descriptions called this "an essentially non-surgical method of treatment." This chapter covers the basic principles of assembling the frames and performing the surgery. Specific methods (as applicable to each limb and bone) shall be discussed next. The most important prerequisite is to have a thorough knowledge of anatomy, surface landmarks and a 3D visualization of the structures within the limb as the pin is passed. This is not as difficult as it sounds and the following drawings and landmarks will make things simpler!

Wire insertion

As the forces are transmitted to the bone by the wires that go across the soft tissues, it is necessary that proper techniques are followed. A thorough knowledge of the cross sectional anatomy of the limb is essential and helps the surgeon to avoid transfixing vital structures. The important guidelines for wire passing are:

A. The wire should be gradually pushed manually until it reaches bone. Once it reaches the bone, it is drilled through both the cortices; once the wire exits out of the rear cortex, it is hammered out through the opposite soft tissues. The drilling should not be done faster than 70 to 100 RPM to avoid thermal necrosis to the bone. It is advisable to pause the drilling frequently to allow the tip to cool down before proceeding further.

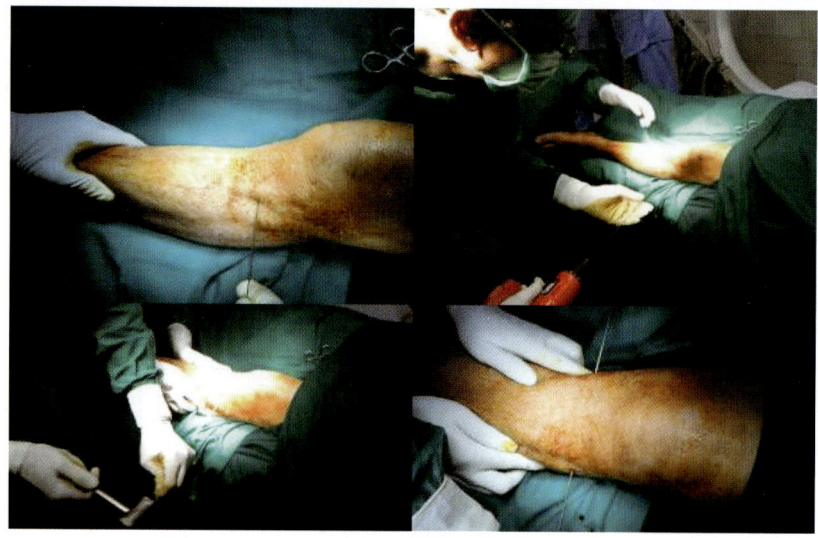

Picture 63: The K-wire is pushed in, drilled through and hammered out.

B. The direction of the wire's passage and its exact level and position are predetermined by the surgeon. I usually locate the neurovascular bundle or palpate the pumping artery. Keeping my thumb over this, I pass my wires at a safe distance (about 2 cm away). The assistant keeps his finger at the exit point and my pin insertion is guided by that.

C. The muscle through which the wire is passing should be positioned at maximum stretch, especially when the ring is close to the joint, to avoid joint contracture. It is logical that this can be achieved only if the muscle is at its maximum length while the wire passes through it. The joint is moved in both directions to achieve this during the wire's passage from one compartment to the other. For example, in the leg, the ankle is dorsiflexed as the wire passes through the posterior compartment and planterflexed as the wire passes through the anterior compartment.

D. The skin must not be stretched or puckered after the pin placement and should rest comfortably around the pin. In lengthening, a part of extra skin may be pulled towards the lengthening area to give a stretch leverage for the skin. An optimum number of wires as absolutely necessary should be passed. As each wire acts as a foreign body in the muscle planes and interferes with the movement, additional wires for increasing the stability of the assembly should be balanced against this risk. In the case of olive wires, a small incision on the skin is important to allow for the passage of the wire.

Ring selection and anchorage of wires to rings

Prior to the surgery, one can keep a ring over the limb to assess the correct size required. As described earlier, the 2 cm distance circumferentially between the inner side of the ring and the patient's limb is mandatory. It is best to pass the wires at one end and attach it to the ring.

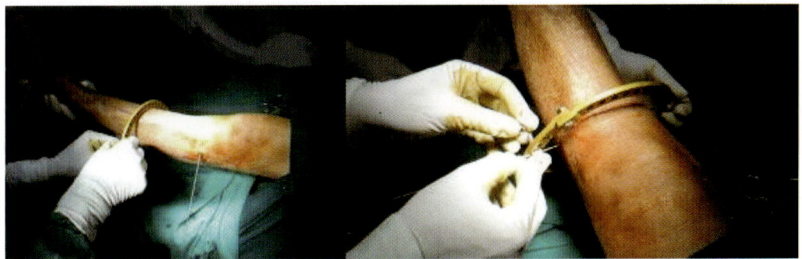

Picture 64: Appropriate sized ring is anchored.

This end of the wire is firmly anchored to one of the holes in the ring with a wire fixation bolt. After tightening the pin, the protruding end is bent and curled off to prevent wire slippage during tensioning. Now the other end of the wire is anchored through the wire fixation bolt without tightening the bolt. The protruding end of each wire is now grasped by a tensioner and tensioned prior to tightening the corresponding bolt.

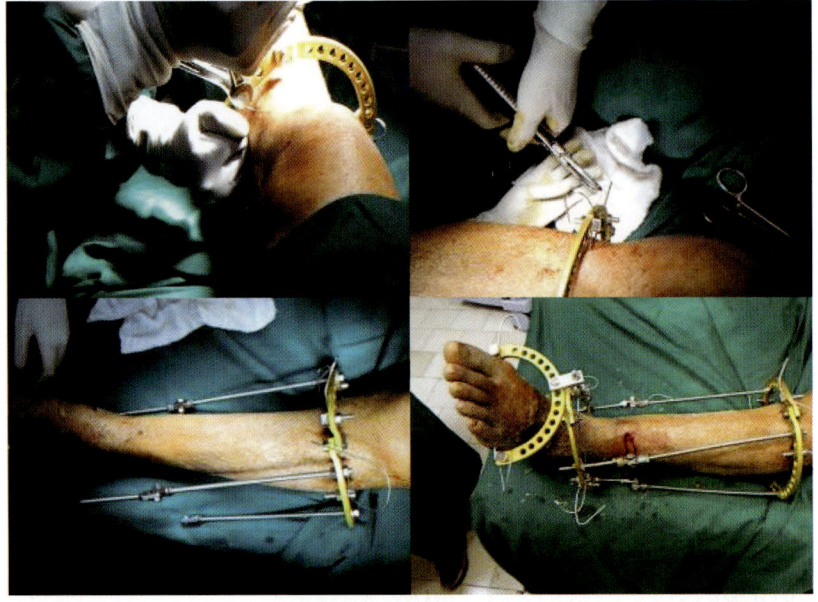

Picture 65: Progressive construct of a frame.

As far as possible, each pair of wires should be balanced with one anchored on the superior surface of the ring and the other to the inferior surface of the ring. One must count the holes to make sure that the wire is straight and is not being unduly bent. The same sequence is followed for subsequent rings.

TYPES OF FRAME CONSTRUCTS AND THE ORDER OF WIRE PLACEMENT

There are many ways to kill a cat. Likewise, a Ilizarov frame can be applied to a limb in different ways. One method is to fix the individual rings, proximal to distal, in a specified order, and anchor them to the tensioned wires driven through the bone. These individual rings are then attached to appropriate hinges and threaded to telescopic rods to complete the assembly. It is only natural that proximal rings have to be tightened before distal rings. This is called a

86

progressive construct, and excellent for a beginner. A large percentage of Ilizarov surgeons use only this method.

The other method is to prefabricate a loose assembly (which is still adjustable), and preoperatively slide it over the limb. This is then evaluated and adjusted according to the individual patient. Once a provisional assembly is finalized, it is autoclaved as one piece. During surgery, it is slid over the limb in one piece before the wire insertion begins. This method is called a *prefabricated construct*. The wires are then anchored to the frame and the assembly built. This method saves intra operative time, but probably a little longer time is spent in preoperative planning and fabrication. *The order of pin placement is not rather important in a progressive assembly, but is the most important step for a prefabricated construct.*

PROGRESSIVE CONSTRUCT RING ASSEMBLY

1. It is preferable to use half rings for all rings except the lowermost ring, where a full ring can be used to advantage, ideally with a couple of additional holes for rods and hinges.
2. Smaller the ring, better the biomechanics. However, too small a ring will occasionally cause an edematous limb to press against it, causing pressure sores. The rule of thumb is to have 2 cm space uniformly between limb and ring.
3. The first ring is the most *proximal metaphyseal ring* and is passed exactly parallel to the joint above it in both planes. A joint line in a live anaesthetized patient is different from the marker lines drawn on a radiograph. It is easy to identify a joint on the operating table and this should be exactly parallel to the first ring. In cases of doubt, a K-wire placed over the skin at the exact joint level, followed by an X-ray gives us the precise joint line.

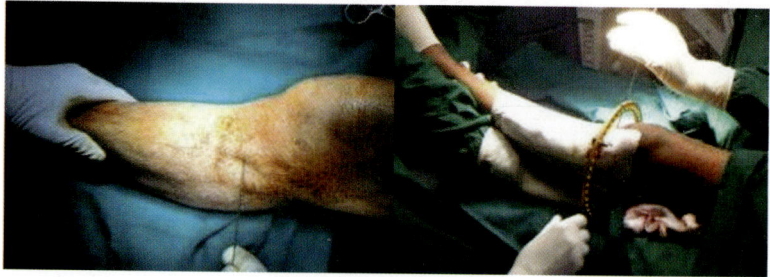

Picture 66: Placement of the proximal ring

4. The second ring is the most distal one, which is fixed parallel to the lower joint, a little above the joint line in the metaphyseal area.

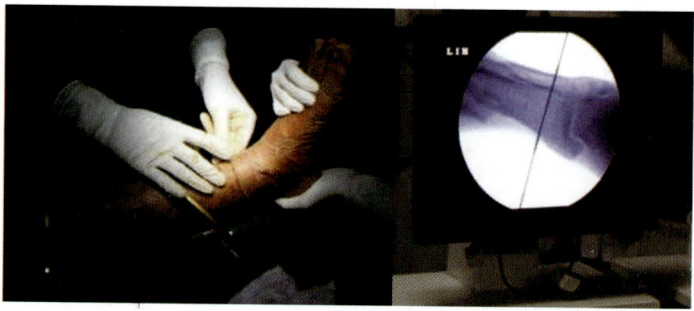

Picture 67: Placement of distal ring, parallel to the joint line.

5. Now short or medium threaded rods are anchored to both these rings, the length of the rods depending entirely on the level of the pathology which is being corrected. To these rods are attached the middle rings, each parallel to the ring it is anchored to.

6. Now these two pairs of rings, each aligned exactly parallel to the joint adjacent to it, would meet at the apex or the deformity or CORA.

7. At this stage, the hinges are applied and additional olive wires, slotted threaded rods or telescopic rods attached to the appropriate points, to complete the assembly.

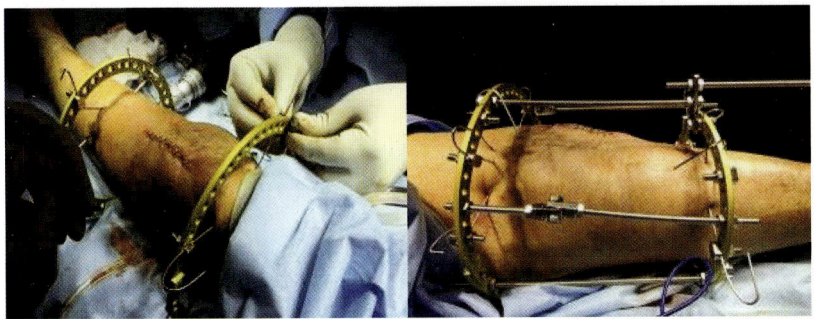

Picture 68: A progressively constructed frame.

PRECONSTRUCTED RING ASSEMBLY:

This is the second way of doing things and saves considerable anaesthetic time, though more time is spent on preoperative fabrication. The patient is examined in the ward preoperatively, and his joint lines and the apex of the deformity marked with a marker pen. A frame is assembled around the limb preoperatively. This is a *loose telescoping adjustable* frame, which has angles matching the deformity or non-union, with hinges or telescopes in the appropriate region. Here the order of wire placements is critical, and the following description and terminology is based on Dr. Jishnu Baruah's simplified prefab construct fixation. For the sake of easy understanding, the following description is for a frame anchored over a deformed tibia.

1. A provisional pre-constructed but telescoping frame is fabricated, with dual connecting rods left loose on both sides. This is preoperatively slid over the patient's limb to ensure that the rings are parallel to adjacent joints and the apex of the actual deformity corresponds to the hinge placement.

2. Each K-wire has a name that indicates its purpose. The first, the *Reference K Wire,* is passed parallel to knee in postero-lateral to antero-medial direction.

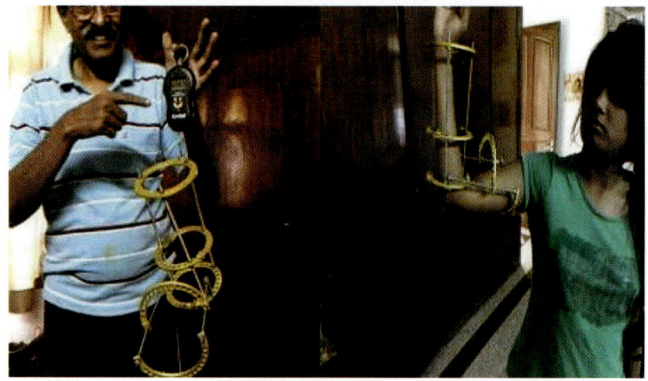

Picture 69: A prefabricated preoperative construct

3. The preconstructed frame is slid over the limb and the most proximal ring is held parallel and flush (but not fixed) to the *Reference K Wire* by an assistant, who also maintains the patella in correct position.

4. The second, the *Rotation K Wire*, is the principal wire controlling rotation. This is passed in the anterolateral to posteromedial direction above the ankle, again ensuring that the direction is exactly parallel to the joint. The distal most ring of the telescoping frame is held flush to this wire by another assistant, who has two important functions at this step: traction and correcting rotation.

5. The next step is spacing and centralization. The surgeon fine-tunes the spaces and tightens the threaded connecting rods. Next comes the important step of clamping both the wires into corresponding holes and tensioning them. (It's better to clamp the anteroposterior distal wire first, then the transverse proximal wire, because empty holes in the anteroposterior regions of bolted half rings are fewer.) After this step, the fixator behaves like a jig and rotation is committed. Shifts and angulations can however be fine-tuned by shifting the bone along the 2 wires, as they are almost at right angles to each other.

6. Second wires at appropriate latero-medial corridors can now be passed and extra connecting rods passed to complete the frame.

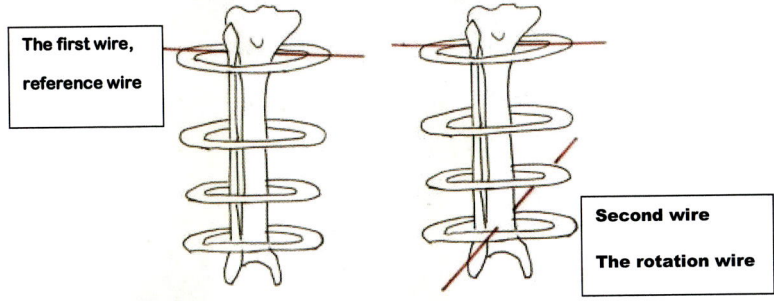

The first wire, reference wire

Second wire
The rotation wire

Picture 70: The reference and rotation K-wires

1. Wires number 3 and 4, called *The Reduction Wires,* are passed after fine-tuning of shifts and angulation on the middle 2 rings. Their sequence may vary, but it is very important that reduction is maintained accurately, while passing these wires. After these are passed and tensioned, further correction is not possible without perimounting the frame. Care is to be taken that the K-wires are flush to rings both at entry and exit as any offset will shift the reduction after tensioning. A clamp inside the selected hole towards the entry can be used to guide the wire; offset on the other side is taken care of by washers and posts.

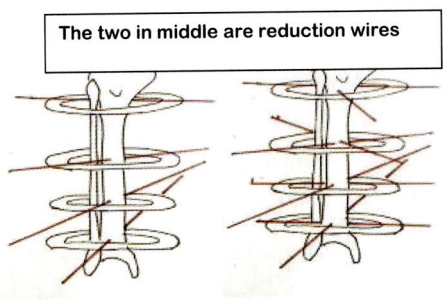

The two in middle are reduction wires

Picture 71: The order of pin placement in a prefabricated construct

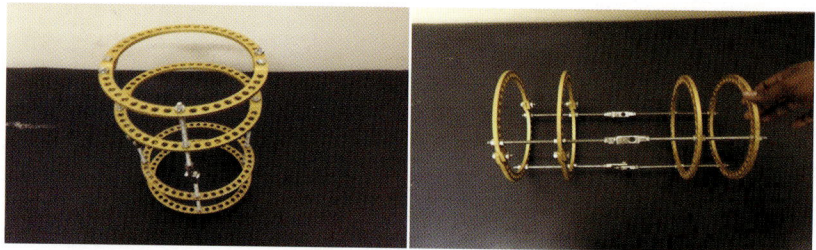

Picture 72: A prefabricated construct with appropriately positioned hinges

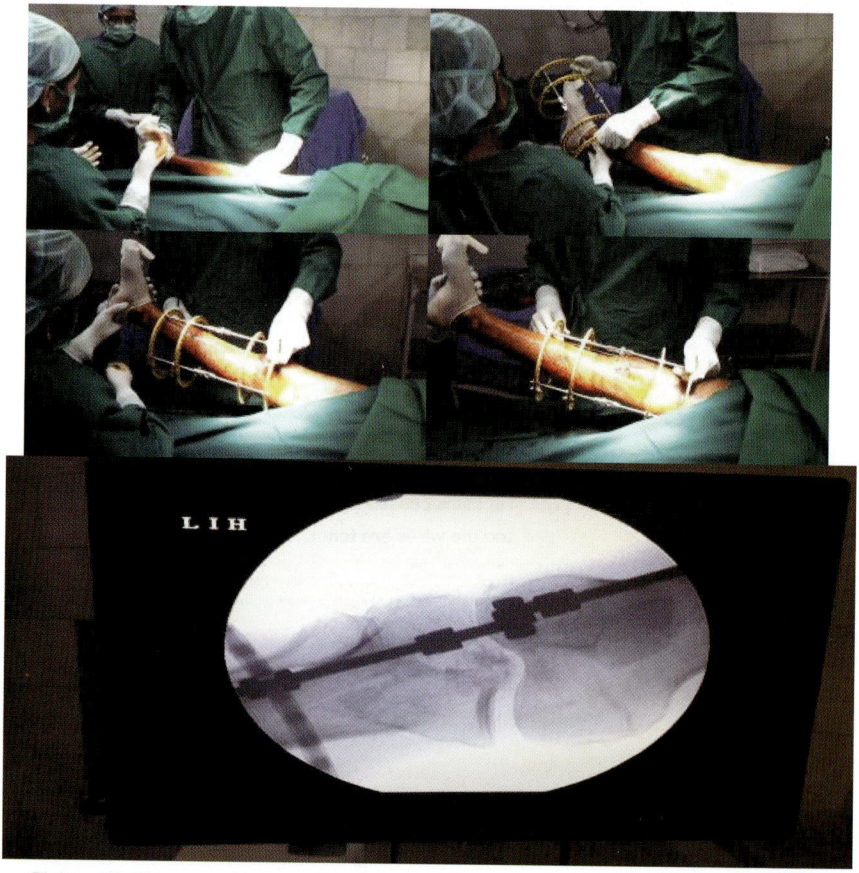

Picture 73: The assembled construct is slid over the limb and the hinges are accurately positioned over the joint line.

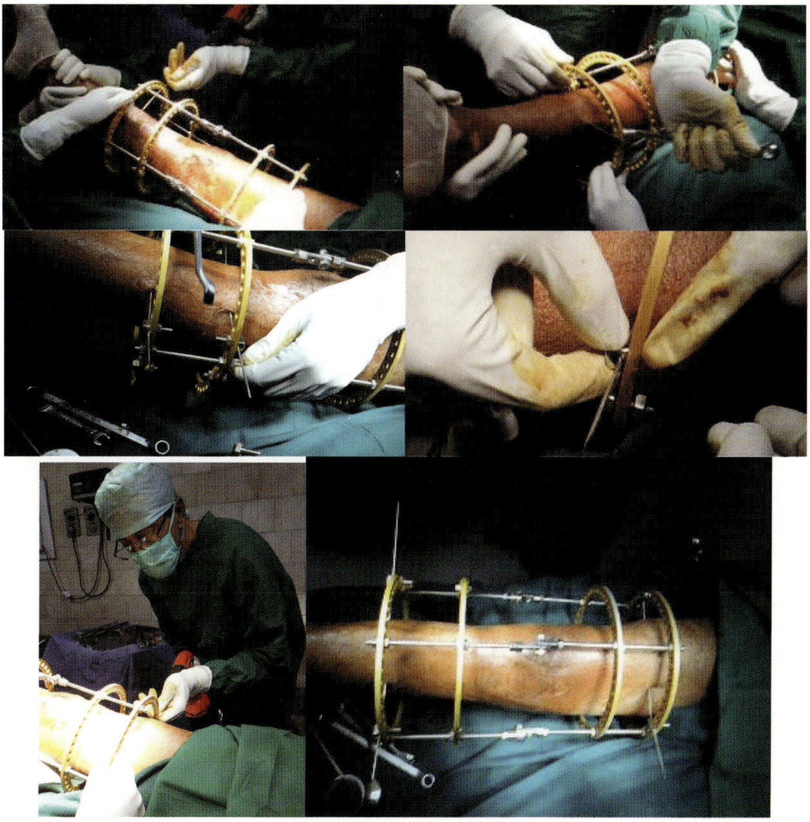

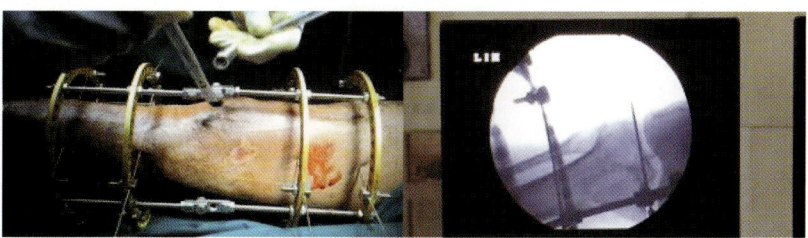

Picture 74: The order of wires. The first set is passed in ML axis. The two terminal rings are first fixed and the wires are tensioned.

Picture 75: The latero-medial wires are now passed for the middle two rings. The location of hinge is adjusted to the precise joint level and checked with a wire placed over skin.

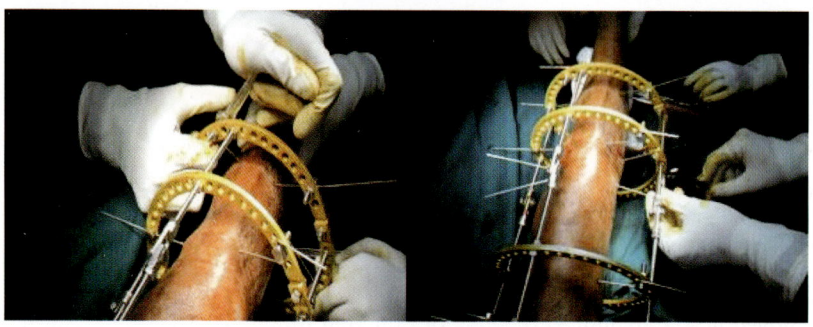

Picture 76: Next set of perpendicular wires is now inserted and tensioned. Olive wires too are inserted at appropriate places

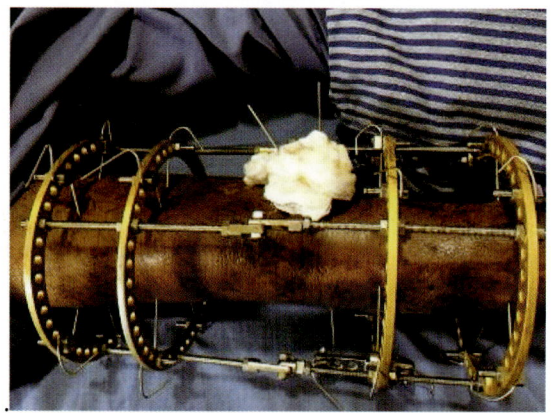

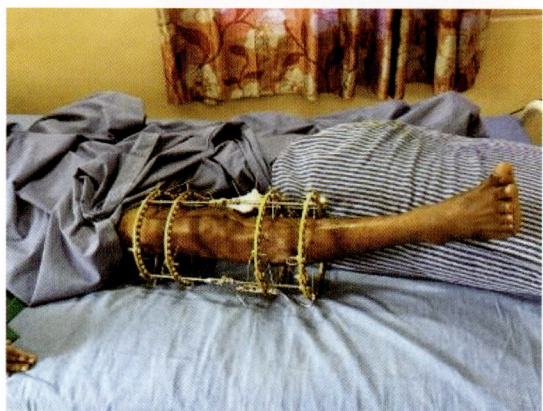

Picture 77: The completed assembly using a pre-fabricated construct.

FINALIZATION OF THE ASSEMBLY

At this stage, one embarks upon additional procedures like clearing of the fracture ends, open or closed reduction of fractures, corticotomy or any other procedure needed for that specific patient. An X-ray is taken at this stage if considered necessary. Appropriate specific details are described in individual chapters. However I shall describe the step of corticotomy because this is employed in a large number of situations ranging from non-unions to elongation.

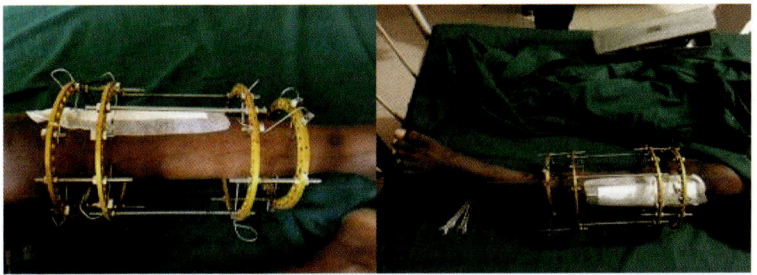

Picture 78: The standard 4 ring tibia assembly.

CORTICOTOMY

This requires a special fish mouth shaped chisel, called the corticotomy chisel. Corticotomy is in fact a low velocity minimum trauma osteotomy without damaging the medullary blood vessels. This is performed through 2, 3, or 4 evenly spaced 6 mm incisions. The bone is reached through each incision and the periosteum cut longitudinally in line with the skin incision. Subsequently, using the corticotomy chisel, the cortex is broken in both directions transversely as far as the limited skin incision will allow. The same steps are repeated through other incisions until a complete section of the cortex is achieved. In some cases, one may have to gently rock or twist the bone to complete the break.

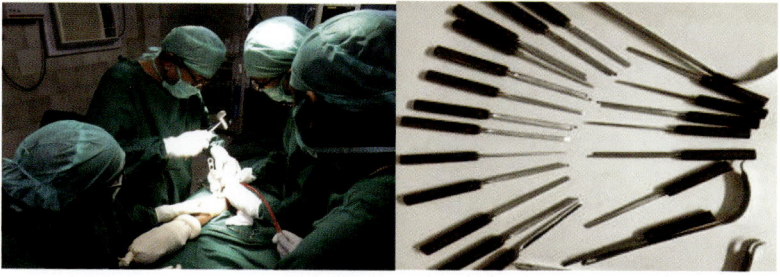

Picture 79: Corticotomy is essentially different from osteotomy.

POST OPERATIVE AND AFTER CARE

The junctions where the pins exit or enter the skin are cleaned thoroughly with an antiseptic solution and an adhesive spray applied. A small gauze piece is stuck here. Corticotomy incisions are usually closed by single skin sutures. Normally no additional paddings or bulky dressings are either needed or required.

REHABILITATION

The patient stays on the frame for weeks or months and it is essential that a preoperative counselling describes the entire process to the patient to keep him or her psychologically prepared. During the immediate post operative period, the patient is encouraged to move the surrounding joints as much as the pain tolerance permits, while attempts are made to make the patient functional as soon as possible. Some patients might be able to get back to school or place of work while on the frame. There have been recorded instances where patients have not only got back to their normal work but have also participated in activities like sports and cycling while still on the frame. The social and physical aspects of the patient on the frame is widely dependent on a large number of factors like the condition for which the frame is applied, the site of application, patient's age, gender, pain threshold, psychological makeup, associated anomalies and diseases, and the enthusiasm and dedication of the trainee surgeon.

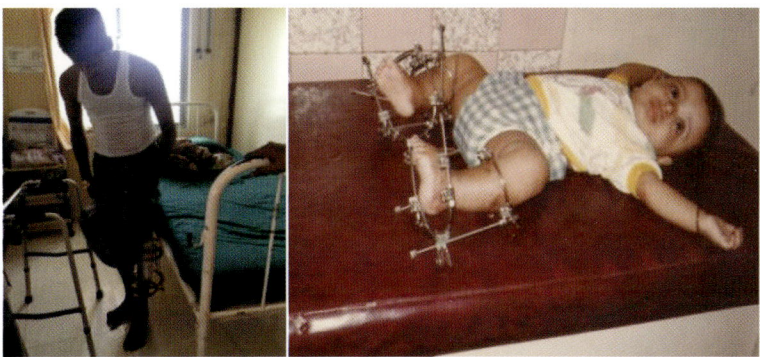

Picture 80: A fit and tight frame is painless and well tolerated.

In my personal experience, children and first time applicants have much better psychological profiles rather than dejected patients with multiple failed surgical procedures on whom this procedure is used as a salvage procedure.

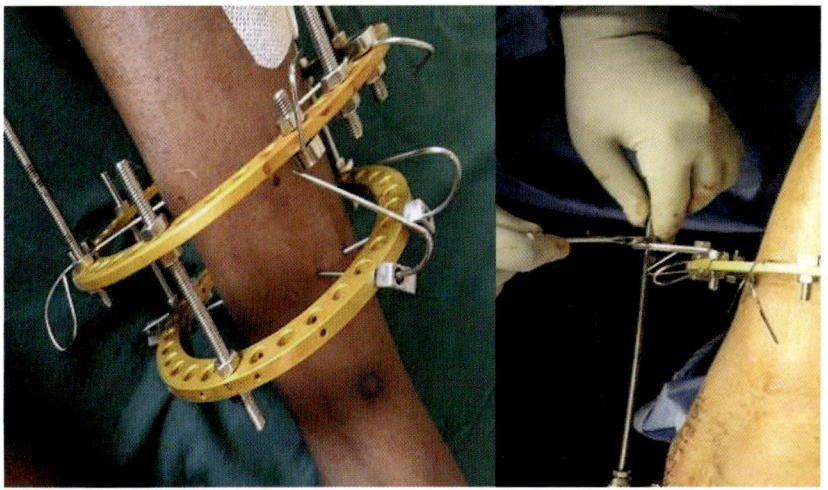

Picture 81: Constant nut turnings and readjustments are essential.

ADJUSTMENTS, LENGTHENING, AND SCREW TURNINGS

In most cases, the lengthening schedule, latency and duration are decided during the course of treatment. Most often, a six hourly distraction protocol is employed. It is thus best to give the spanners to the patients themselves. The first few steps are performed by the surgeon or the physiotherapist, followed by the patients themselves under the supervision of the physiotherapist. By the time the patients are discharged, they have learned the techniques and are capable of doing it at home. During periodic reviews and after follow ups, a decision is taken on the basis of clinical and radiological response as to a speed and extent of distraction. In cases of complicated deformity corrections, it may be preferable to retain the patients in hospital with corrections performed under direct supervision until the desired effect has been achieved.

The Magic of Pin Placements

The one single factor that separates a well versed Ilizarov surgeon from a beginner is the accuracy and confidence of wire placements. Apart from the biomechanical rules that mandate a near right angle placement, the anatomical consideration is only one: *Thou shalt not impale a nerve or vessel.*

It is an easy matter to learn the surface markings of the areas of pin placement. It is quite fortunate that vessels and nerves travel together for most of the part as a neurovascular bundle. The thumb or a finger palpates the vessel as the pin is carefully passed straight up to the bone. The assistant keeps his finger at the exit point and the surgeon slowly drills until he has passed both cortices. The drill is detached at this point and the joints above and below manipulated to achieve muscle stretch. The wire is then hammered out till it stretches the skin. By equalizing the tension all around, the skin is gently pushed in.

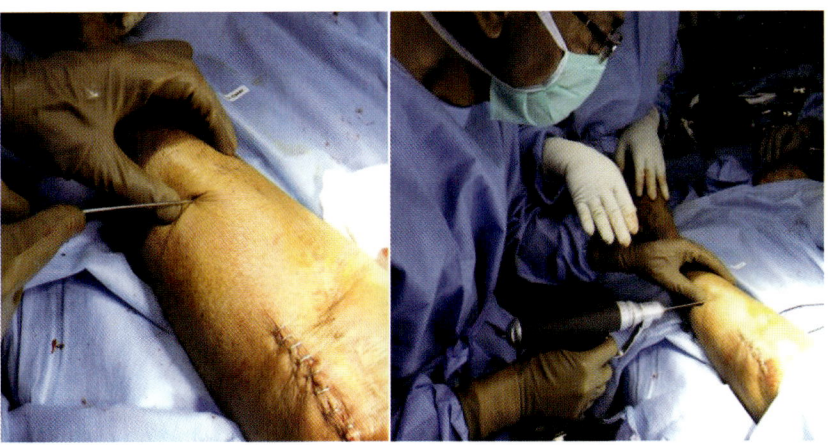

Picture 82: Pin insertion

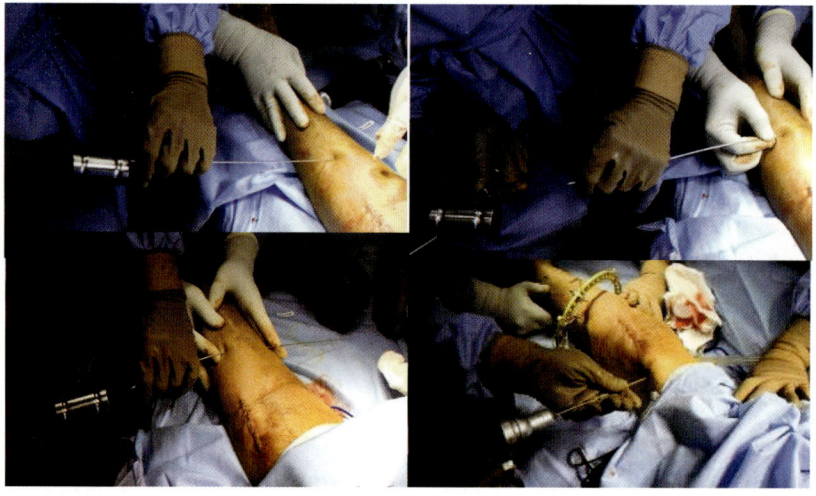

Picture 83: Pin is pushed to the bone, drilled through it, and hammered out.

In subsequent chapters, I shall deal with each extremity and limb individually. It is extremely easy to recollect our anatomy from medical college days and imagine the 3D and cross sectional views as we pass the wires. At this point, I would like to add that it is actually very difficult to impale a nerve or vessel even deliberately as they tend to fall back, allowing the wires to pass above them.

Once you have mastered the art of proper and accurate wire placement, the rest automatically falls in place. **It is very important to remember that though Ilizarov is a versatile, forgiving and correctable system, the only step which cannot be corrected during the course of management is the wire insertion. This has to be done correctly and 100% accurately the very first time, else it would result in another visit to the operation theatre and a second anesthetic.**

Pin placements in the foot

Metatarsal pins

In most tibial fixations, the foot tends to go into equinous during the post operative period. To avoid this, many surgeons routinely pass a metatarsal pin and use a half ring to keep the foot plantigrade. In addition, a metatarsal pin is essential in most foot deformity corrections. Lateral-to-medial or medial-to-lateral, the metatarsal heads and necks are safe zones. It is essential to pass the wire individually through each metatarsal, ensuring that none is left behind. If even one metatarsal head is left un-impaled, it will bunch the foot, causing neurovascular compromise. Only a half ring can be used at the metatarsal area, because the foot needs to be unencumbered to allow walking. But if this half ring is supported by a single wire alone, there is nothing to prevent a side-to-side shift, or even regular rocking and shifting post operatively, causing severe discomfort to the patient. I have mentioned earlier, and am repeating again: *A tight stable frame is a pain free frame. Every loose pin is an agony and misery.*

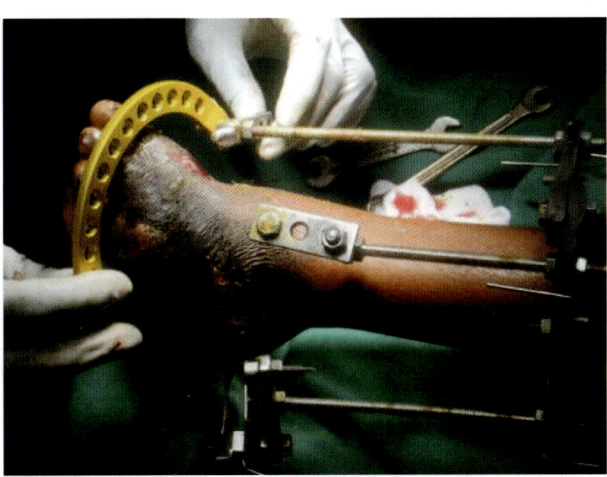

Picture 84: Pin placement in metatarsals.

. The metatarsal half ring

One method to stop the side-to-side shift is by fixing a 3.5 mm Shanz screw to the first metatarsal head from the dorsal side. A single Shanz pin is adequate to prevent side-to-side shifts. Purists may disagree and point out that this deviates from Ilizarov's all-wire concept. The other solution for preventing side-to-side shift is by using 2 olive wires, 1 from each side. The distance between the parallel wires should equal the distance between 2 holes on the half ring. Each olive is tensioned to its metatarsal and these dual wires give as much (or more) stability than a wire and a Shanz screw.

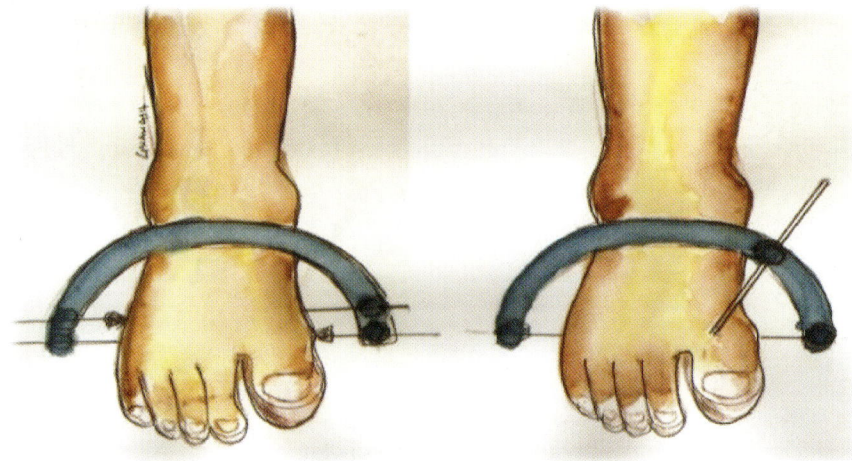

Picture 85: Metatarsals need one Shanz pin and one wire or two crossed olive wires.

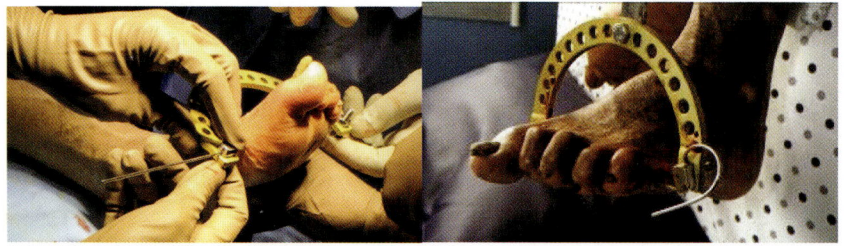

Picture 86: Two olives or a wire and a Shanz pin are used to prevent lateral shifts.

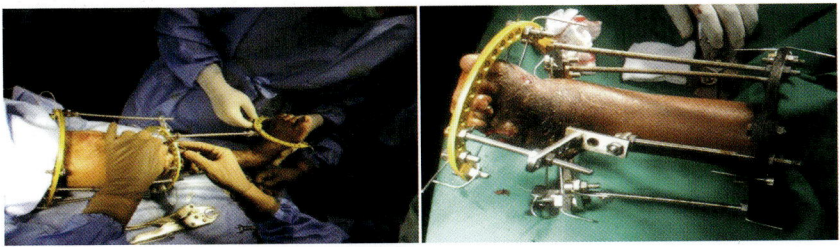

Picture 87: The wire should pass through all metatarsal heads.

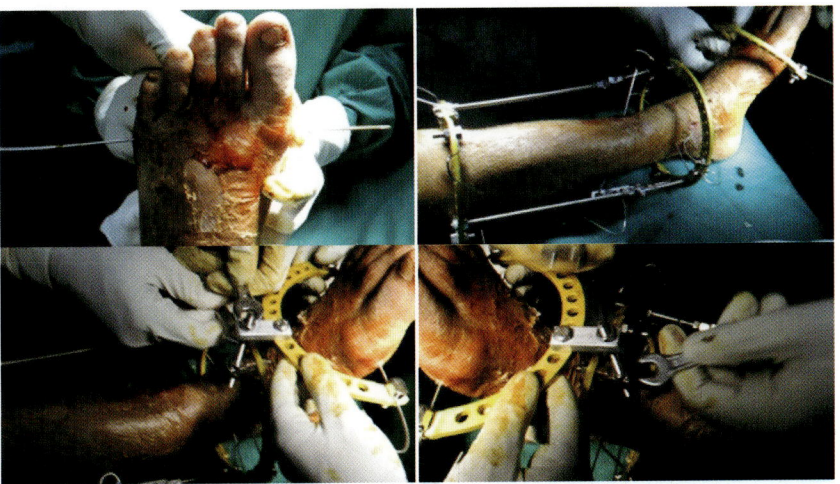

Picture 88: Steps for a metatarsal half ring

CALCANEAL PINS

The calcaneum is more or less subcutaneous bone, so it is easy to palpate areas medially and laterally for pin entry and exit points. We have to be careful not to go close to the maleoli. A finger placed below either medial or lateral maleolus protects the neurovascular bundle. The entire calcaneum behind this is a safe area for pin insertion. Here also, only a single half ring alone is needed to allow a plantigrade ground touching foot. To prevent side-to-side movements of the half ring on a single wire, one can either insert a Shanz screw from posterior to anterior, or use 2 olive wires, with the olives compressing the calcaneum from both sides. Occasionally even three pins can be inserted into the calcaneum for increased stability and to avoid use of Shanz pins.

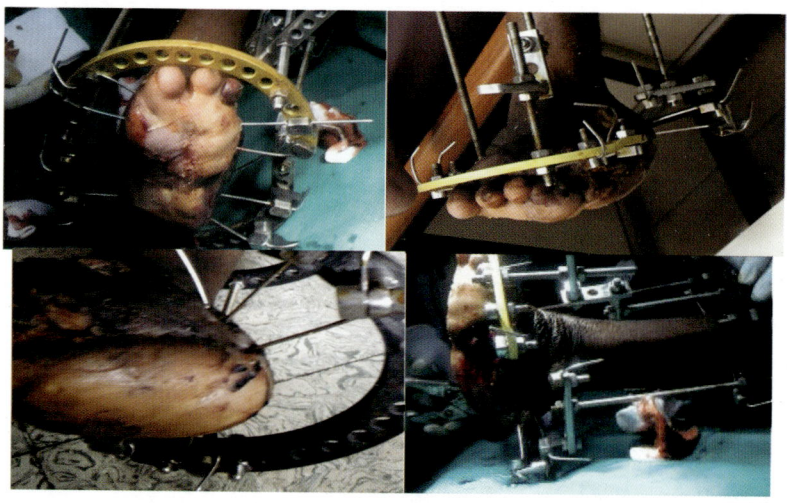

Picture 89: Calcaneal ring with appropriately placed pins

MID FOOT PINS

These are not usually required and the application of forces between metatarsal heads and calcaneum is enough to correct most deformities. However, in certain rocker bottom feet (with inverted arches), it becomes necessary to pull the mid foot dorsally. Under these situations, a pin transfixing the metatarsals at their mid shaft level is required. Here we have to go from medial to lateral. The shaft of the first metatarsal is subcutaneous in the dorso medial direction. It is here that the skin is impaled to reach the bone. Once the bayonet tip touches the bone, it is slightly lowered to get the direction right and drilled across so that it emerges from the lateral side of the fifth metatarsal. Midfoot half rings too require additional stabilization, either by a metatarsal Shanz pin from dorsal side or the use of two opposite olive wires to prevent lateral shift.

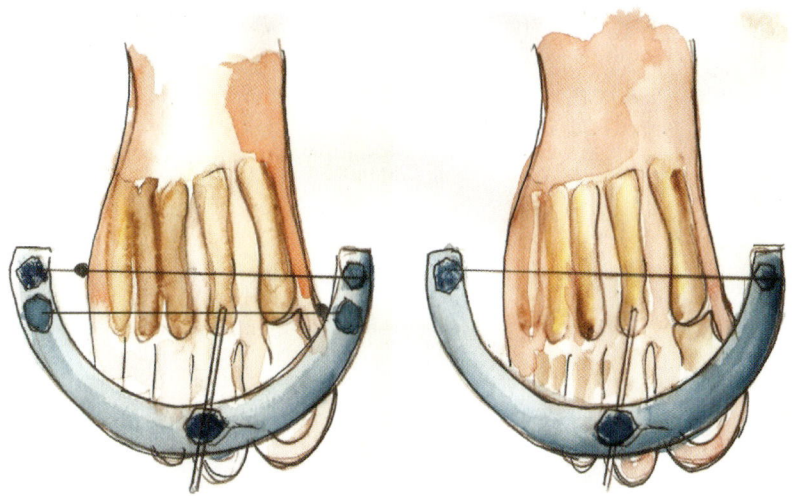

Picture 90: Pins in the mid foot area. Two opposite olives or a right angled Shanz gives stability.

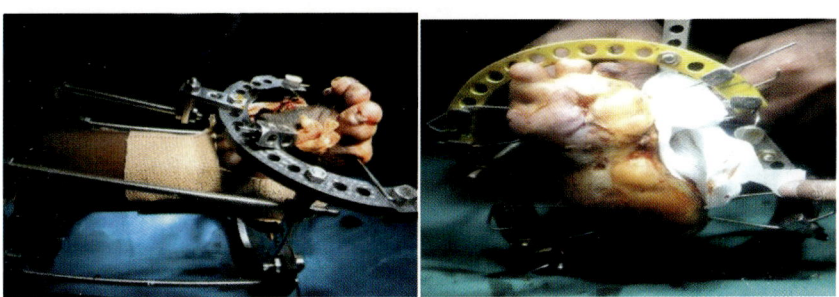

Picture 91: Mid foot pin

Direction of half rings in the foot

1. *All calcaneal rings will lie parallel to the ground or floor as the patient keeps the foot down.*

2. *Most metarsal rings are positioned at right angles to the floor on the dorsal aspect. Occasionally a challenging foot deformity may demand a half ring to*

be placed parallel to the floor. In such cases it is essential to give sufficient toe clearance.

Pin placements in tibia and fibula

Tibia is a superficial bone throughout; its anterior surface can be felt from anteromedial tibial plateau superiorly to medial maleolus inferiorly. The two neurovascular bundles traversing vertically down are the anterior tibial/ deep peroneal nerve anteriorly and tibial nerve/ posterior tibial vessels posteriorly. Saphenous nerve and great saphenous vein lie dead posterior. As shown by the cross sectional drawings below, it is apparent that both these neurovascular bundles lie in the space anterior and posterior to the interosseus space between the tibia and fibula. The anterior tibial vessel is palpable in its middle, but the posterior tibial artery is deep below the calf muscle and not easily felt. Thus it is essential to remember the safe corridors and pass the wire accordingly.

An easy way to describe the points of pin insertion is the CLOCK METHOD. Dead anterior is 12 O'clock. Dead posterior is 6 O'clock. Medial and lateral are 3 or 6 O'clock depending on the side of the limb. In the following descriptions I will stick to the clock analogy, rather than using the Latin names of blood vessels and nerves, because I believe that a 3D anatomical visualization is far more important than knowing all the Latin names of vessels and nerves. Some drawings are made by me, others copied from anatomy text books. The following points should be kept in mind while inserting pins into tibia:

In lower tibia, it is possible to get a good bony contact between medial and lateral maleoli. Most neurovascular structures are either anterior or posterior. So safe corridors are from anterio medial to posterio lateral. The photos below show the safe corridors.

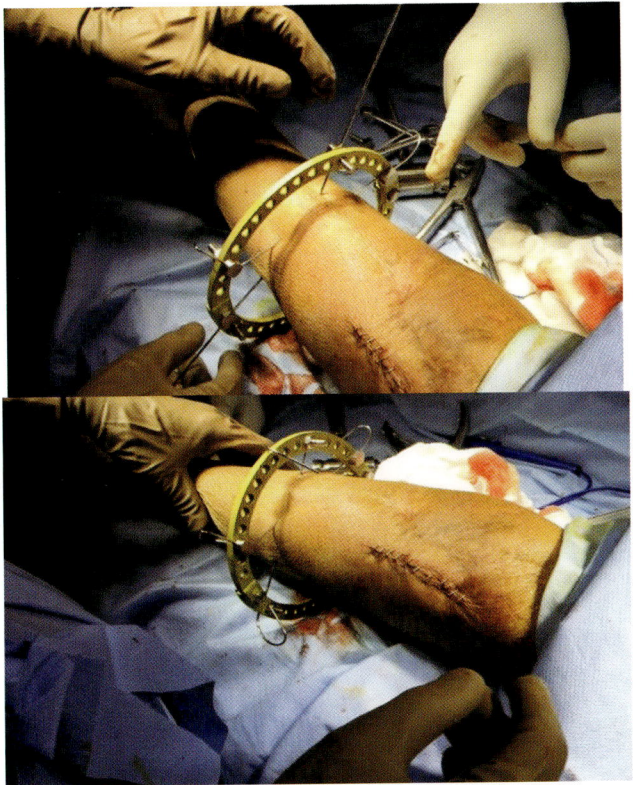

Picture 92: Pin placement in lower tibia

1. Extra safe corridors are available in the anterio posterior direction, so long as you are aware of the posterior neurovascular bundle location. From these photographs, it would be clear that safe corridors for lower tibia will be between 8 and 11 O'clock entry and 2 to 5 O'clock exit. The 8 to 12 O'clock wire can be used for tibial fixation alone.

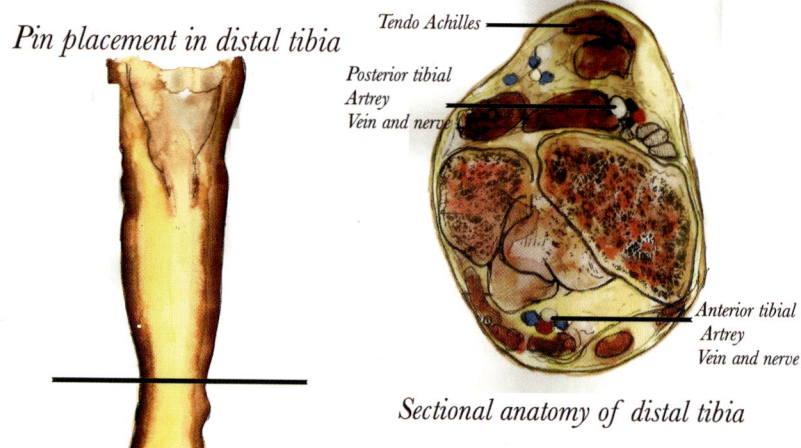

Pin placement in distal tibia

Tendo Achilles

Posterior tibial Artrey Vein and nerve

Anterior tibial Artrey Vein and nerve

Sectional anatomy of distal tibia

Picture 93: The safe corridors for pin placement in lower tibia

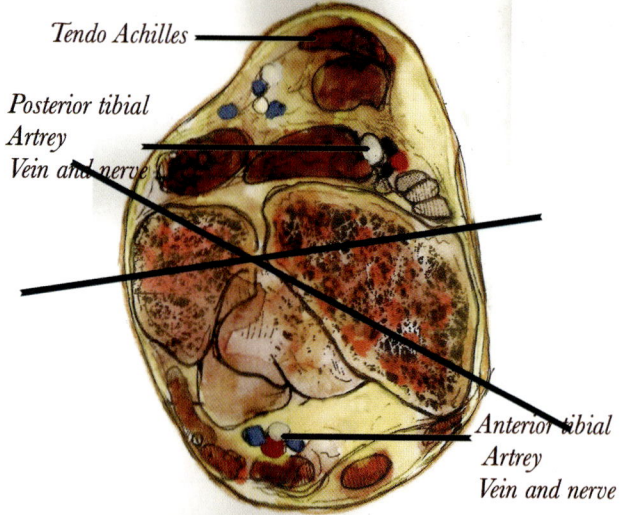

Tendo Achilles

Posterior tibial Artrey Vein and nerve

Anterior tibial Artrey Vein and nerve

Pin placement in distal tibia

Picture 95: The sequence of pin placement in lower tibia

.2. The following photographs show the sequence of pin placement in lower tibia.

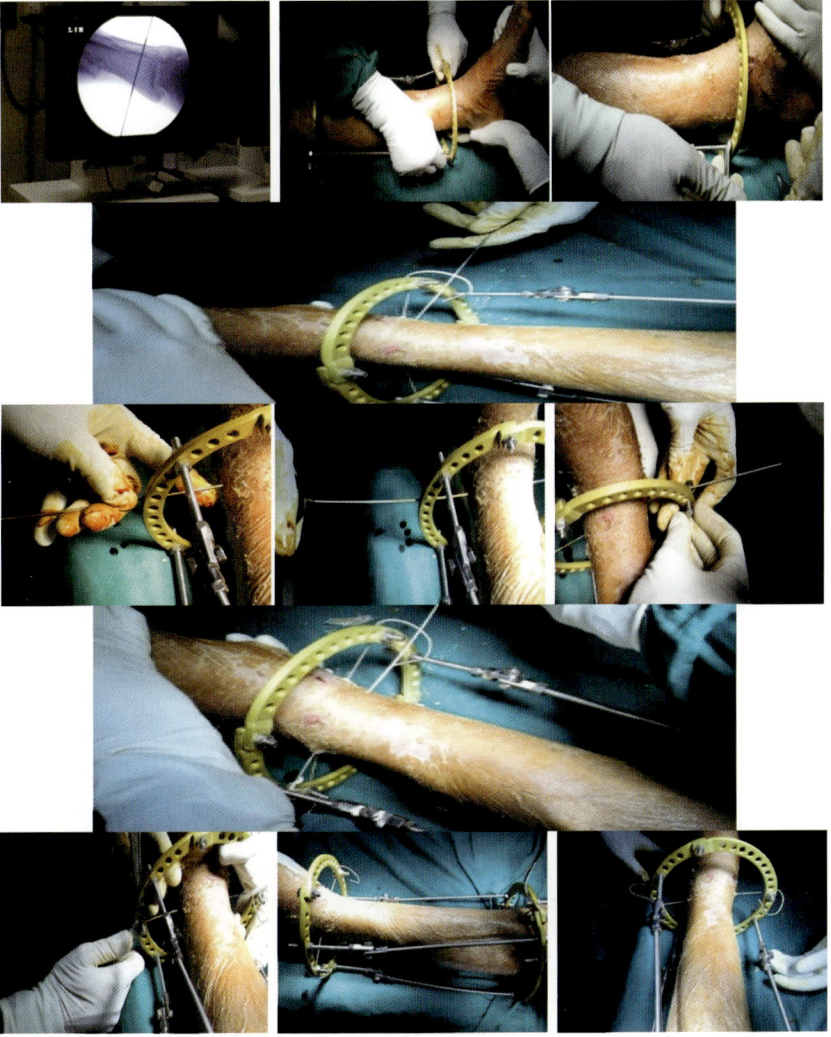

Picture 94: The sequence of pin placement in lower tibia

3. In lower third of tibia, the safe points are entries between 9 and 11 O'clock with exits between 1 and 5 O'clock.

4. If you go a little higher. the entry and exit points change only slightly. Here all 8 to 11 O'clock pins get a wide corridor for entries, so long as you keep only the tibia as your centre point. Only in 9 to 9.30 pin would you be able to transfix both the tibia and fibula. However, from this level onwards, it is enough if tibia alone is fixed.

Pin placement in mid tibia

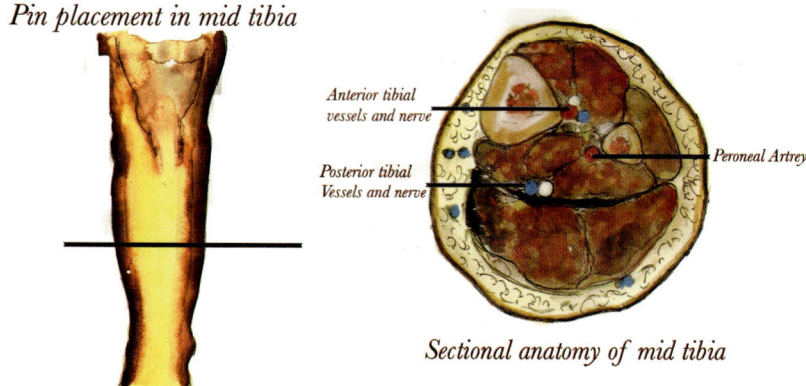

Sectional anatomy of mid tibia

Picture 96: Pin Placements and safe corridors in middle to upper third of tibia

5. The pictures below show operative photos of pin placements in middle to upper tibiae.

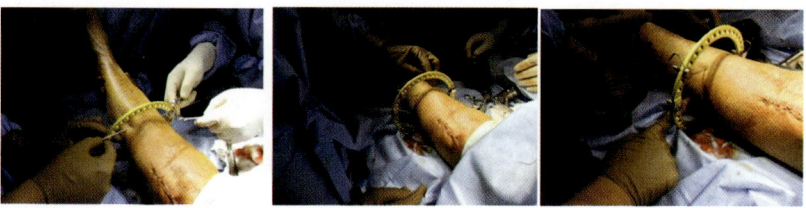

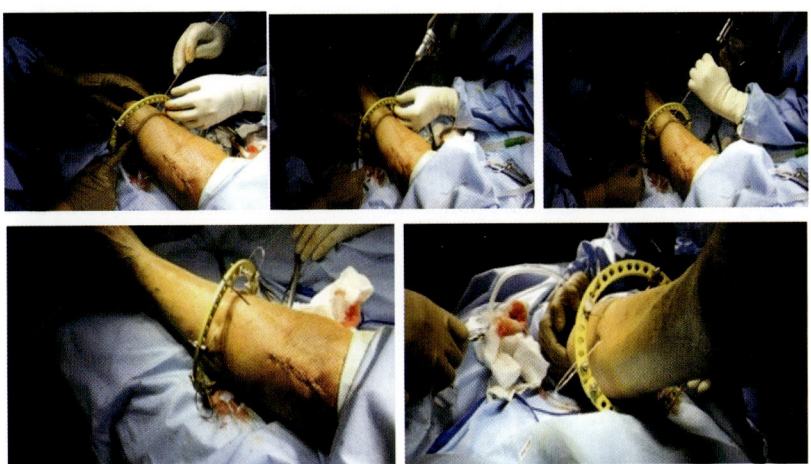

Picture 97: Pin placement in middle and upper tibia

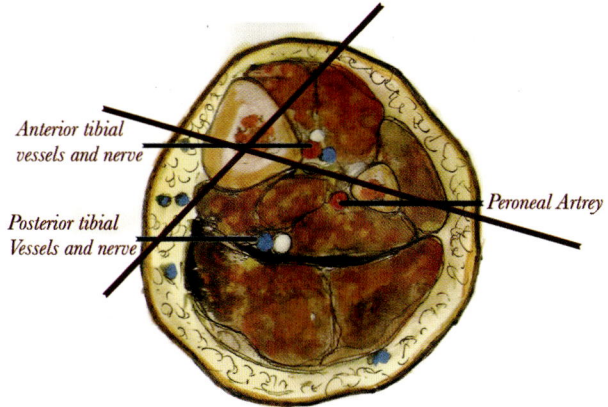

Anterior tibial vessels and nerve

Posterior tibial Vessels and nerve

Peroneal Artrey

Wire placement in mid tibia

6. In upper tibia, the side-to-side wires are passed from lateral to medial. The area above tibial tuberosity is safe so long as one keeps in mind the lateral popleteal nerve. In the antero posterior direction, one must avoid the vessels

and nerves in the popleteal fossa. Exit points beyond the hamstrings forms safe corridors.

Pin placement in proximal tibia

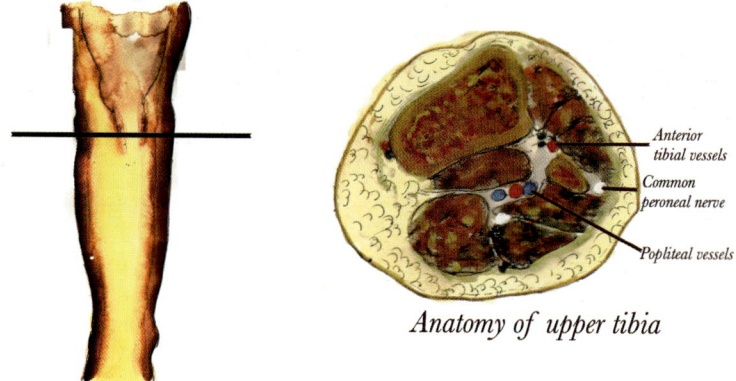

Anatomy of upper tibia

Picture 98: Sectional anatomy of upper tibia.

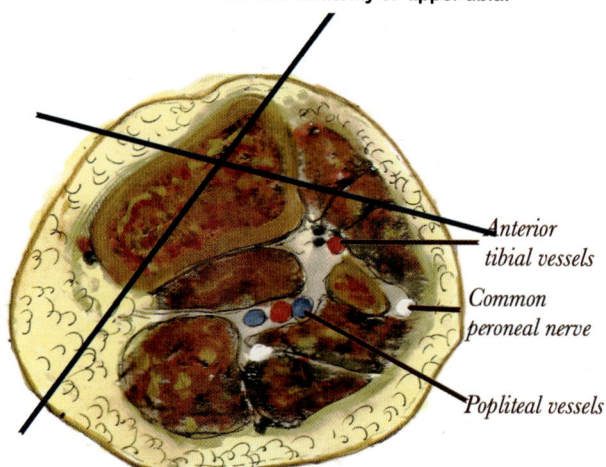

Pin placements in upper tibia

7. The following photographs show the surgical steps of pin placement in upper tibia at tibial condylar levels.

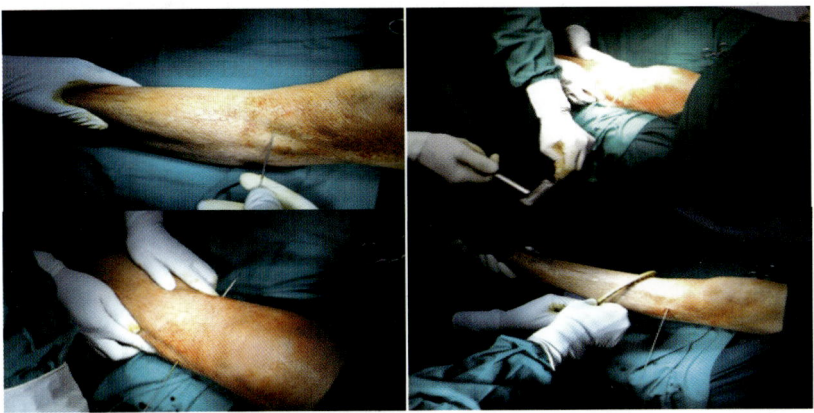

Picture 99: The pin is pushed to the bone, drilled across, tapped through and then anchored to the wires.

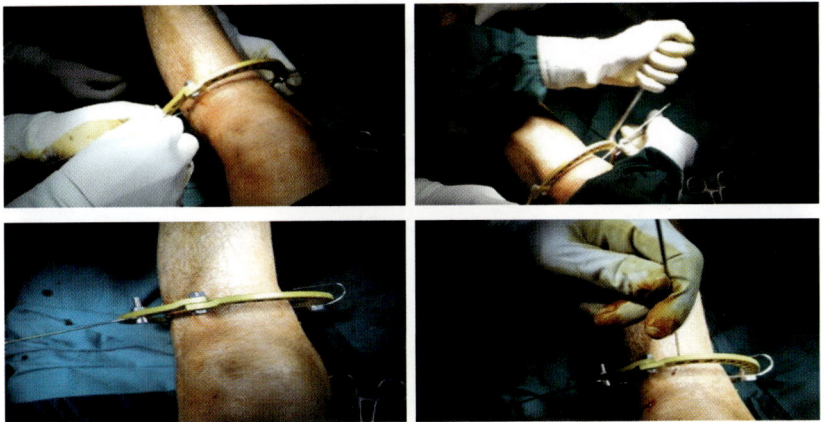

Picture 100: Each pin is tensioned before the next right angled pin is inserted.

In all situations, we must remember:

1. The ring closest to each joint lies exactly parallel to that joint in both planes.

2. The rings next to these are parallel in both planes to their adjacent rings.

3. Wires can be passed at almost any level throughout the length of tibia.

Pin placements in Femur

Immediately above the patella, at the level of suprapatellar pouch, the femur lies anteriorly, with the quadriceps tendon above it. Just behind the femur lie the popleteal structures, separated by semimembranosis.

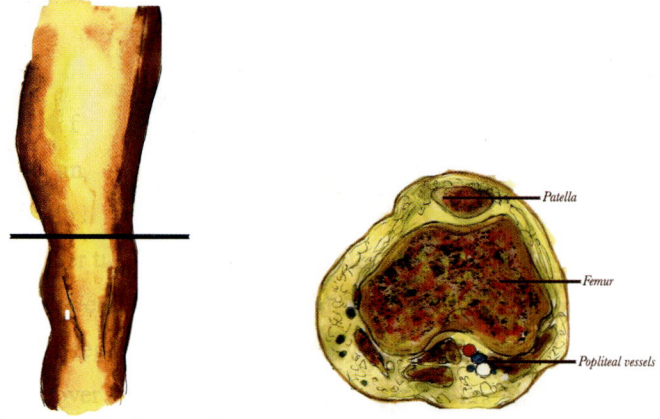

Pin placement in lower femur   *Sectional anatomy of distal femur*

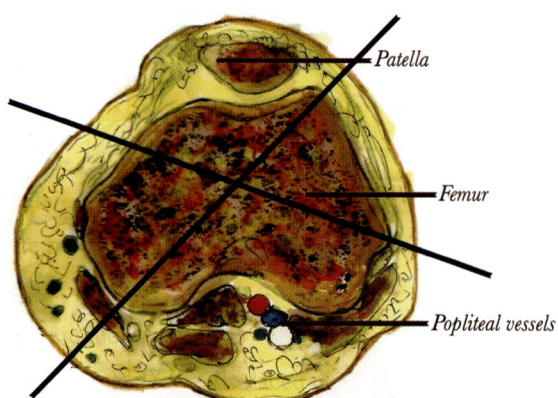

Pin placement in distal femur

Picture 101: Safe corridors for pin placement in lower femur

Here the entry points can be between 8 to 11 O'clock positions, while the exit points will emerge around 2 to 4.30.

The following intraoperative photographs show the pin placements in lower femur.

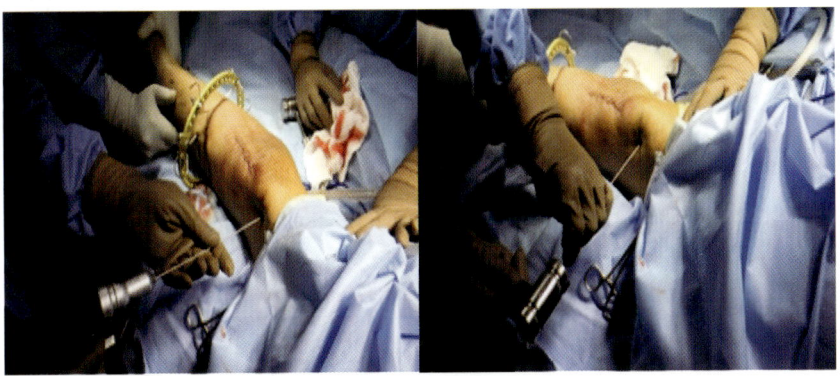

Picture 102: Pin placement in lower femur.

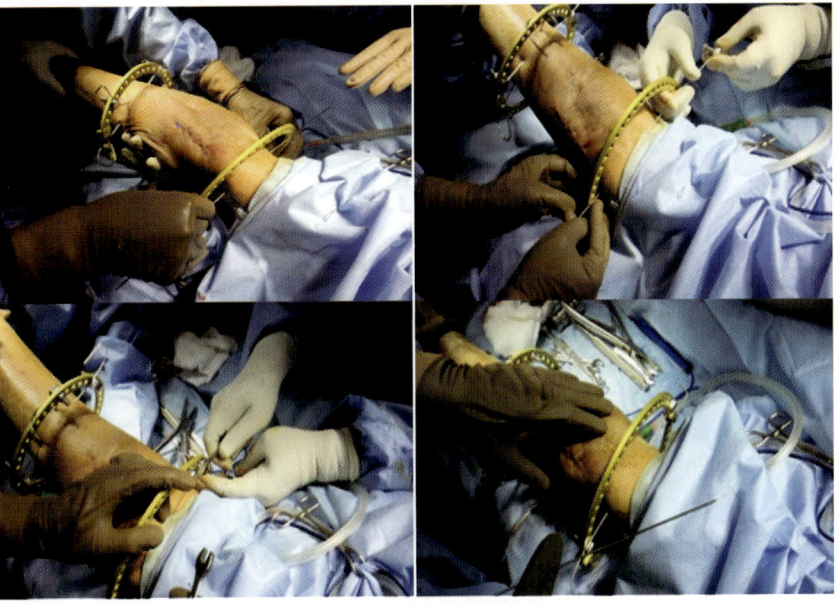

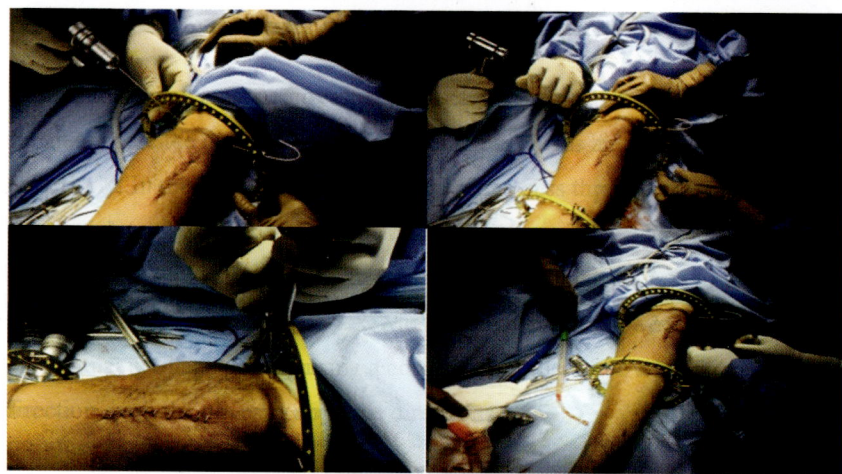

Picture 103: Sequence of ring fixation in distal femur. It may not always be possible to get a 90/90 spread. Some compromise has to be done.

In the mid thigh, the femoral artery and saphenous nerve are within the adductor canal medially. The sciatic nerve is dead posterior to the femoral shaft. Thus 9 to 3 O'clock and 12 to 6 O'clock are the dangerous areas to be avoided. Entry points at 10 and 11 O'clock are pretty safe exiting at 2 or 5 O'clock.

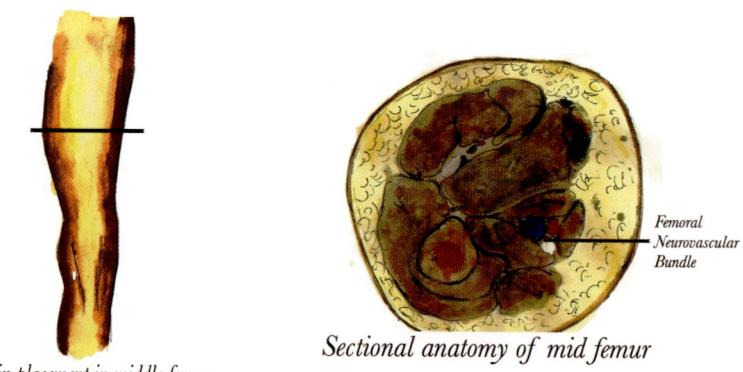

Pin placement in middle femur

Sectional anatomy of mid femur

Femoral Neurovascular Bundle

Picture 104: Pin level and surface anatomy in mid thigh

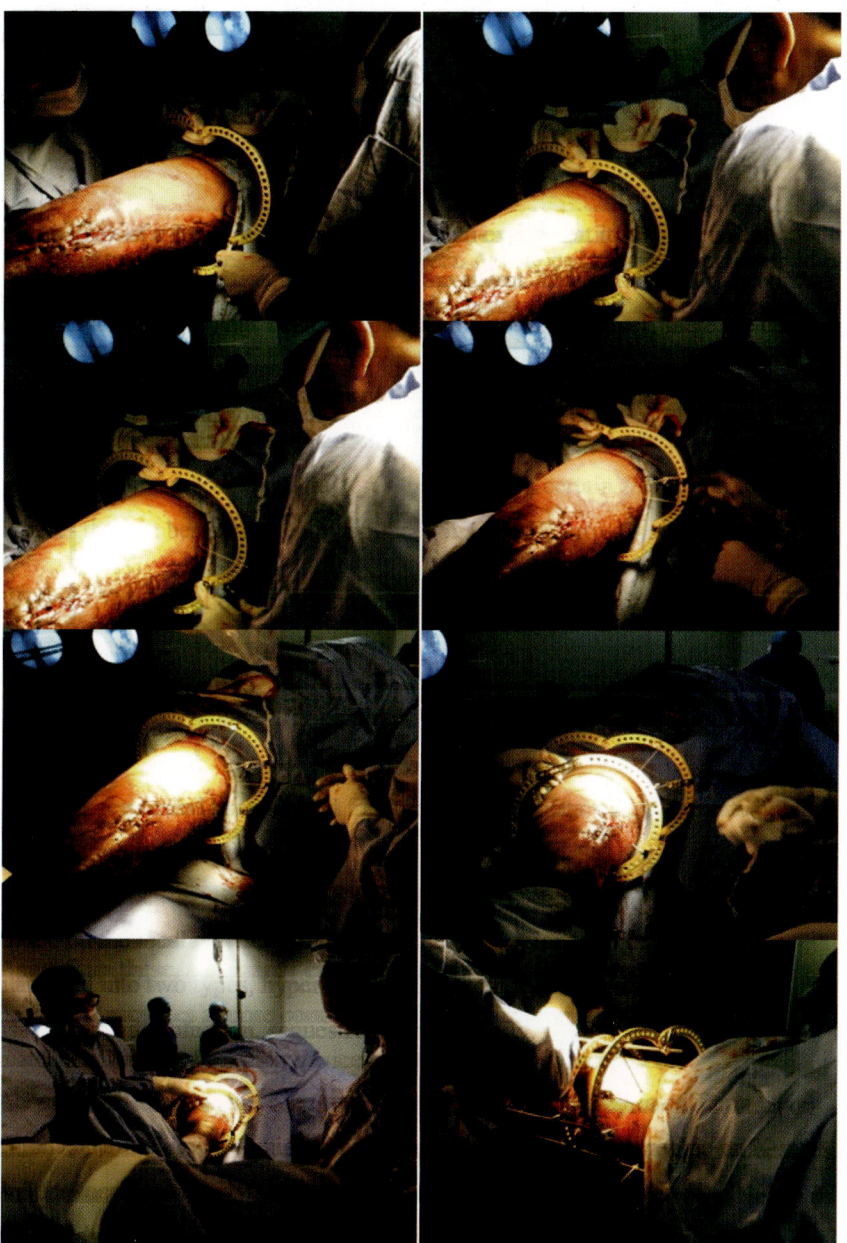

Picture 105: Pin placements in mid thigh.

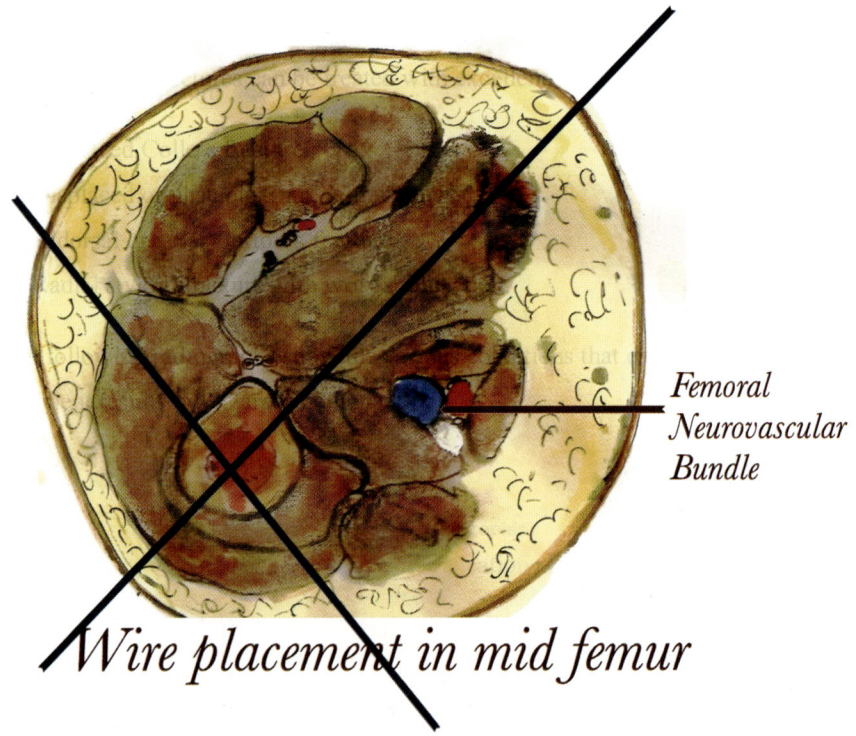

Femoral Neurovascular Bundle

Wire placement in mid femur

Proximal femur is only accessible to pins between 10 to 12 O'clock entries with 12 to 6 O'clock exits. Even 2 pins in this axis do not give a sufficient spread for a stable fixation. This can be augmented either by olive wires or by Shanz pins.

Though Ilizarov purists almost always use crossed wires augmented by olive wires and get a fairly stable assembly, for beginners it is forgivable to use one or two Shanz pins. I use and recommend Shanz pins only for proximal humerus and proximal femur.

118

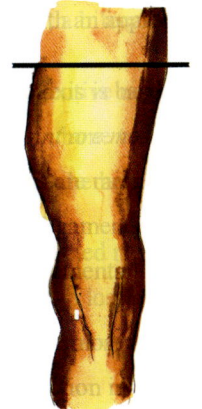

Pin placement in upper femur

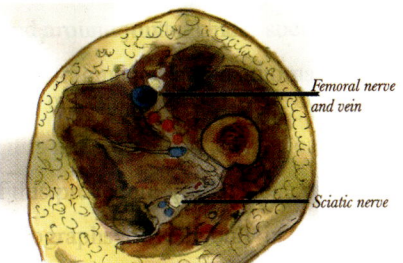

Sectional anatomy of upper femur

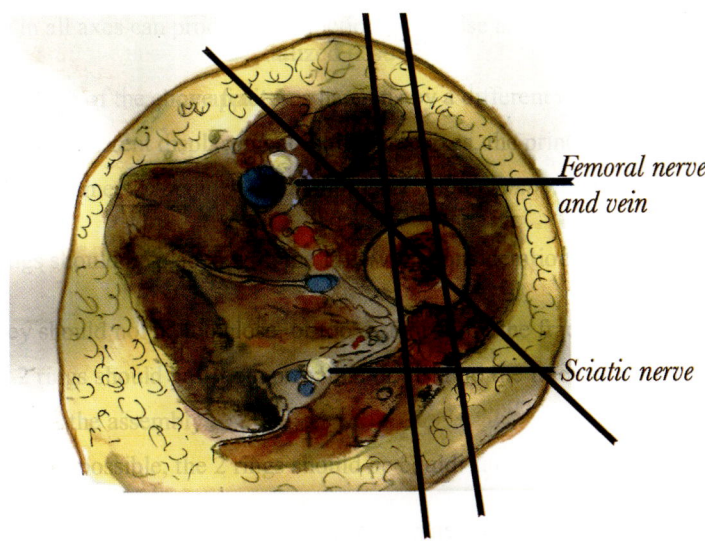

Pin placement in upper femur

Picture 106:   Safe corridors for proximal femur. A Shanz pin may be needed laterally

Pin Placement in Metacarpals

The pins are driven through the head of metacarpals, a little below the joint line. One can go down up to the upper one-fourth of the metacarpals. Occasionally, two parallel olive wires, one from medial to lateral, the other from lateral to medial, will give additional stability. The exit and entry points are subcutaneous and easily palpable. The pin is first pushed to the bone, drilling started, and paused at exit. It is then gently tapped with a hammer till it gets to the next bone. Drilling is begun once again. In this manner, it is ensured that the wire passes through all the metacarpal heads at the same level.

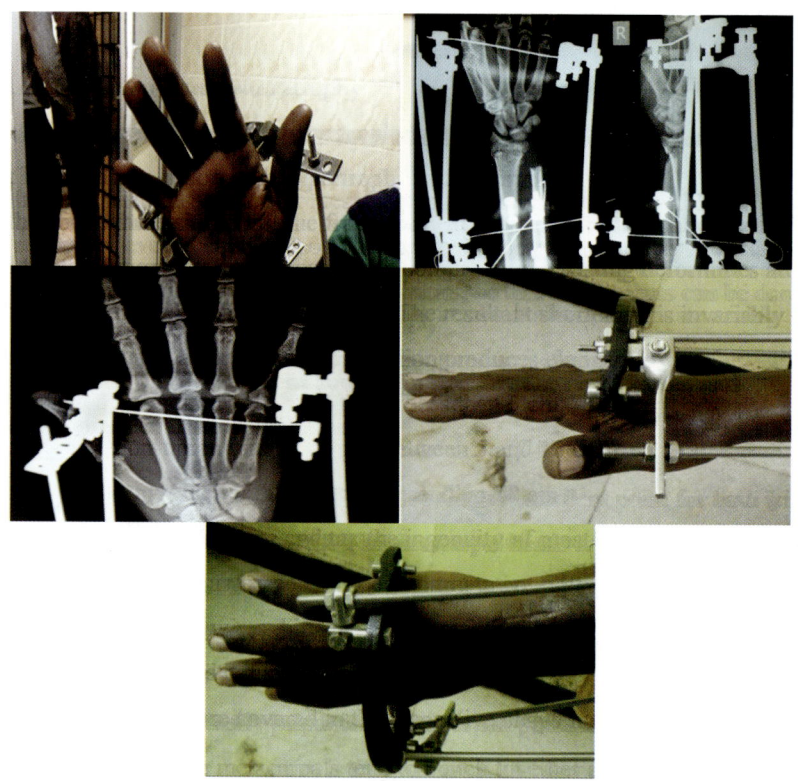

Picture 107: Pin placement in the metacarpal region

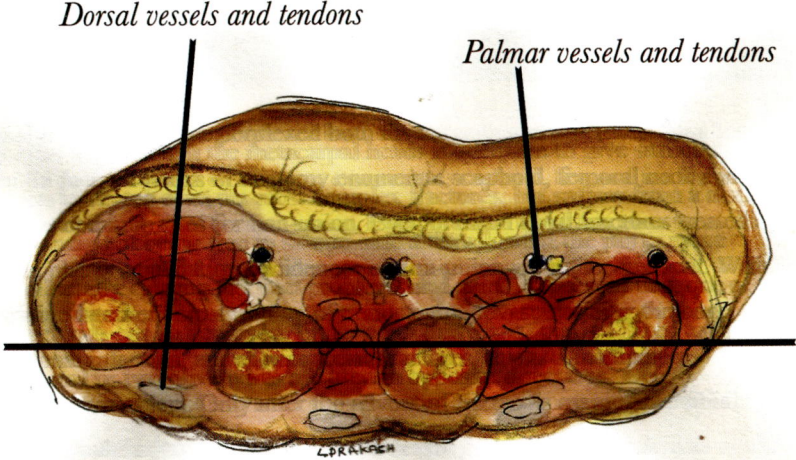

Dorsal vessels and tendons

Palmar vessels and tendons

Pin placement in the metacarpal region

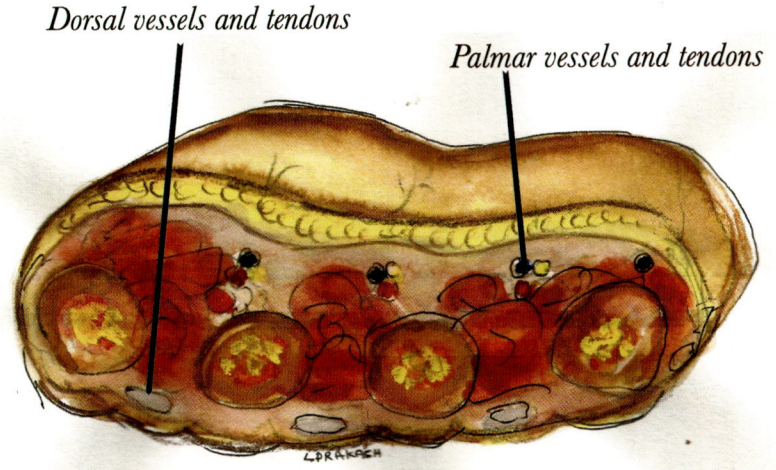

Dorsal vessels and tendons

Palmar vessels and tendons

Sectional anatomy of the metacarpal region

Pin placements in the forearm

Distal forearm just above the wrist

At the level of distal radioulnar syndesmosis, the radial neurovascular bundle lies laterally and the ulnar neurovascular bundle medially. Both these are superficial and can be palpated with ease. Thus the mediolateral safe corridors would be dorsal to both these neurovascular bundles. In the dorsovolar axis, we have to carefully palpate the flexor tendon bunch, relax them and negotiate the wire without a drill after it has passed the volar cortex. Though an exact 90/90 wire placement may not be possible, a decent position can be invariably obtained.

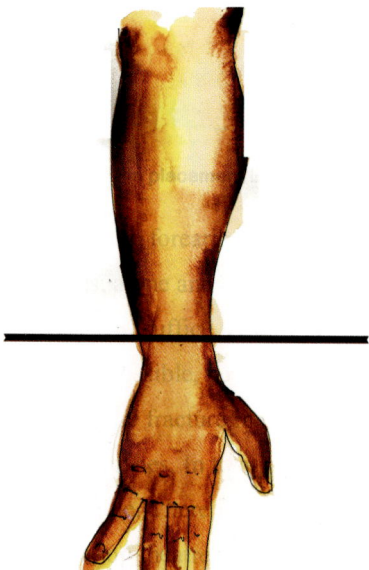

Pin placement in lower forearm

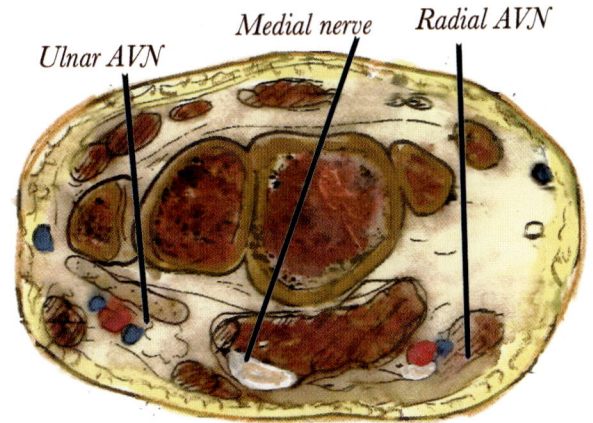

Sectional anatomy of distal radius and ulna

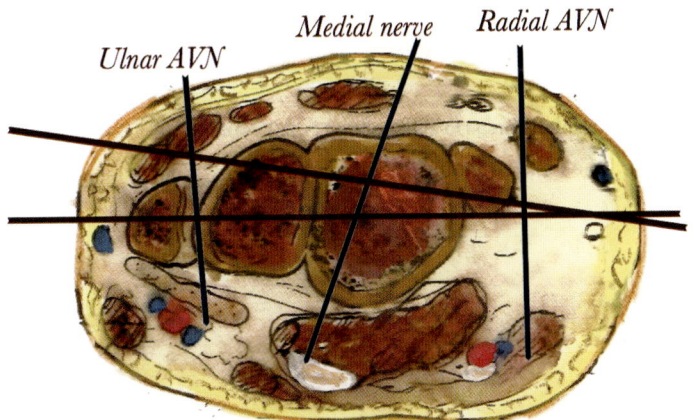

Pin placement in distal radius and ulna

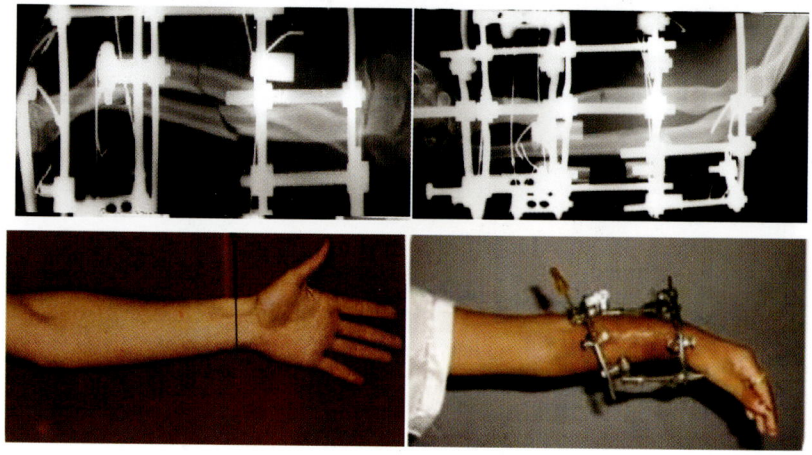

Picture 108: Safe corridors and wire placement in the lower forearm

Pin placements in the middle forearm

Here we have to use a primary bone bi-fixation strategy. (By the way, this is a phrase that I just coined!) In distal forearm, radius is usually the primary bone, whereas in upper forearm, closer to elbow, radius becomes a little slender as ulna flares to make a good hinge joint with lower humerus. Thus ulna becomes the primary bone in the upper forearm. Unless we are treating a single bone pathology necessitating pin placements in one specific bone, the usual practice is to pass one wire transfixing both bones, while the right angled wire impales only the primary bone of that area. Here the flexor carpi radialis is the palpable landmark. We must remember that the two important structures lie on either side of it. Radial to FCR (lateral) lies the radial neurovascular bundle, while ulnar (medial) to it is the median nerve. Flexor carpi ulnaris is the other landmark, as the ulnar neurovascular bundle travels along it. Thus, at this level both bones are transfixed by a single wire only in the mediolateral direction. Safe corridors however exist for both bones to individually allow two wires through each of them. The following pictures demonstrate this point.

Occasionally, one can use a olive wire and a 3.5 Shanz pin in the dorsal aspect, so that the vulnerable structures in the volar aspect are not put to risk.

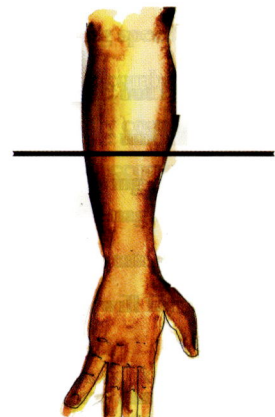

Pin placement in middle forearm

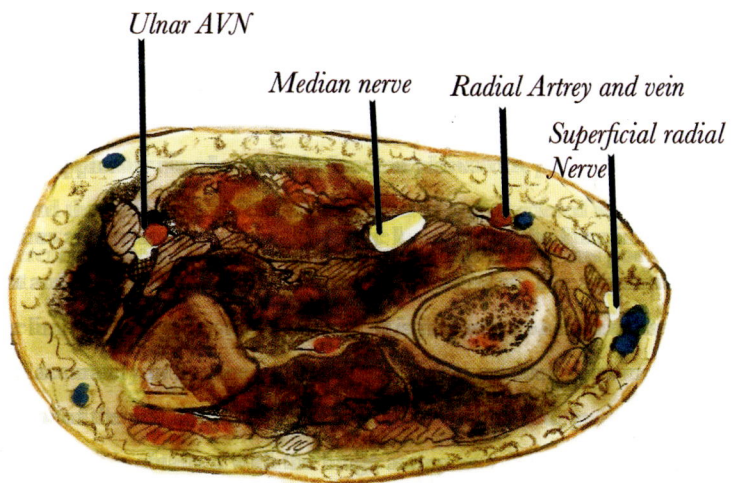

Sectional anatomy of mid forearm

Picture 109: Safe corridors for pin placement in middle forearm

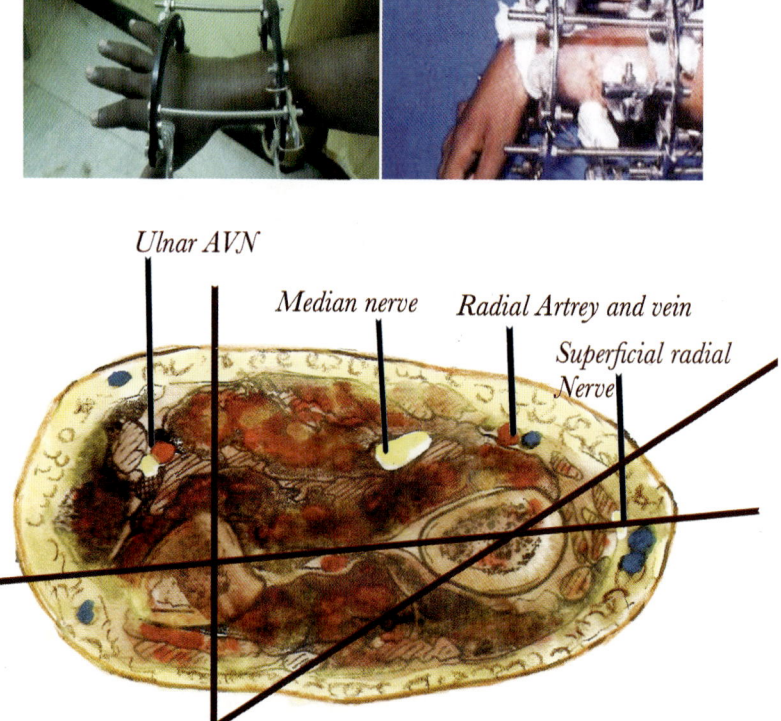

Picture 110: Wire passage in the middle forearm

Pin placements in upper forearm close to elbow

At this level, the ulnar artery has separated from ulnar nerve and moves laterally. The median nerve is anterior to radius separated by flexor profundus. Between brachioradialis and pronator teres lie the radial artery and superficial radial nerve. So here it gives a safe corridor from medial to lateral to trasnsfix both the bones. Isolated radial and ulnar wire transfixations can be done avoiding the above structures as displayed in the following photographs.

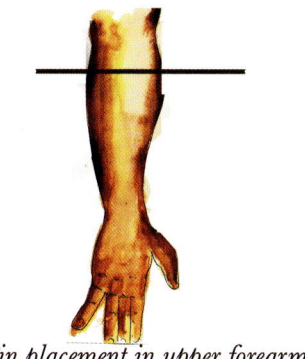

Pin placement in upper forearm

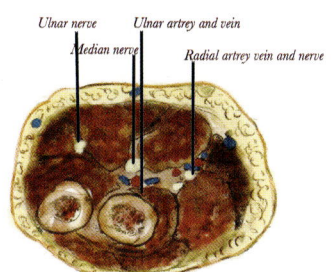

Sectional anatomy of upper forearm

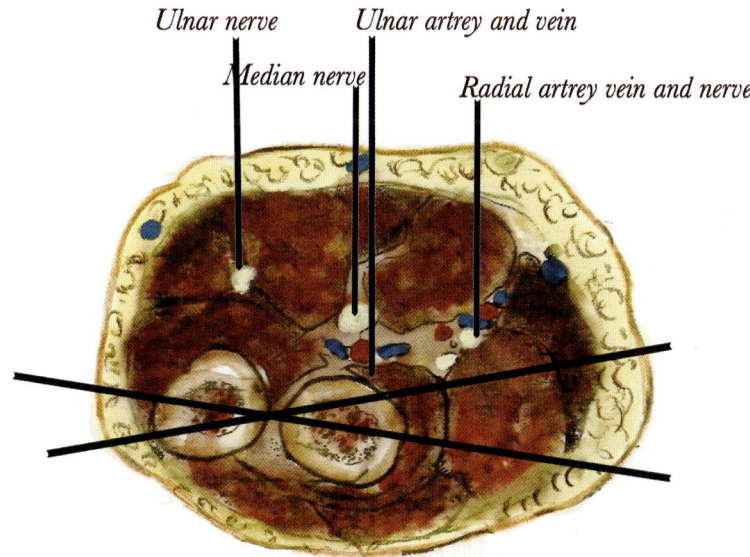

Pin placement in upper forearm

Picture 111: Safe corridors for pin passage in upper forearm

Pin placements in the arm

Pin placements in the lower arm

Just above the elbow, the humerus is triangular in cross section and becomes cylindrical as it progresses higher. In the sulcus between biceps and brachialis lies the neurovascular bundle consisting of brachial artery, vein and median nerve. The radial nerve is lateral to brachialis, while the ulnar nerve rests on medial border of triceps. The pins are to be passed appropriately as seen in the following photos.

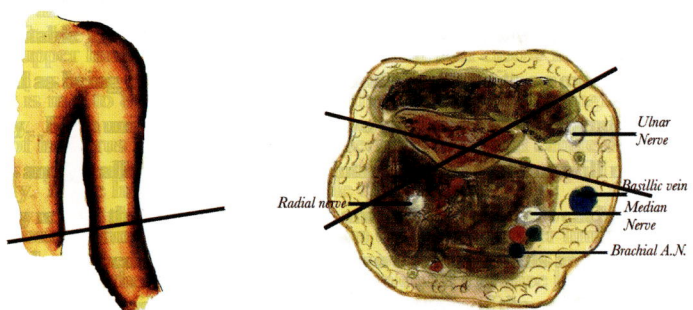

Pin placement in lower humerus   *Pin placement in of lower humerus*

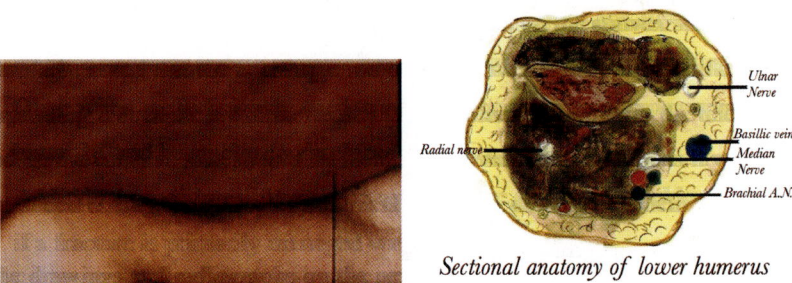

Sectional anatomy of lower humerus

Picture 112: Safe corridors for pin passage in the lower arm

At this level, many surgeons prefer to pass a Shanz pin posteriorly through the triceps. Though this makes the surgeon's life a little easier, it does not conform to the principles of original Ilizarov, and many purists only recommend an all wire ring at this level. The clinical photographs below show the ring position at this level and the direction of wires.

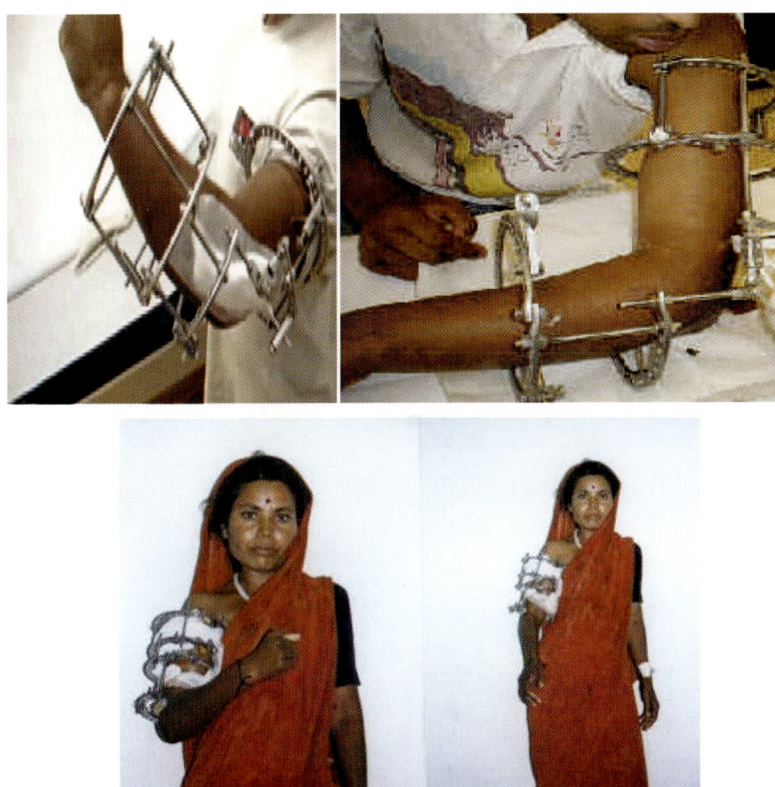

Picture 113: Ring position and wire direction in lower humerus

Pin placements in the middle arm

This is a fairly easy and uncomplicated level to pass wires through, because at this level, all the neurovascular structures except the radial nerve are medial.

The radial nerve is more or less dead posterior, lying between the lateral head of triceps and brachialis. Thus, by avoiding the anterio posterior corridors, we can have enough area for placing two or more pins.

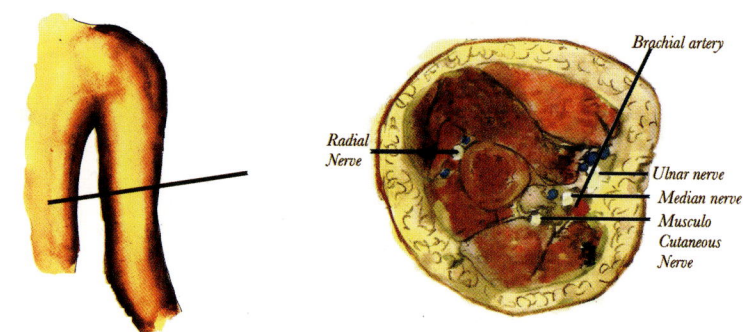

Pin placement in middle humerus   *Sectional anatomy of mid humerus*

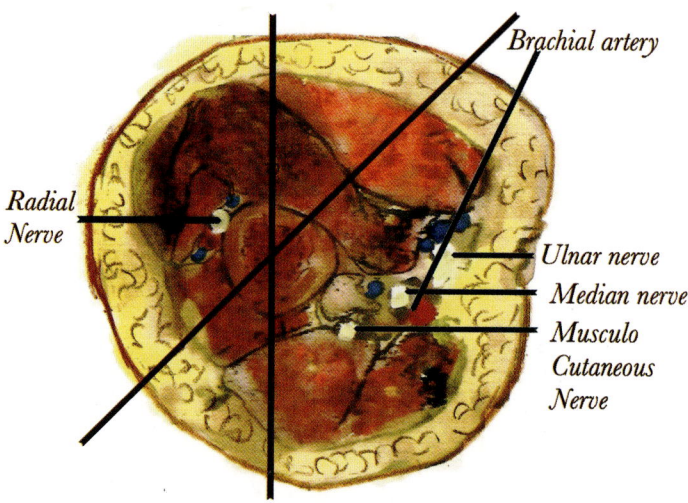

Pin passage in mid humerus

Picture 114: Safe corridors for pin passage in middle arm

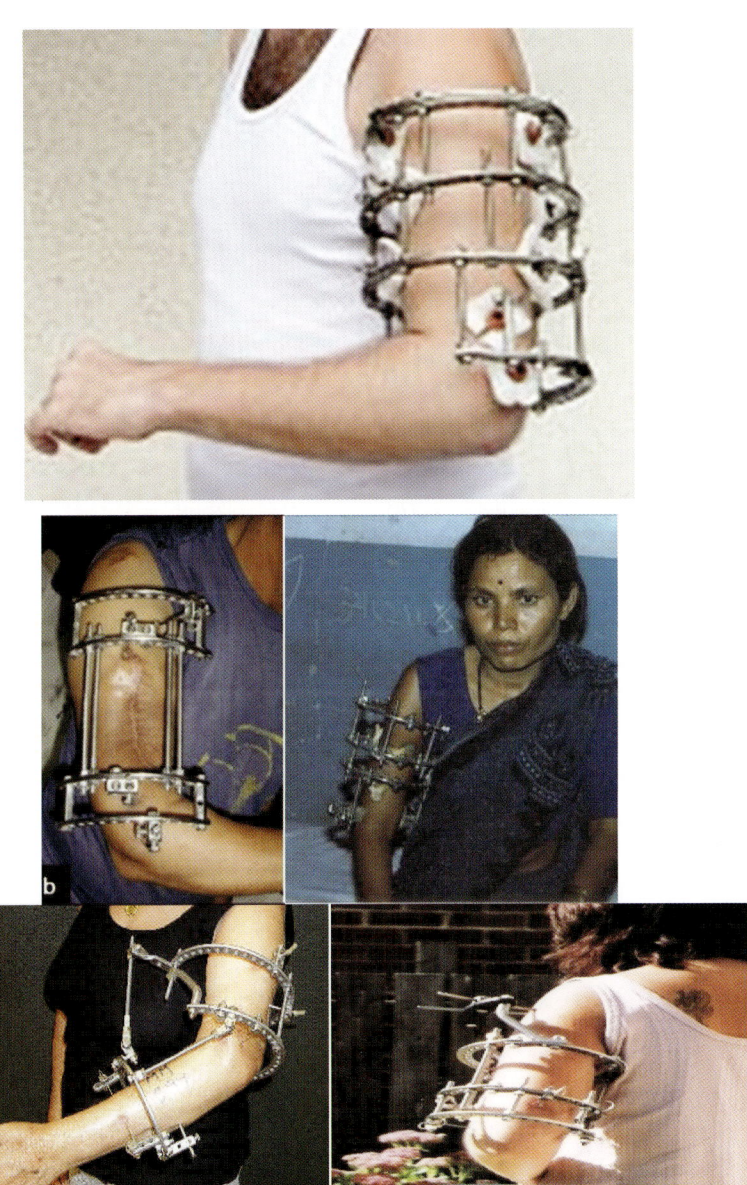

Picture 115: Clinical examples of ring placement in mid humerus

Pin placements in the upper arm near neck of humerus

Around this level, most neurovascular structures are present medially. This is the area where the deltoid almost encircles the humerus anteriorly, laterally and posteriorly. In this area, pins in the sagittal plane pass through safe corridors. No mediolateral pin placement is permitted. In these areas, one might elect to use a humeral arch, and use a Shanz screw or two from the lateral to medial, stopping short of the medial cortex. Most Ilizarov purists however get away without using Shanz pins by using a couple of parallel olive wires in the AP direction, with the olives in opposite directions.

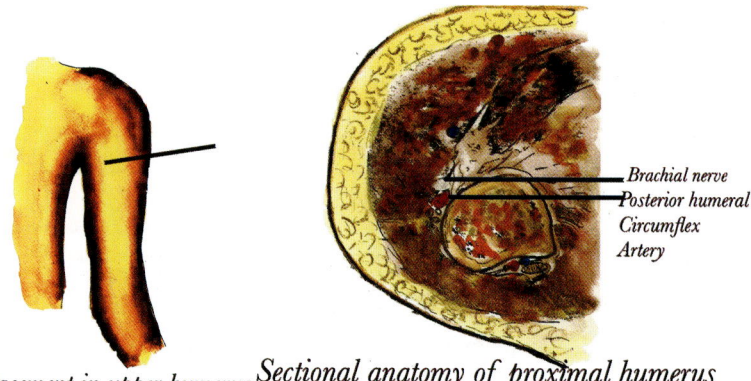

Pin placement in upper humerus *Sectional anatomy of proximal humerus*

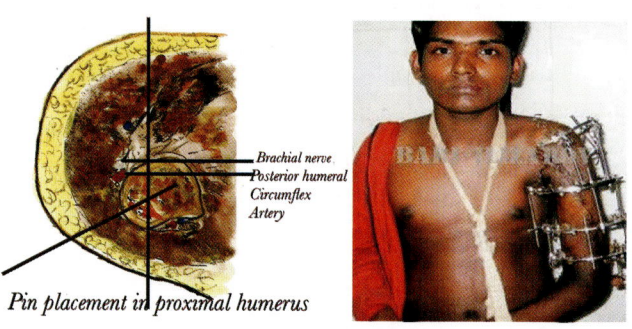

Pin placement in proximal humerus

Picture 116: Pin passage in the upper arm

Ilizarov Fixator in Primary Closed Fractures

There are two extremes to the above subject. At one end are those surgeons who believe that there is no place for Ilizarov in primary treatment of fractures, while at the other end are those who find applications of this system in most fractures. If you are a student or practitioner of this fascinating science and art, you should tread the middle path, just as I do. Ilizarov is not routinely indicated as a primary treatment for closed fractures, but there are certain fractures and injuries that are best managed by application of an Ilizarov fixator.

With my 30 years of experience in this system, I have found that the following fractures really do well with Ilizarov:

1. Comminuted, displaced, or complex (bag of bones) fractures around the wrist
2. Multi-segmental comminuted fractures of long bones where accurate open reduction is a challenge
3. Intraarticular fractures around knee

Apart from these, an Ilizarov can be applied to practically every fracture, because it provides a more comfortable immobilization than a plaster, and matches all internal fixation devices in stability and dynamism of immobilization. However compared to the *fix and forget* approach of plates or nails, an Ilizarov system needs constant monitoring by the surgeon and demands compliance of a bulky alien object protruding from the patient's body. Hence its use should be selective and appropriate.

Comminuted, displaced, or complex fractures around wrist:

The following fractures can be treated with excellent results.

1. Displaced Colle's fracture
2. Displaced or unstable Smith's fracture
3. A dorsal or volar Barton's fracture
4. Radial styloid fracture with wrist subluxation.

The following radiographs show the various conditions that can be treated with excellent results by Ilizarov methods.

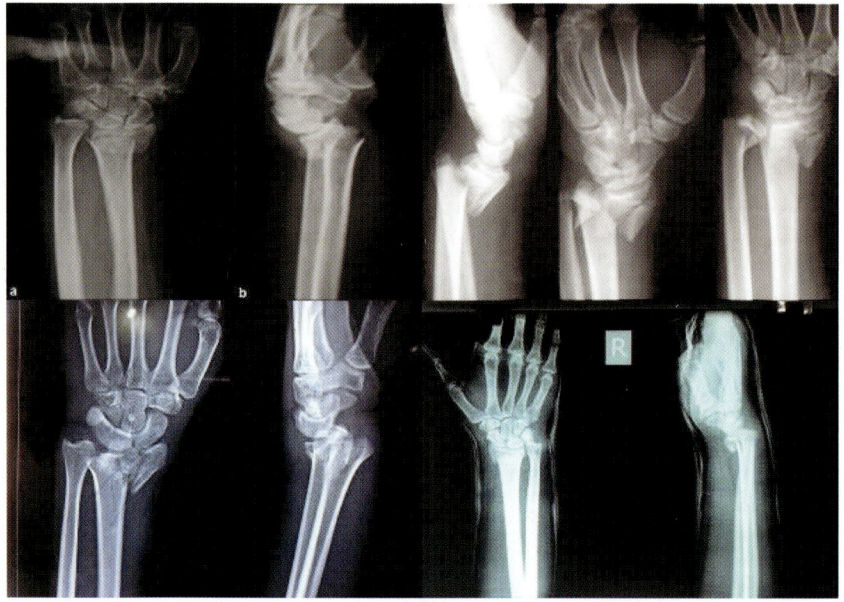

Picture 117: Fractures that can be treated with excellent results with Ilizarov methods

The principles are fairly straightforward. Called *ligamentotaxis,* it involves transfixing bones on either side of the fracture and distracting them in the correct direction, until the fracture falls in place. If any additional fragment remains splayed or displaced, it is quite an easy matter to pull it in the correct direction with an appropriately placed olive wire.

Ligamentotaxis is based on the sound scientific principle that *the ligaments that bind the joint are most often stronger than the bones they anchor.* Thus dislocations are rarer than fractures in and around joints. Under such situations, with intact ligaments, just pulling apart the fragments should automatically align the fragments.

However, the most important aspect of this procedure is to achieve precise and perfect reduction in all three planes. Radiographs are seen only in two dimensions; AP and lateral. The rotational element usually has to be imagined. It is essential to remember this during placement of pins so that appropriate hinges in all axes can produce a reduction as precise as desired.

Though each of the above fractures happens by a different mechanism and produces a different displacement in the three axes, the principles of treatment remain the same. *An accurate reduction and stable immobilization.*

The rings should be placed with the following considerations in mind

1. They should not be too close, or too distant from, the fracture site. Ideally the 2 rings should be 10 cm proximal or distal to the fracture giving a 20 cm span for the assembly.
2. As far as possible, the 2 rings should be equidistant from the fracture to allow a balanced application of forces.
3. The hinges are placed at the fracture level and not the joint level, because more than early wrist mobilization, our aim is to get the reduction right in 3 dimensions and retain it in a stable position for 3 to 4 weeks until the fracture becomes stable and sticky.

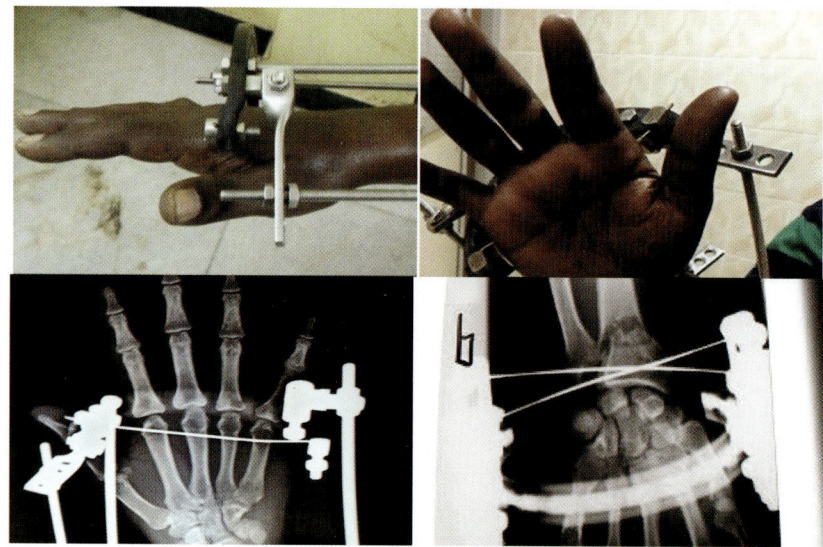

Picture 118: Hinges should be positioned at fracture level and not the level of wrist joint.

4. In fresh fractures, the easier method is to first perform a reasonable reduction, even accurate if possible by closed means, then apply the fixator with full regard to biomechanical positions, so that adjustments can be done when needed.

The following wire placement zones will provide the right forces and precise points of their application.

1. *Head or neck of metacarpals.* These provide an excellent point for both wire placement and distraction axis. The metacarpal heads are usually located approximately 8 to 12 cm from the wrist joint in an adult. Wire passage through this area is considerably easy because whether the wires are passed medial to lateral or vice versa, both the entry and exit points, being subcutaneous, are easily palpable. An important point to be kept in mind at this time is that the metacarpals tend to bunch together and this shifts their axis from a fairly straight line to a curved one. In such a situation, it's quite

easy to miss 1 or even 2 heads. It is therefore important to ensure that the palm is kept flat without curving and the K-wire should impale each bone at the same level in the anterioposterior axis.

A single wire through the metacarpal heads is adequate to give sufficient traction to stretch even the most complex fractures, but suffers from a distinct disadvantage of being free in side-to-side axis, allowing the pin to move mediolaterally causing pin tract problems and pain. To prevent this, one of the two methods can be deployed. Either a 3.5 mm Shanz pin is affixed to the first metacarpal or two olive wires are used in opposite directions.

A full ring at this level will prevent full finger movements, which goes against the very purpose of the surgery; thus only a half ring is used. I personally prefer crossed olives, though I have occasionally got away with a single K wire.

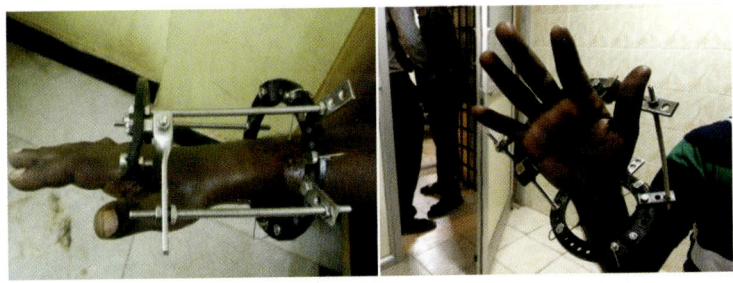

Picture 119: A simple three wire assembly is most often adequate.

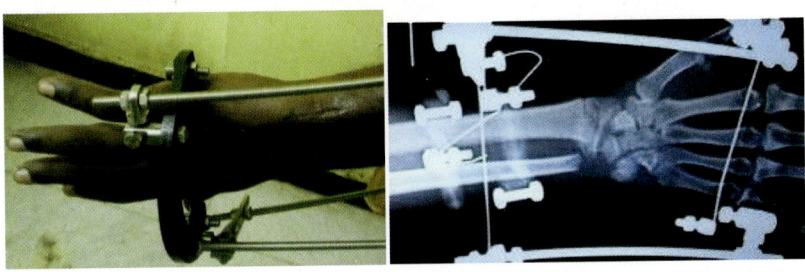

Picture 120: Ligamentotaxis corrects the most displaced and complex deformities.

2. *Mid Shaft of forearm*: Around 10 cm from the wrist is the mid forearm. As radius is the major component of the wrist joint, it is enough if two crossed wires are passed through radius, and one of these transfixes the ulna as well. This would mean that a medio-lateral pin would pass through shafts of both radius and ulna, while the anterio-posterior pin would pass through radius alone. Obviously we would use a full ring at this level, and one should ensure that the axis of wire placements allows the rings to be positioned in the correct sagittal axis.

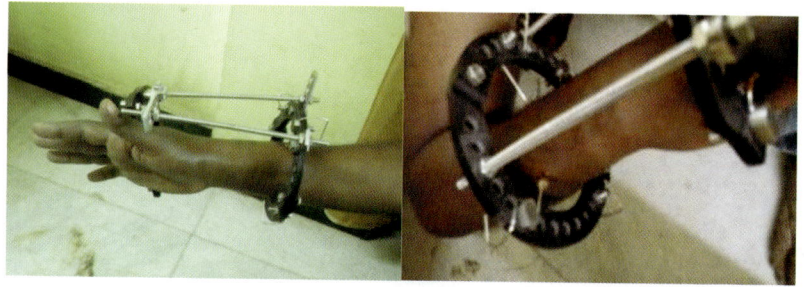

Picture 121: Pin placement in middle forerarm.

For fractures around the wrist, the forearm ring need not be placed above mid forearm. So in most situations, a one and a half ring assembly with four pins or three pins and a Shanz screw will suffice. After this, the fracture is reduced and closed to the maximum extent possible, before deciding on the hinge placements. The aim is to pull the fracture in the direction opposite to its existing deformity in all three planes. In treating such fractures, a 100% reduction is achieved on the table. There is no question of accepting a less-than-perfect reduction in the operation theatre with an intention of gradually correcting it post operatively. This simply does not happen in this situation.

The following sequence of pictures shows a Smith's fracture treated by ligamentotaxis.

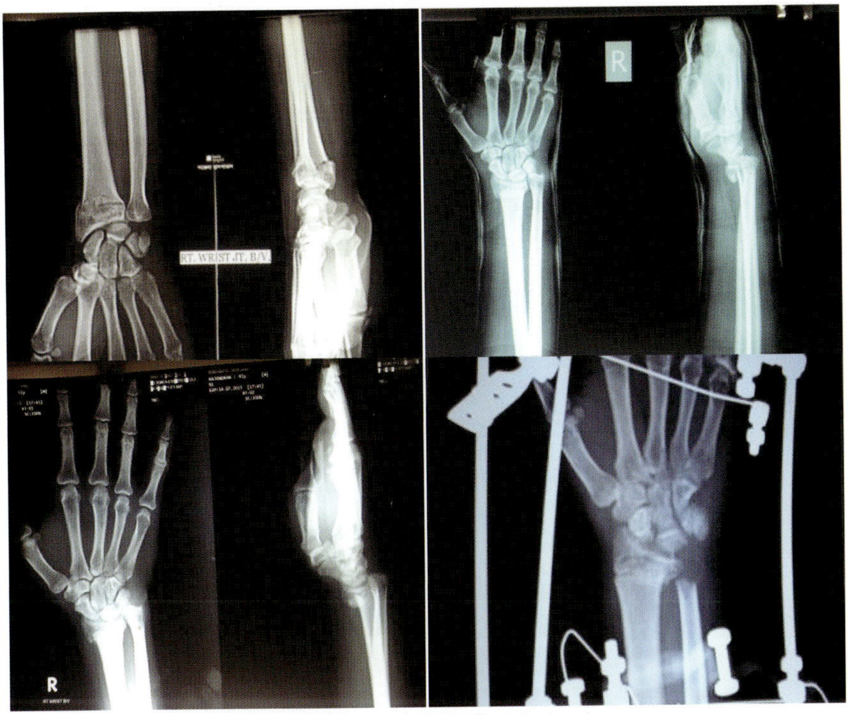

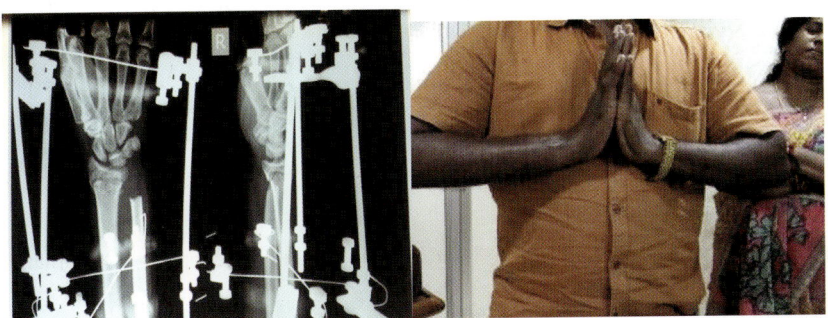

Picture 122: The sequence of ligamentotaxis.

Picture 123: Results of Smith's fracture treated by ligamentotaxis

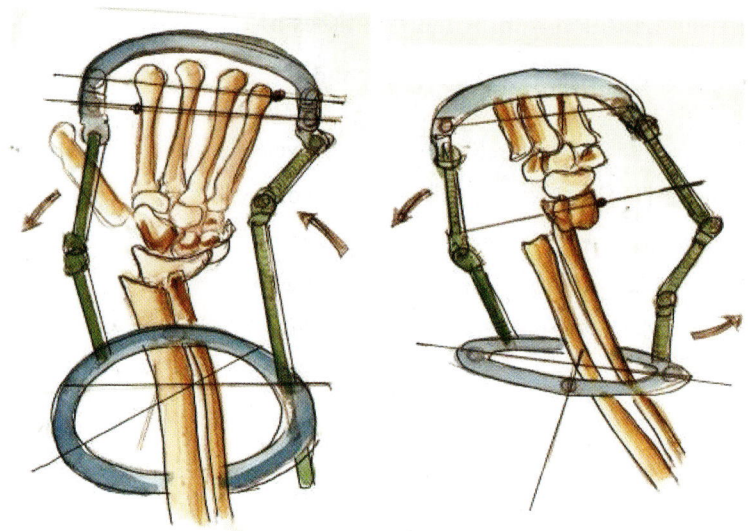

Picture 124: Various wrist fractures and the appropriate frame constructs

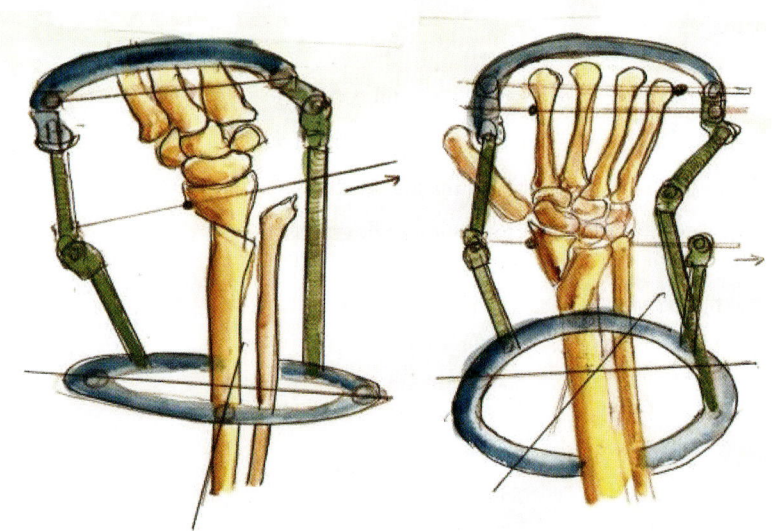

Picture 125: Various wrist fractures and the appropriate frame constructs

Multi-segmental comminuted fractures of long bones where accurate open reduction is a challenge

With modernization and increasing speed, high velocity trauma is becoming increasingly frequent. Likewise, a combination of lateral shear, torsion and violent angulation produces grossly comminuted fragments, usually segmental. These fractures in themselves are accompanied with massive internal soft tissue damage, tear of perisoteum and damage to medullary vessels. In addition, the fracture is suffused in fracture haematoma, which will eventually form the nidus, around which future callus will form.

Open reduction and plate fixation is likely to disrupt the blood supply more, and cause delay in union. Likewise, an intramedullary nail too will cause iatrogenic vascular disruption, resulting in delayed or non-union. In addition, such hypovascular areas are prone to infection due to extensive soft tissue stripping and damage.

Of course, if the fracture is open, it would naturally limit the role of internal fixations, and Ilizarov is one of the best external fixators, provided the open wounds and their plastic surgical management is not interfered with by the circumferential fixator. The following radiographs illustrate this point.

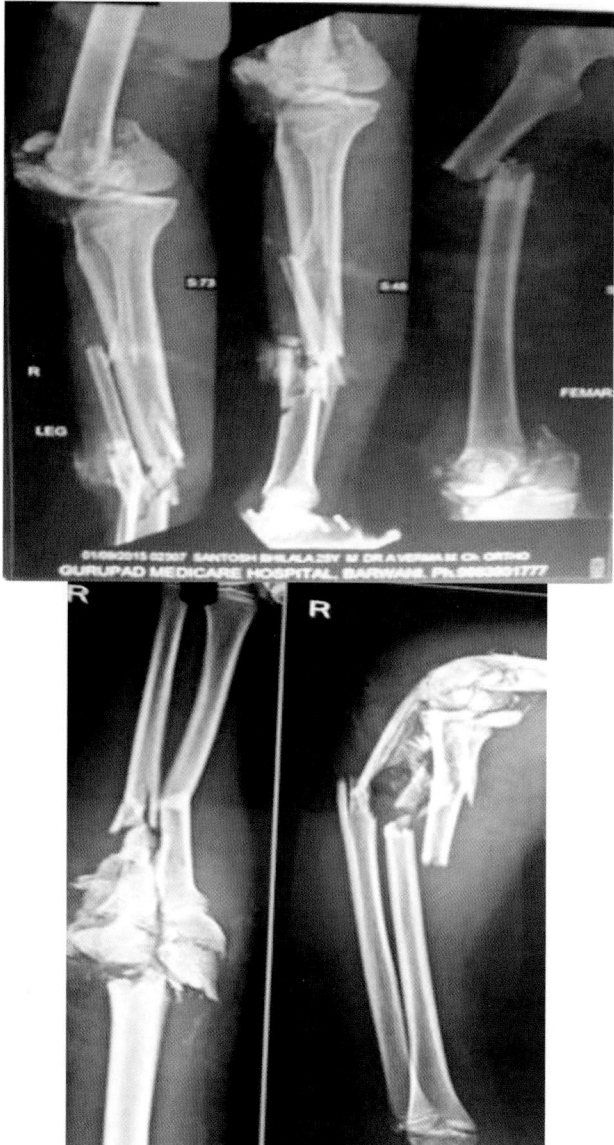

Picture 126: In the above types of cases, Ilizarov is the method which probably provides the best solution.

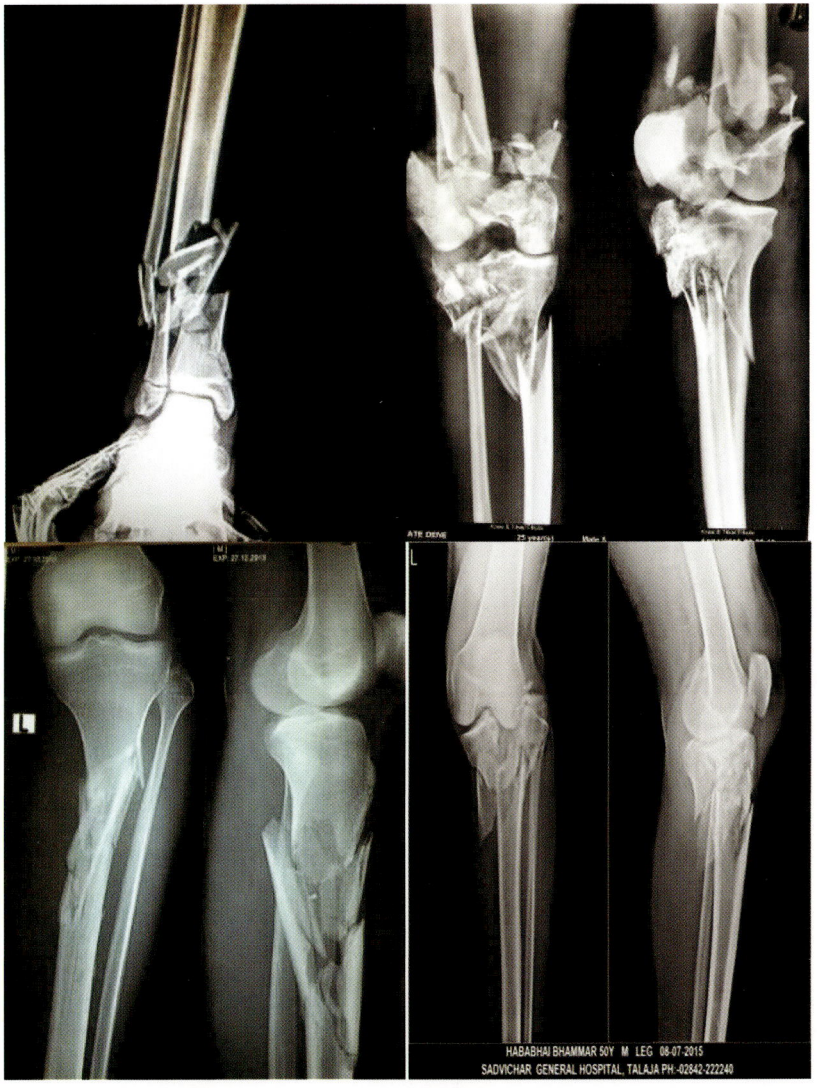

Picture 127: In the above types of cases, Ilizarov is probably the best method.

In all these cases, the following points are very important:

1. The limb has to be pulled out to the correct length. One must take accurate preoperative measurements of the opposite limb, and using flexible scales or an autoclaved wire coil and a stiff steel scale, measure the limb intra-operatively, to ensure that it is exactly the same length.

2. It is essential to remember the bony landmarks and the correlation of the joints above and below, to ensure that there is no mal-rotation. For lower limb, an imaginary line starting from the inguinal region at the femoral artery, representing the head of femur, passes over the centre of patella, crosses the tibial tuberosity and touches the second toe.

3. In the upper limb, with the wrist in supination and elbow in extension, the elbow is in 6 to 8 degrees valgus, and the two lines of this angle begin from head of humerus proximally, and the second finger and centre of wrist distally. These lines join in the middle of the elbow.

4. The proximal ring should lie 7 to 10 cm beyond the upper limit of the fracture, while the distal ring should be an equal distance below the lowest fracture.

5. Hinges should be applied at the joint level. But in the initial stages, these hinges are bolted tight and remain static hinges. After a few weeks when the fracture becomes sticky, mobilization can begin at the hinges gradually.

6. Olive wires are judiciously used to pull together fragments, compress a butterfly, and bring close a displaced obliquity.

7. Additional procedures like corticotomy or bone grafting are seldom needed if a fracture is primarily managed with Ilizarov apparatus.

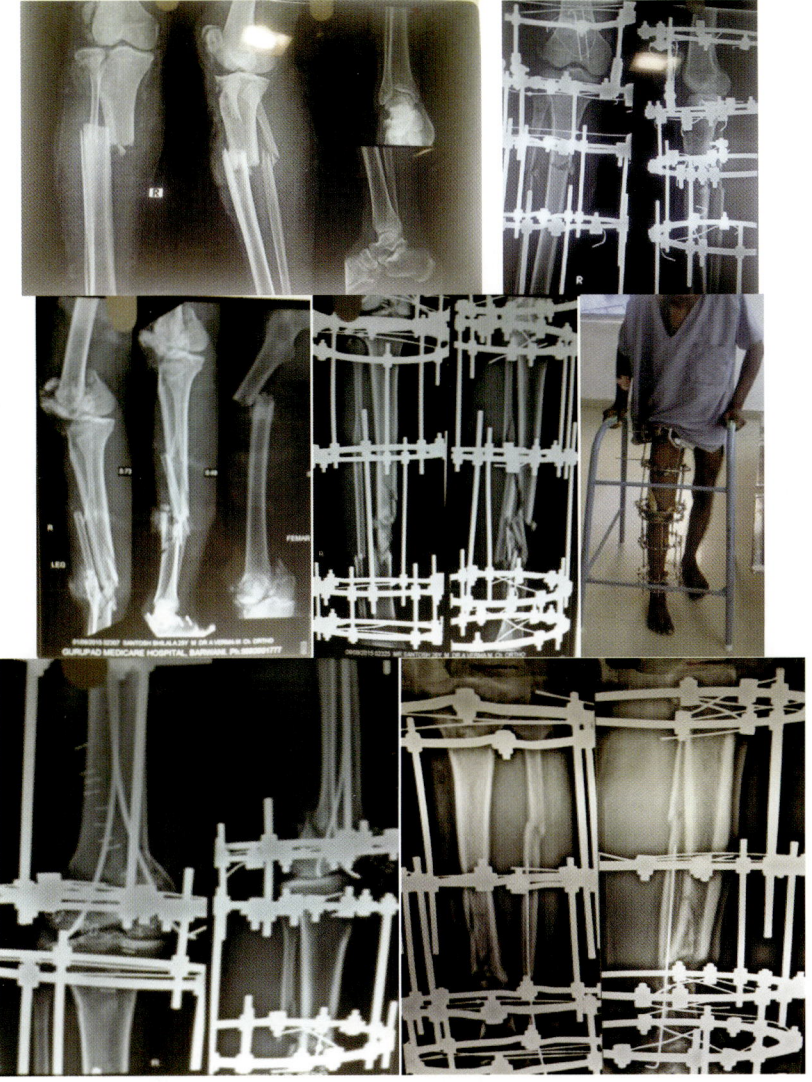

Picture 128: Ipsilateral fractures of femur and tibia managed with Ilizarov system

Intraarticular fractures around the knee joint:

Ilizarov apparatus and methods are extremely useful in the following injuries around the knee joint:

1. Depressed, splayed or shattered tibial plateau or tibial condyle fractures
2. All patterns of lower and supra condylar femoral fractures with an articular extension
3. Associated fractures of the patella
4. The following are the important parameters for treating such fractures:

   a. The limb has to be pulled out to the correct length. It is essential to remember the bony landmarks and the correlation of the joints above and below, to ensure that there is no mal-rotation. An imaginary line from the inguinal region at the femoral artery, representing the head of femur, passes over the centre of patella,. The second line crosses the tibial tuberosity and touches the second toe. These two lines should be in 5 to 7 degrees valgus.

   b. The proximal ring should lie 5 to 7 cm beyond the upper limit of the fracture, while the distal ring should be an equal distance below the lowest fracture.

   c. Hinges should be applied at the joint level. But in the initial stages, these hinges are bolted tight and remain static hinges. After a few weeks, when the fracture becomes sticky, mobilization can begin at the hinges gradually.

   d. Olive wires are judiciously used to pull together fragments, compress a butterfly, and bring close a displaced obliquity.

   e. Bone grafting may occasionally be needed in a depressed fracture where olive wires are incapable of pulling the plateau up because of deformation due to compression of cancellous bone.

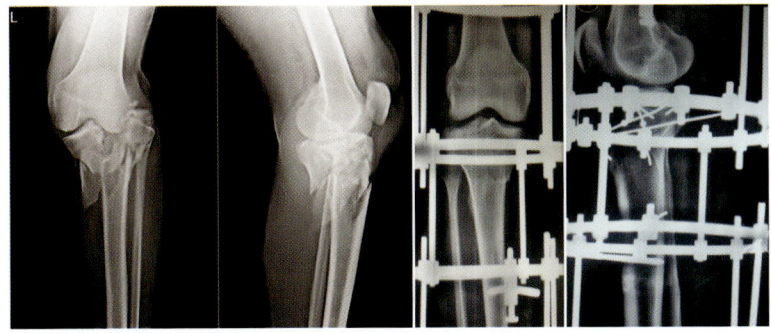

Picture 129: Tibial plateau fracture corrected by Ligamentotaxis.

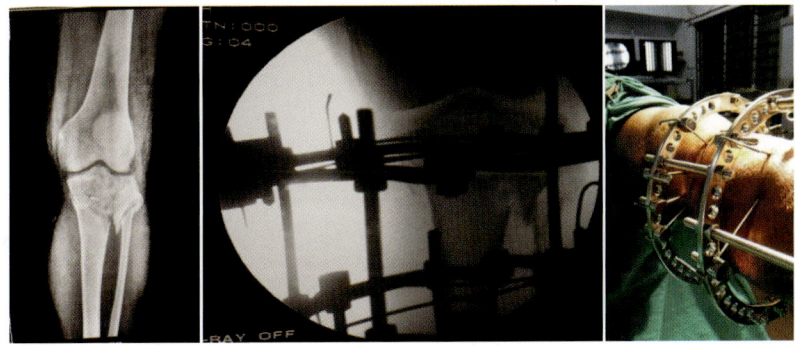

Picture 130: Tibial plateau fracture corrected by Ligamentotaxis.

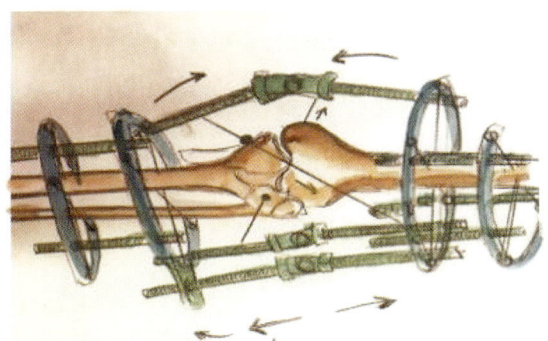

Picture 131: Sample construct for fractures around the knee joint.

147

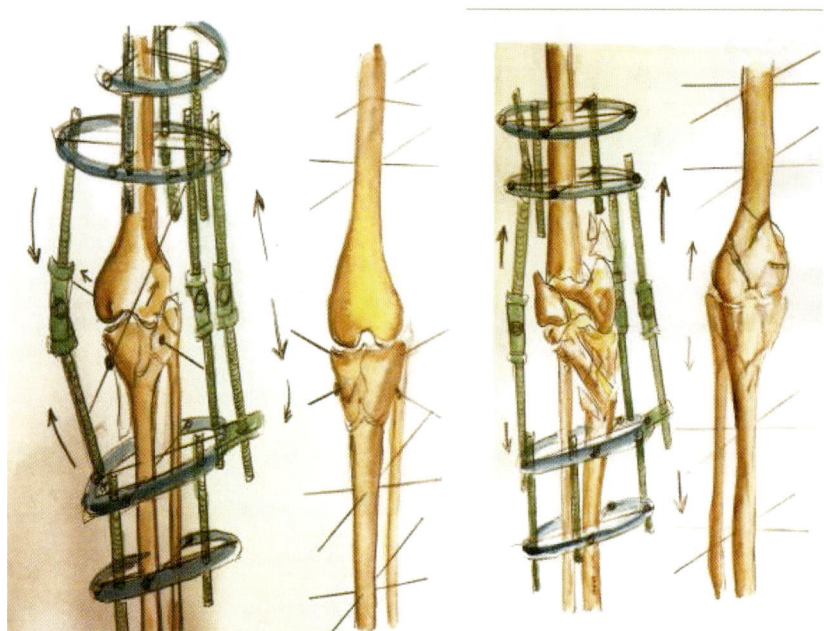

Picture 132: Different constructs for fractures around the knee joint.

Classification and treatment of Non-Union

If the union of a fracture is delayed to such an extent that it will not unite without surgical invention, it is called a non-union. This definition (propounded over the last century) has been accepted as the norm. However, there are certain grey areas. A delay in consolidation for periods beyond the surgeon's and patient's patience is also termed as a non-union.

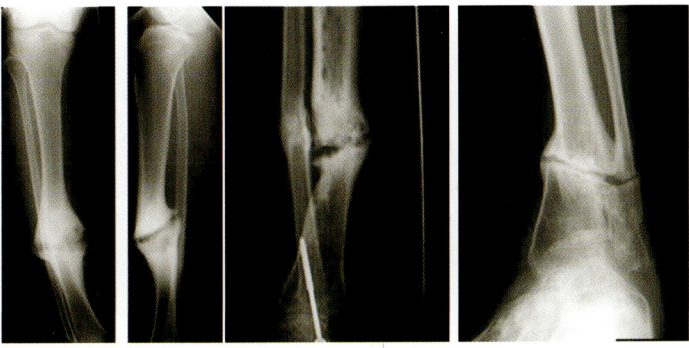

Picture 133: Non-unions can be mobile or stiff

CLASSIFICATION OF NON-UNIONS

Based on the local condition of the fracture, non-unions can broadly be classified into two types, hypertrophic and atrophic. Either of these may be associated with infection, sequestrum, or deformity.

According to Ilizarov there are two broad types of non-union; a stiff non-union and a mobile non-union. The stiff non-unions are hypertrophic on X-ray and the local vascularity is not compromised. This can be converted into union by eliminating shear stresses and augmenting compression distraction stresses.

A mobile non-union showing atrophy in an X-ray will need a proximal corticotomy for bone stimulation and a compression on the non-union site to lead to consolidation.

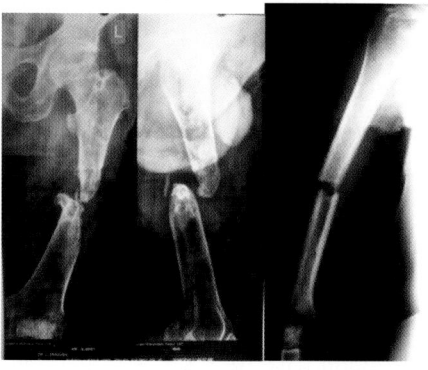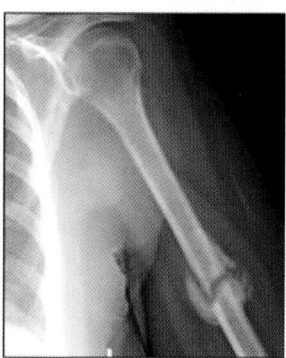

Picture 134: Non-unions can be atrophic or hypertrophic

Catagni of the ASAMI has evolved a classification based on treatment parameters. He has divided them in two groups, one describing non-union situations and the other describing treatment modalities

I have simplified Catagni's classification, and this was published in the earlier edition of my book. I have divided the non-unions into two types: infected and infection free. One is atrophic, two and three hypertrophic and four to six have bone gaps.

Type A non-unions are those without infection. Here the aim of treatment is fracture union alone.

A1: Non-infected mobile non-union. This needs a corticotomy distraction associated with fracture compression.

A2: Non-infected stiff hypertrophic non-union without deformity. This requires primary distraction followed by compression.

A3: Hypertrophic non-infected non-union with deformity. This needs primary distraction and secondary compression along with deformity correction. The deformity can be corrected either with hinges, transverse wires or olive wires.

A4: Non-infective non-union with bone defect of up to 5 cm. This will require a corticotomy, a bifocal expansion followed by compression of the non-union

A5: Non-infective non-union with bone defect exceeding 5 cm. In this case, a corticotomy, bone transport and fracture compression are needed. Occasionally, to accelerate the healing time, a two level corticotomy may be done.

A6: Non-infected non-union exceeding 10 cm with local scarring. Due to extensive bone loss and local scarring, it is not possible to do the bone transport using transverse wires. Here crossed olive wires are used to increase the surface area.

Type B non-unions are those with infection. The basic principles are essentially the same as with Type A, but to eliminate infection, it is best if the fracture site is opened, all the dead and devitalized tissue removed, sequestrectomy performed and the frame applied.

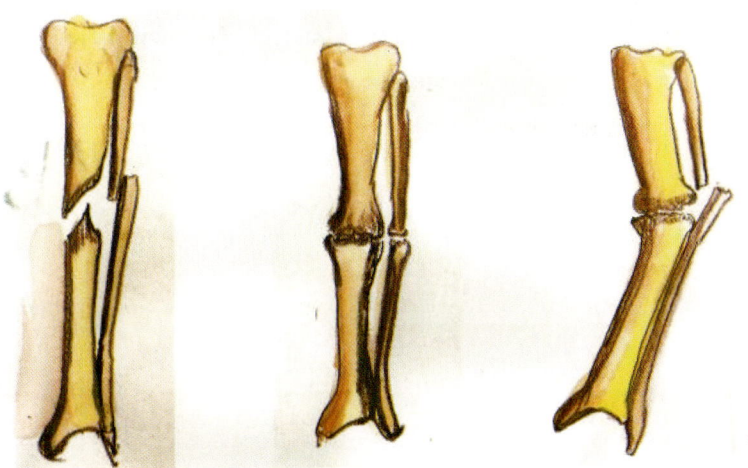

Picture 135: Type A1, A2 and A3 non-unions

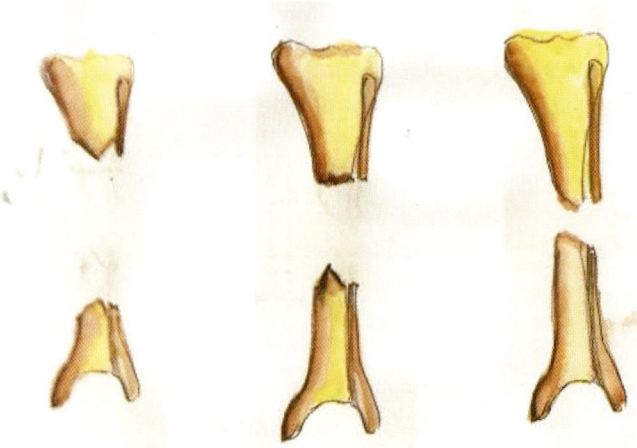

Picture 136: Type A4, A5 and A6 non-unions

B1: Infected non-union with atrophy

B2: Infected non-union with hypertrophy without deformity

B3: Infected non-union with hypertrophy and deformity

In the above three situations, the fracture is exposed, unhealthy bone resected and the two fragments are opposed with compression. Existing deformities are corrected taking minimal bone wedges. The resultant shortening is invariably less than 5 cm and a corticotomy distraction produces elongation.

B4: Infected non-union with bone gap of less than 5 cm

B5: Infected non-union with bone gap between 5 and 10 cm

B6: Infected non-union with bone gap exceeding 10 cm

These are complex problems and tax the ingenuity of most surgeons. Each case has to be individually assessed and specific treatment protocol planned.

Judicious use of olive wires, hinges, posts, corticotomy, monofocal distraction, bifocal distraction, and compression are deployed to achieve results. Details of specific applications are covered in the respective chapters.

Non-Union of Tibia

Tibial non-unions have perplexed both the surgeon and anatomist for a long time. In fact, all books of anatomy enumerate scaphoid, femoral neck and distal tibias as common sites for non-union. Even in distal tibial fractures treated by simple plaster application, incidences of non-union are rather frequent. With operative intervention, stripping of periosteum, devascularizing the bone, occasional infection, and in compound fractures, this is a much more challenging problem. Only after the advent of Ilizarov's magic have tibial non-unions been brought from a refractory to manageable condition. I have simplified the classification of Tibial non-unions and the **Prakash classification** with the treatment modalities for various types is described below. Type A non-unions are *non infected* or those in which the infection has been eliminated, while type B non-unions are those which still have *infection* or are pouring pus.

Type A1

This refers to non infected mobile atrophic non-union. The cause for non-union is atrophy of the bone and deficiency of biological stimulus at the fracture site. This is the classical bone end atrophy with minimal callus. A 4 ring assembly is required with 1 proximal metaphyseal ring, 1 distal metaphyseal ring, and 2 central rings about 2 cm away from the non-union site on either side. A fibular osteotomy is necessary. As shown in the diagram, the treatment modality is a corticotomy between rings 1 and 2 with distraction and a compression between rings 2 and 3. The following drawings and radiographs show this clearly.

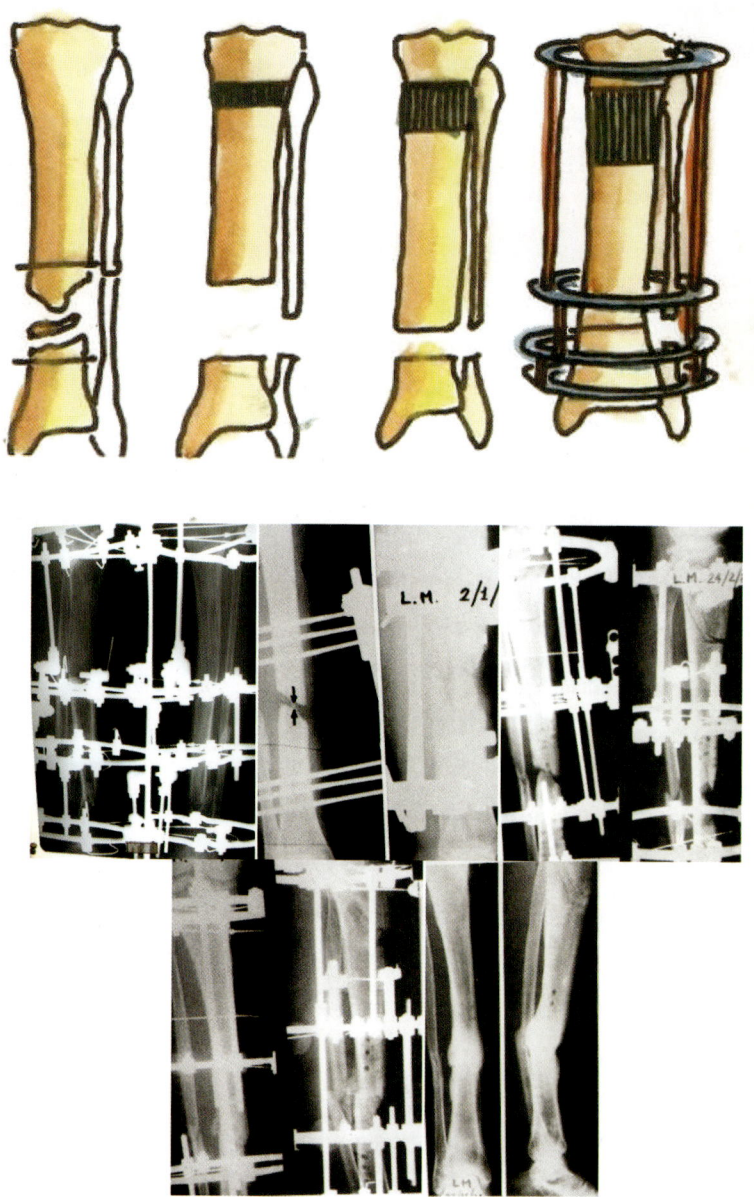

Picture 137: Type A1 non-unions treated by compression with corticotomy distraction

Type A2

This refers to a non infected stiff hypertrophic non-union without deformity. Preoperative radiological evaluation is done to see if the segments are congruent and if stability can be achieved by direct linear compression. In case it is apparent that linear compression cannot be achieved due to incongruence of the fragments, one must plan to use olive wires for stabilizing the fragment. A 4 ring assembly is used with 2 peripheral rings in the metaphyseal region and 2 central rings on either site of the fracture. Use of olive wires to increase stability is optional. Here a corticotomy is not needed and Ilizarov compression/ distraction/ compression scheme is followed. The fracture site is compressed for the first week, followed by distraction for a period of 10 to 20 days, which will stimulate osteogenesis. Subsequently, compression is applied for a period of 2 to 3 weeks. This is called the shock absorber, telescoping effect, or the *piano accordion effect.*

In case the bone ends are not congruent or are not in a compactable position, the alternative method is to open the fracture site and freshen the fracture ends to make them congruent. At this stage, it is prudent to excise all sclerotic and avascular bone and reshape the ends in such a manner that compression will not cause a slippage. A primary compression is applied at the fracture site and a proximal corticotomy is performed which will have two functions. Firstly, the corticotomy will increase the blood flow by over 300% and stimulate bone healing and callus transport. Secondly, distraction at the corticotomy site will allow us to equalize the limb length.

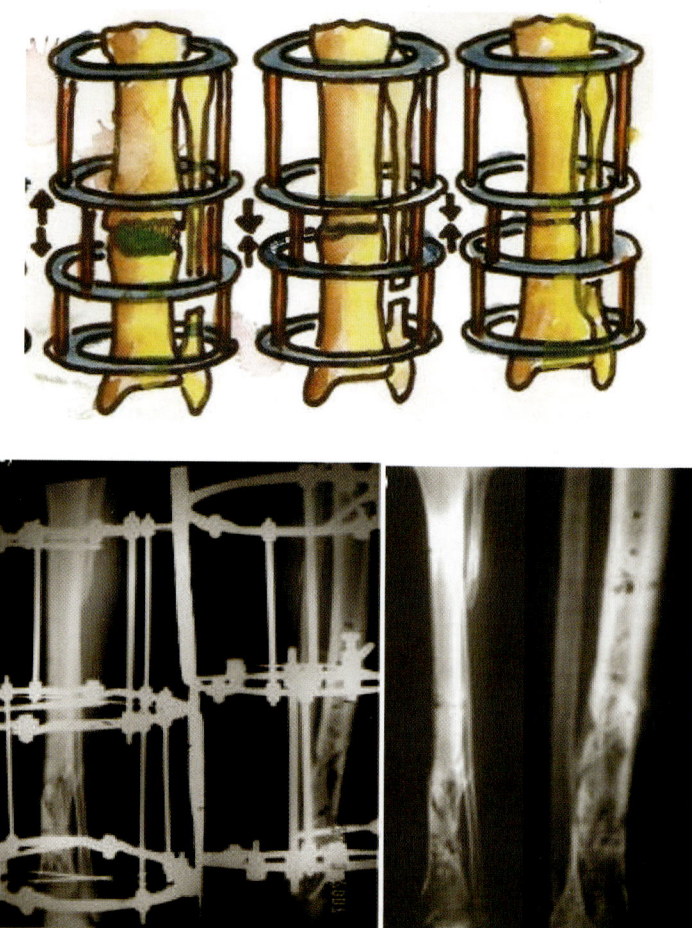

Picture 138: Piano accordion effect for A2 non-unions.

One has to be extremely careful to ensure that the bone axis in both planes is properly studied, and no deformities are produced during the course of treatment. A tibia is a curved bone, while all threaded rods are straight. In these cases, we don't usually need to incorporate the foot in the frame unless the non-union is in the lower fourth of tibia. If so, a metatarsal ring will prevent the equinus that usually accompanies distraction at the corticotomy site. Tibia being a subcutaneous bone, wire placements seldom cause troubles and one should strive to achieve an all-wire construct, rather than using Shanz pins.

Type A3

Here the non-union is hypertrophic but is associated with deformity. The aim of the treatment is not only to achieve union, but also to correct the deformity. There are three methods for achieving correction:

1. Correction with hinges

2. Correction with olive wires

3. Correction with transverse wires and telescopic rods

CORRECTION WITH HINGES:

A four ring apparatus is prefabricated prior to the surgery based on the patient's leg measurements and a pre-operative radiographic assessment. It is important to locate the placement of the hinges in relation to the non-union. The assembled apparatus may be sterilized as one piece.

Olive wires are passed perpendicular to the long axis of the knee in the proximal segment and long axis of the ankle in the distal segment. The apparatus is slid over the limb and the wires are anchored. It is important to ensure that the hinge is placed accurately in the line of the deformity. By gradual screwing or unscrewing of the nuts located on the opposite threaded rod, gradual correction of the deformity is obtained with the hinge acting as a fulcrum. Once the axis has been corrected, the hinges are substituted for threaded rods and the now-stable assembly is subjected to axial compression.

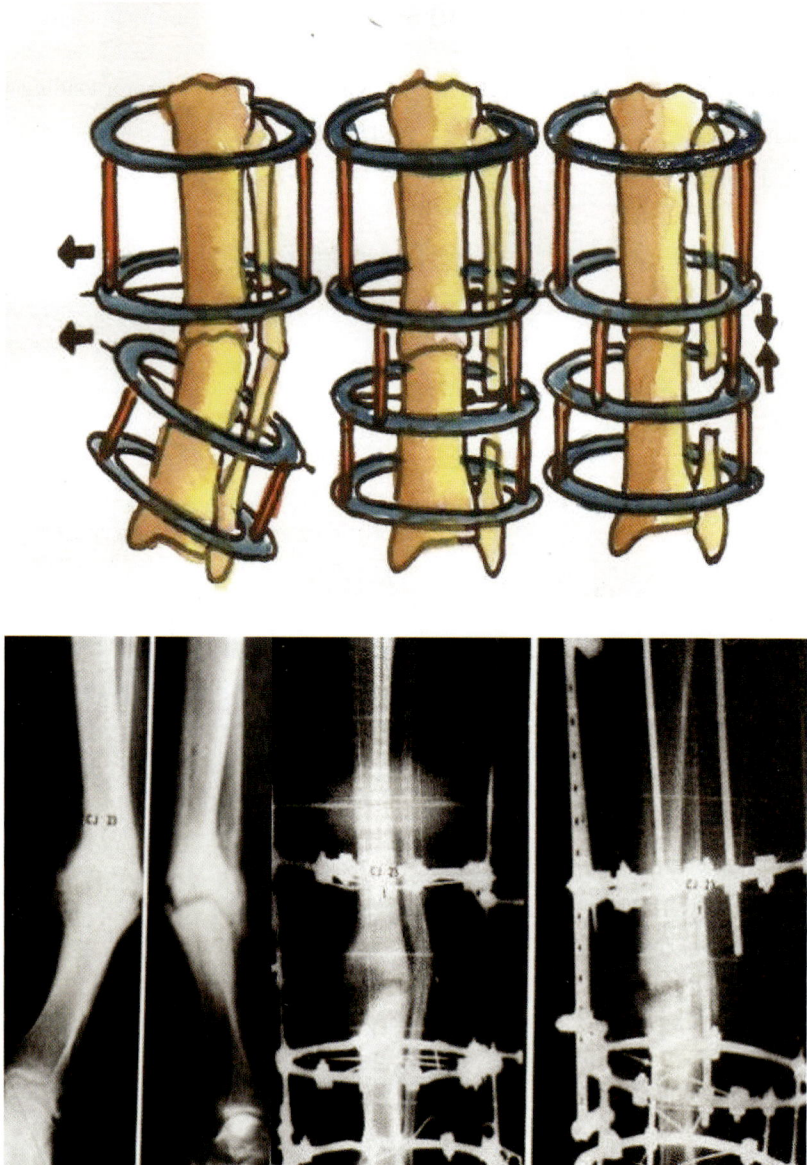

Picture 139: A3 non-union corrected with hinges.

CORRECTION WITH OLIVE WIRES:

If the deformity is less than 15 degrees, olive wires placed in four point loading will achieve corrections. The wires are placed under gradual tension to a slotted threaded rod.

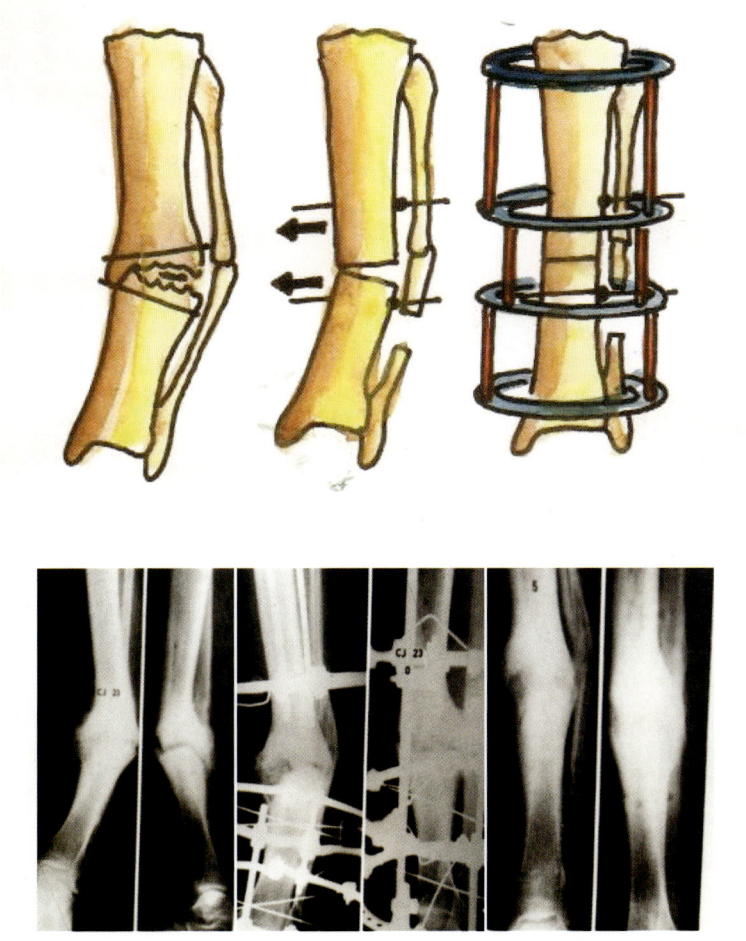

Picture 140: A3 Non-unions corrected with olive wires

The extent of deformity is calculated preoperatively by full length X-rays in two planes. Once the post operative radiograph shows that the deformity has been fully corrected, the slotted rods are changed for standard threaded rods, and a compression regime is commenced. On occasions, when the callus at the fracture site is less, a compression/ distraction/ compression schedule can be tried. This piano accordion manoeuvre is a wonderful method to stimulate bone formation at both the fracture and corticotomy sites.

CORRECTION WITH TRANSVERSE WIRES AND TELESCOPIC RODS:

This is suitable for severe angulations and stiff non-unions. The limb is visualized as being composed of two separate linear units on either side of the deformity. Each unit requires a simple two ring assembly perpendicular to the long axis and parallel to the adjacent joints. The two systems will now accurately reflect the angular deformity and are connected to each other with hinges in the desired axis of correction. Two telescopic rods are now connected, one to the concave side and other to the convex side of the assembly.

Correction is obtained by gradual expansion of the telescopic rod on the concave side and compression of the telescopic rod on the convex side. It should be noted that the telescopic rod on the convex side is affixed after fully expanding it because it will be needed to be shortened. Similarly the telescopic rod on the concave side should be fixed in maximum contraction as it will be expanded during the course of treatment while the deformity is being corrected.

The drawings and radiographs on the next page show the frame construct for achieving the results by telescopic rods and transverse wires.

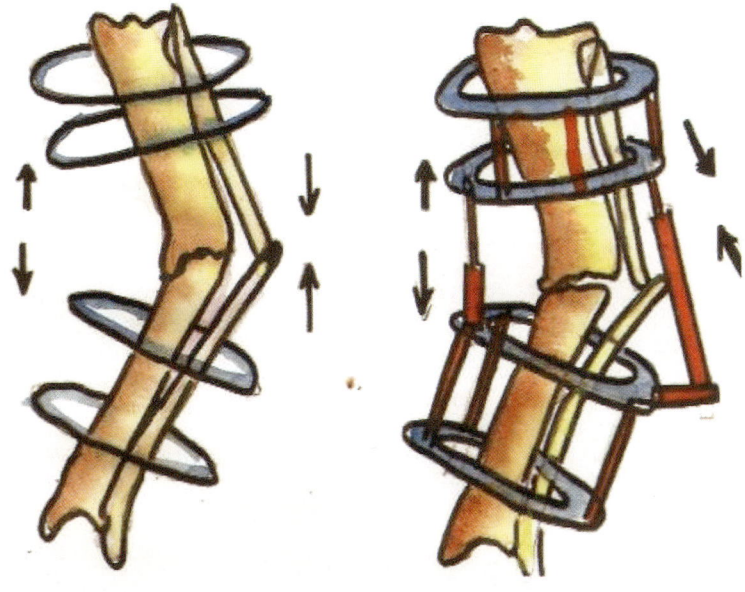

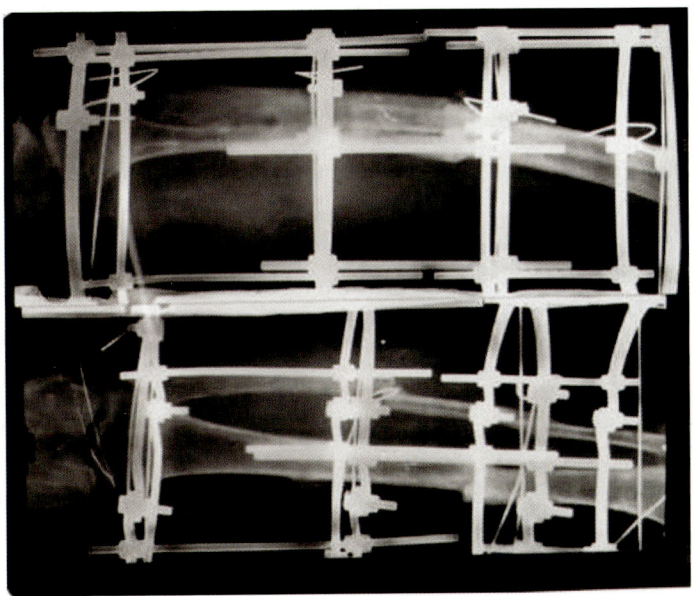

Picture 141: A3 non union correction with telescopic rods.

Type A4

Here, the gap between the ununited fragments is up to 5 cm. The recommended treatment is:

1. Fibular osteotomy
2. Direct compression of the fracture site after freshening the edges, resulting in a measurable shortening
3. A four ring assembly with two distal and two central rings
4. A corticotomy distraction with a gradual lengthening to correct the exact amount of shortening that has resulted from the compression of the bone fragments
5. Axial compression of the fracture site, followed by frame dynamization

6. Full weight bearing and return to function from day one stimulates union, vascularity and osteogenesis.

7. As the acute docking is five centimeters or less, the tissue bunching is not a great problem. However the most important step in this case is to freshen the ends to make them exactly fitting into one another, end to end, and ensure that after docking, all the deformities in anterio-posterior, side to side, angular and rotational; are fully corrected and the tibia is in near anatomical shape and position, exactly similar to the normal side, except for the shortening consequent to docking.

8, A properly applied frame ensures that no deformities are produced while the corticotomy site is distracted.

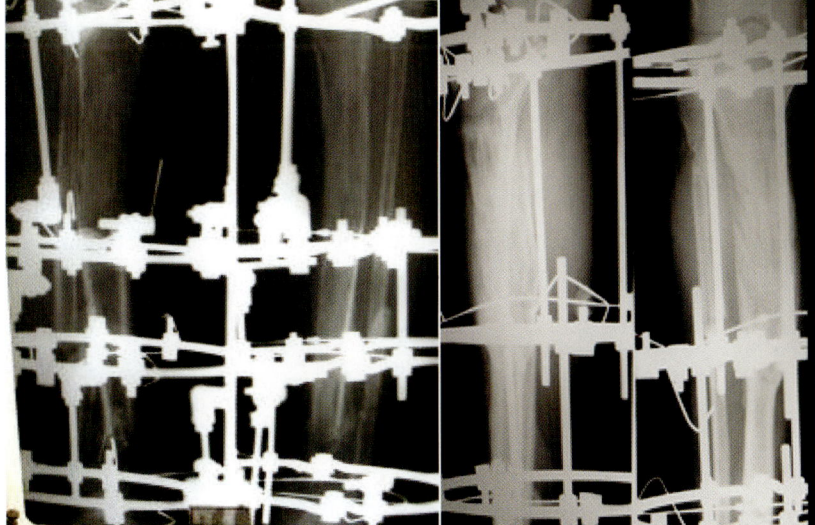

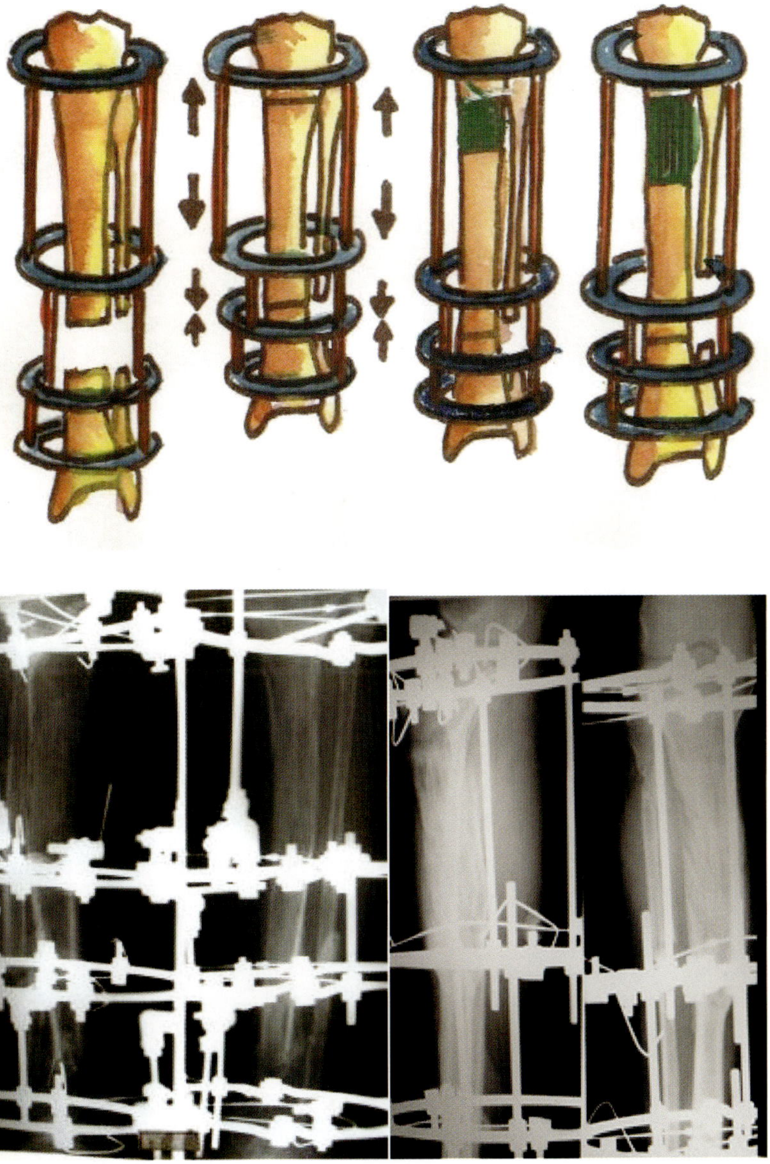

Picture 142: A4 non-union treated by acute docking and corticotomy elongation

Type A5

In this case, the gap between the fragments is between 5 and 10 cm. The method preferred is to preserve the length of the limb along with the bone gap and perform a bone transport procedure. The following steps are employed:

1. Fibular osteotomy
2. A 4 ring assembly with 2 peripheral and 2 central rings is used. The central rings are fixed in such a manner that the gap is retained and the length of the limb is kept equal to the that of the other limb.
3. Rings 3 and 4 are stabilized using short threaded rods.
4. Long threaded rods are employed for connecting ring 1, 2 and 3. A corticotomy is performed between rings 1 and 2.

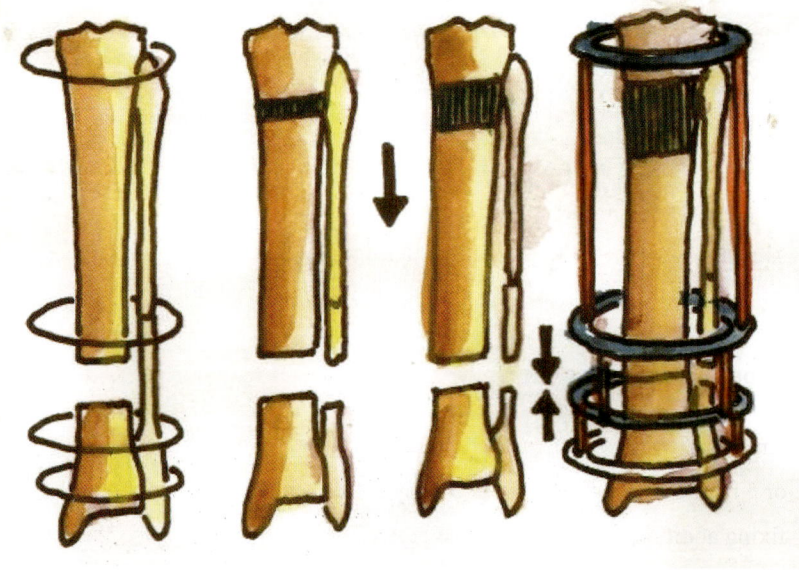

Picture 143: Bone transport in A 5 non union.

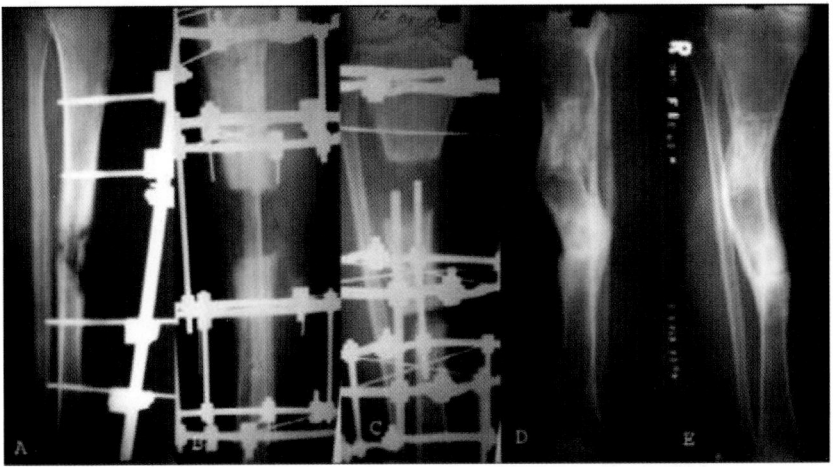

Picture 144: Method of treating A5 non-union with bone transport

5. By moving ring 2 downwards in a gradual manner, lengthening is achieved at the corticotomy site. At the same time, the bone fragment moves downwards along with ring 2, gradually reducing the gap at the non-union site.

6. Once the gap has been reduced, a compression distraction protocol is employed to progress to bone union.

7. In this method, we usually transfix one half of fibula with wires, while the other part is left free to allow an unfettered tibial elongation.

Type A5 (Alternative method)

An alternative method would be bifocal transportation with rings. A standard 4 or 5 ring assembly is used. Occasionally, the terminal rings can be reinforced by fixing additional pins through the posts. The following are the steps of bifocal transportation:

1. Ring 1 and 4 are applied at both ends of the tibia and rings 2 and 3 on either side of the gap.The entire assembly is connected by multiple short threaded

rods while the gap is retained and the length of the limb is kept equal to the other side.

2. Fibular osteotomy is performed.

3. Two corticotomies are performed, one between rings 1and 2 and the other between rings 3 and 4.

4. Expansion is performed at both the corticotomy sites, thereby moving ring 2 away from ring 1, and ring 3 away from ring 4. This will bring rings 2 & 3 closer, thereby gradually reducing the bone gap.

5. Once the ends are apposed, a compression distraction protocol is deployed to lead to union and consolidation.

6. After satisfactory radiological union, the frame is dynamized till clinical union before fixator removal.

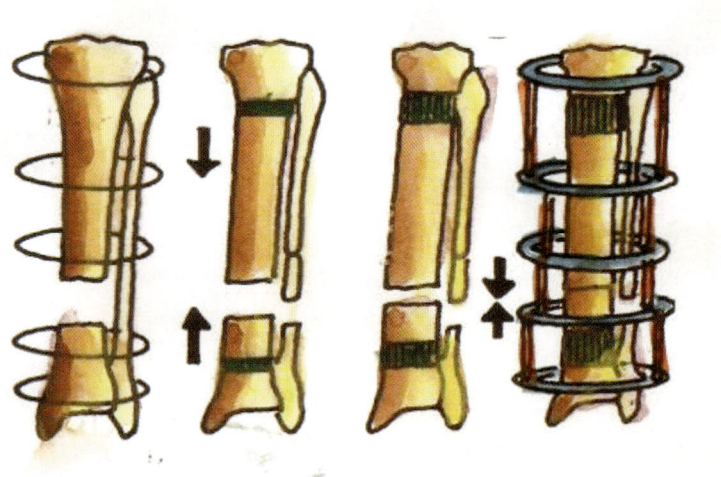

Picture 145: Bifocal transport in A5 non union.

Type A6

These are non infective non-unions with gaps in excess of 10 cm. Here, the bone transport is achieved by means of olive wires.

1. A pair of crossed wires is inserted in the upper part of tibia and brought out on the opposite side. The 2 wires are now fixed to a ring. Long threaded rods are attached to this ring.

2. A second ring is slid across these rods up to the site of non-union.

3. The third and fourth rings are located distal to the non-union with the third kept as close as possible to the non-union and the fourth close to the ankle. The distal rings are fixed to the tibia by 2 wires each.

4. 2 crossed olive wires are inserted longitudinally and connected to the middle ring which was free until now.

5. A corticotomy is performed between rings 1 & 2.

6. By moving ring 2 towards ring 3 by gradual distraction, regenerate is formed between rings 1 and 2, resulting in elongation and the fracture gap gradually diminishes.

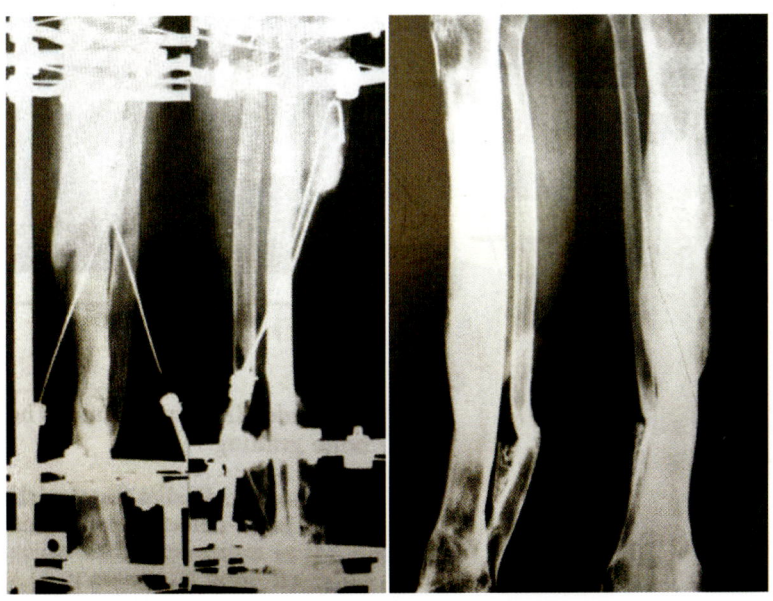

Picture 146: Type A6 treated by cross olive wire bone transport

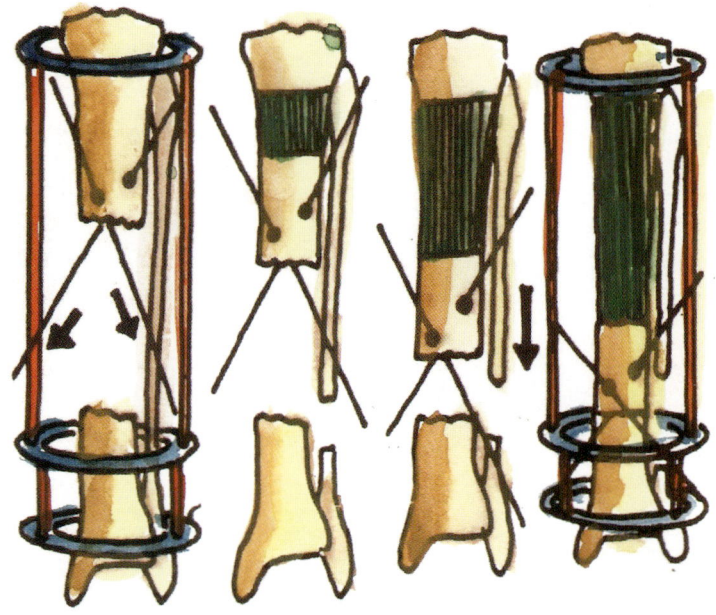

Picture 147: Bone transport with crossed olive wires in A6 non union.

Type B1

1. Here one will have to open the fracture site and excise all dead bone and refashion the fracture ends before frame application.
2. A 4 ring assembly is utilized with 1 proximal metaphyseal ring, 1 distal metaphyseal ring and 2 central rings about 2 cm away from the non-union site on either side.
3. A fibular osteotomy is necessary as shown in the diagram; the treatment modality is a corticotomy between rings 1 and 2 with distraction and compression between rings 2 and 3.

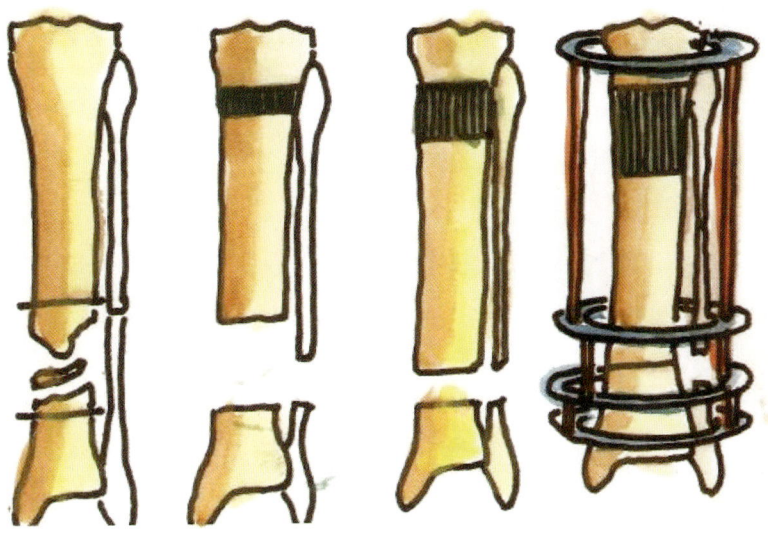

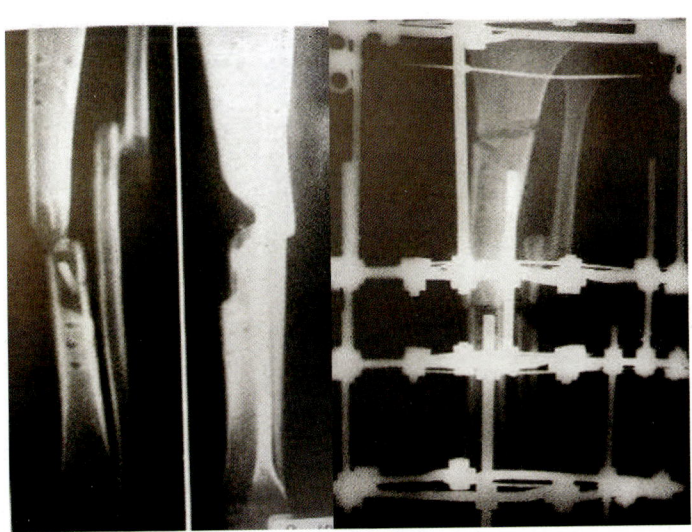

Picture 148: Type B1 non-union treated with corticotomy and compression

Type B2 and B3

These are infected stiff hypertrophic non-unions with or without deformity. There is no bone gap or deficiency. Pre-operative radiological assessment is done for two important factors:

1. Presence of any sequestrate or dead bone.
2. Evaluation of the bone ends to see if they are congruent and if stability can be achieved by direct linear compression. If linear compression cannot be achieved due to incongruence of the fragments, one must plan to use olive wires for stabilizing the fragment.

B2 Non-unions:

There is no deformity in these and a 4 ring assembly is used with peripheral rings in the metaphyseal region and 2 central rings on either site of the fracture. Use of olive wires to increase stability is optional. Here a corticotomy is not needed and Ilizarov compression/ distraction/ compression scheme is followed, unless one does a sequestrectomy which leaves a large gap.

1. For the first week, the fracture site is compressed, followed by distraction. This process will stimulate osteogenesis.
2. Subsequently, compression is applied for a period of 2 to 3 weeks.
3. In case the bone ends are not congruent or are not in a good position, the alternative is to open the fracture site and make them congruent. A primary compression is applied at the fracture site and proximal corticotomy is performed which will have two functions. Firstly the corticotomy will increase the blood flow and stimulate osteogenesis to the entire bone and secondly the corticotomy can be distracted to compensate for any loss of length that has occurred due to refashioning of the bone edges.

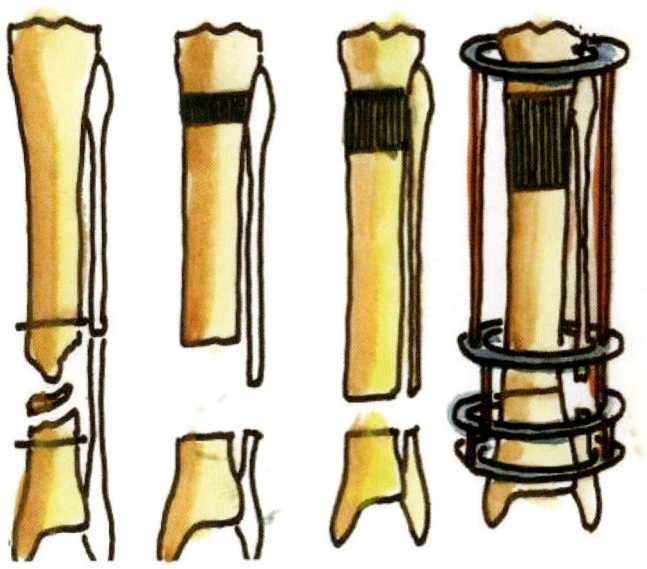

Picture 149: Frame construct for B2 non unions. Resection, compression, corticotomy and ellongation.

B3 Non-unions: These are stiff infected non-unions with deformity. The aim of the treatment is to correct the deformity and produce union. There are three ways of achieving correction:

1. Correction with hinges

2. Correction with olive wires

3. Correction with transverse wires and rods

Hinge correction

1. For a hinge correction, a four ring apparatus is pre-fabricated prior to the surgery based on the patient's leg measurement and a pre-operative

radiographic assessment. It is important to locate the placement of the hinges in relation to the non-union. The assembled apparatus may be sterilized as one unit.

2. Olive wires are passed perpendicular to the knee in the proximal segment and long axis of the ankle in the distal segment. The apparatus is brought over the limb and the wires anchored.

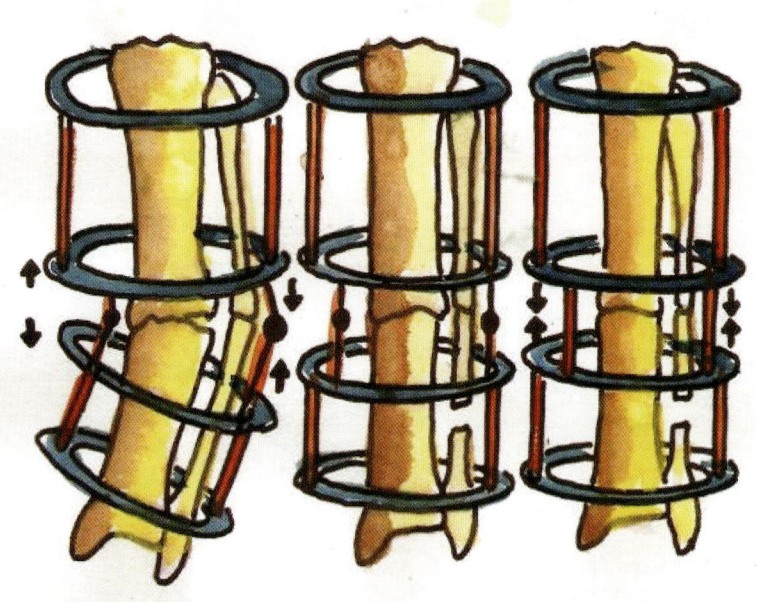

Picture 150: Hinge correction of a B3 non union.

3. It is important to ensure that the hinge is placed accurately in the line of the deformity. By gradual screwing or unscrewing of the nuts located on the opposite threaded rod, gradual correction of the deformity is obtained with the hinge acting as a fulcrum.

4. Once the axis has been corrected, hinges are substituted for threaded rods, and the now-stable assembly subject to axial compression.

Olive wire correction

1. This is used when the deformity is less than 15 degrees.

2. Olive wires placed in four points of contact will achieve corrections.

3. The wires are placed under gradual tension to a slotted threaded rod.

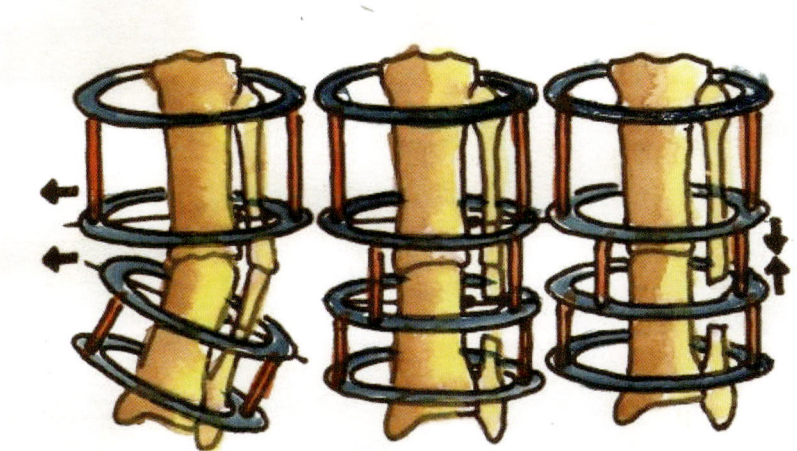

Picture 151: Frame for correction of B3 deformities with olive wires.

Transverse wire and telescopic rod correction:

This is indicated and suitable for severe angulation and a stiff non-union.

1. The limb is visualized as being composed of two separate linear units on either side of the deformity. Each unit requires a simple two ring assembly perpendicular to the long axis and parallel to the adjacent joints.

2. The two systems now accurately reflect the angular deformity and are connected to each other with two hinges in the desired axis of correction.

3. Two telescopic rods are now connected, one to the concave side and other to the convex side of the assembly. Correction is obtained by gradual expansion

of the telescopic rod on the concave side and compression of the telescopic rod on the convex side.

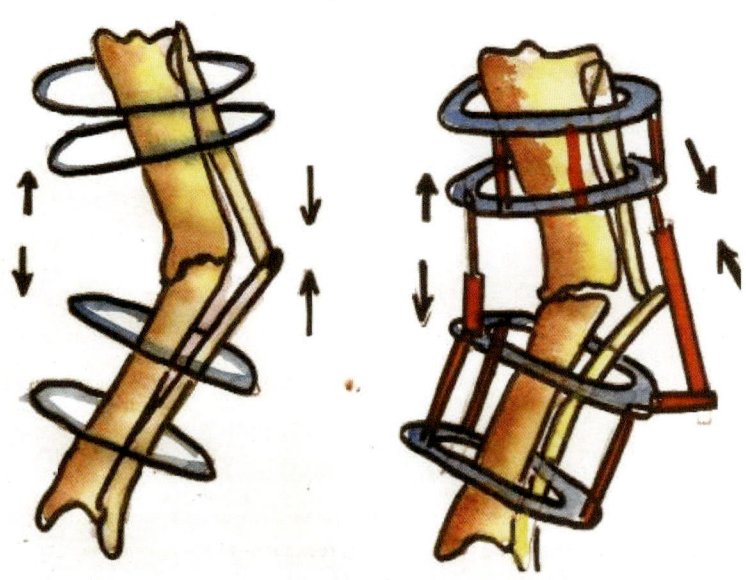

Picture 152: Schematics for correction and treatment of B3 non unions with telescopic rods and transverse wires.

4. It should be noted that the telescopic rod on the convex side is affixed after fully expanding it, because this will be need to be shortened. Similarly, the telescopic rod on the concave side should be fixed in full contraction because this will be need to be expanded during the course of treatment while the deformity is being corrected.

5. Instead of using a telescopic rod on the convex side, one may use a long plate affixed with hinges which will allow for tilt of the axes of the rings while the telescopic rod placed on the concave side will achieve correction of the deformity

Type B4

Here the gap between the non-unions is up to 5 cm along with an existent infection.

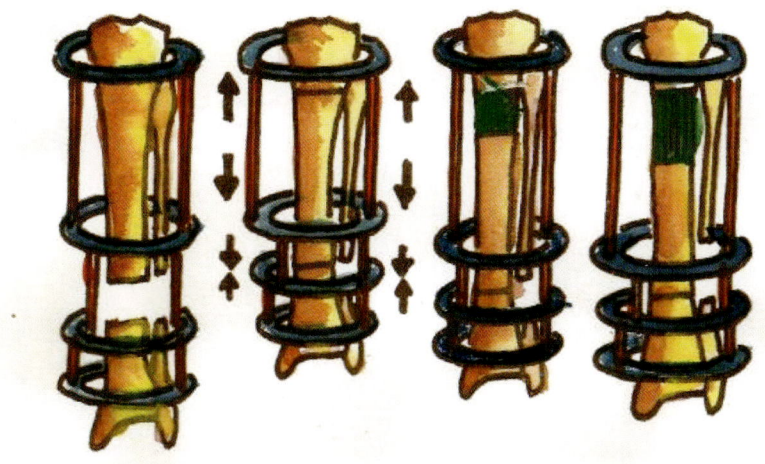

Picture 153: Treatment of B4 non unions by resection of infected segment, acute docking and corticotomy.

The first step is a meticulous and thorough clearance of the non-union ends until fresh healthy bone is visualized. At this stage, if the gap is more than 5 cm, the protocol for B5 is used. If the gap is 5 cm or less, the following steps are applicable:

1. Direct compression of the fracture site, resulting in a measurable shortening.
2. Fibular osteotomy with a four ring assembly with two peripheral and two central rings.
3. A corticotomy distraction with a gradual lengthening to correct the exact amount of shortening that has resulted from the compression of the bone fragments with an axial compression of the fracture site.

Type B5

In this case, the gap between the fragments is between 5 and 10 cm and there is a coexistent infection. The infected bone is removed and all sequestrate and unhealthy bone littles are excised. The bone ends are trimmed to produce a congruent shape capable of being compressed. The desirable method is to preserve the length of the limb along with the bone gap and perform a bone transport procedure. The following are the steps employed:

1. Fibular Osteotomy
2. The 4 ring assembly has 2 peripheral and 2 central rings. The central rings are fixed in such a manner that the gap is retained and the length of the limb is kept equal to the normal side.
3. Rings 3 and 4 are stabilized using short threaded rods.

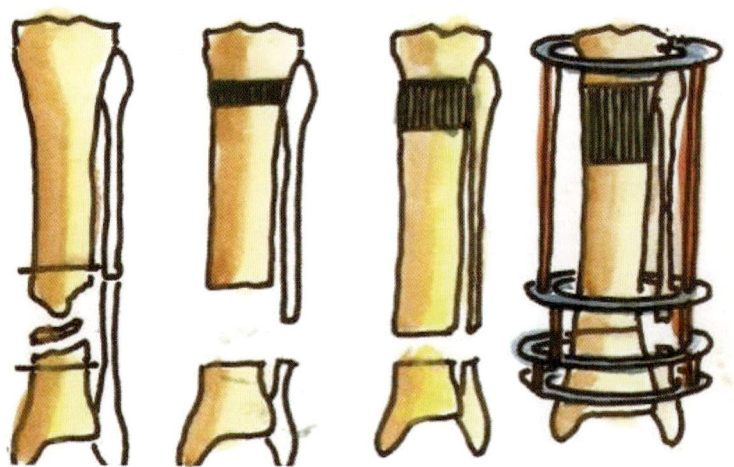

Picture 154: Treatment strategy for B4 non unions.

4. Long threaded rods are employed for connecting ring 1, 2 and 3. A corticotomy is performed between rings 1 and 2.

5. By moving ring 2 downwards in a gradual manner, lengthening is achieved at the corticotomy site. At the same time, the bone fragment moves downwards along with ring 2, gradually reducing the gap at the non-union site.

6. Once the gap has been reduced, a compression distraction protocol is employed to lead to bone union.

7. The radiograph below shows the complete sequence of this procedure.

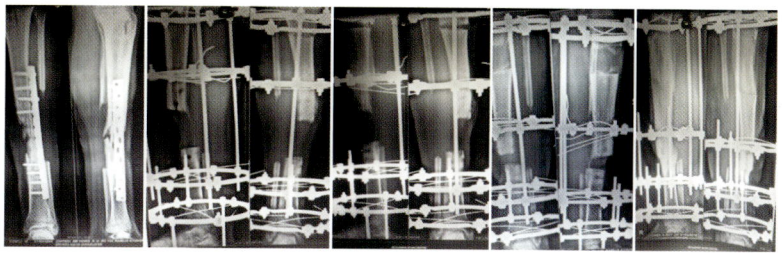

Picture 155: A B4 tibial non union treated by bone transport.

Alternatively, a bifocal transportation with rings can be done. A standard 4 or 5 ring assembly is used. Occasionally, the terminal rings can be reinforced by fixing additional pins through the posts. The following are the steps of bifocal transportation:

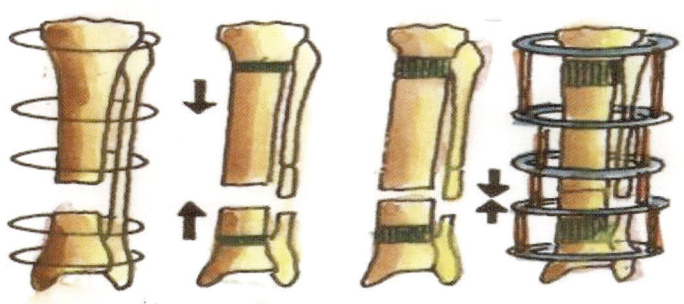

Picture 156: Assembly for a bifocal transport in B4 non union.

1. Ring 1 and 5 at both ends of the tibia and rings 2 and 3 on either side of the gap. Occasionally we can add an extra ring in the longer segment for better control while distracting.

2. Entire assembly parts are connected by multiple short threaded rods while the gap is retained and the length of the limb is kept equal to the other side.

3. Fibular osteotomy is performed.

4. Two corticotomies are performed, one between rings 1 and 2 and the other between rings 3 and 4.

5. Expansion is performed at both corticotomy sites by moving ring 2 away from ring 1 and ring 3 away from ring 4. The above scheme of operations will bring rings 2 and 3 closer, thereby gradually reducing the bone gap.

Type B6

These are infected non-unions with a gap in excess of 10 cm. These have been difficult problems, taxing the patience of orthopaedic surgeons for many many years. With the advent of the Ilizarov system, it has no doubt become possible to manage these cases, but this is not an easy matter and a lot of associated factors like skin condition, muscle and tendon loss, tethering and adherence have to be taken into consideration. At times, it may be essential to perform plastic surgery procedures in the form of full thickness flaps prior to Ilizarov frame fixation. Here the bone transport is achieved by means of olive wires.

1. A pair of crossed wires is inserted in the upper part of tibia and brought out on the opposite side. The 2 wires are now fixed to a ring. Long threaded rods are attached to this ring.

2. A second ring is slid across these rods up to the site of non-union.

3. The third and fourth rings are located distal to the non-union with the third kept as close as possible to the non-union and the fourth close to the ankle. The distal rings are fixed to the tibia by 2 wires each.

4. 2 crossed olive wires are inserted longitudinally and connected to the middle ring which was free until now.

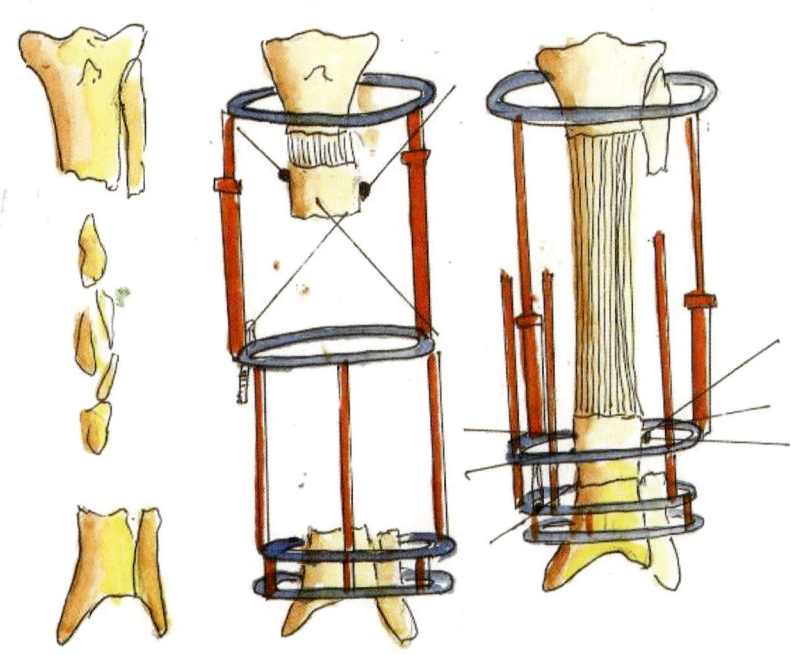

Picture 157: Schematics for bone transport with olive wires for massive bone loss and long segment transport.

5. A corticotomy is performed between rings 1 and 2.

6. By moving ring 2 towards ring 3 by gradual distraction, regenerate is formed between rings 1 and 2, resulting in elongation and the fracture gap gradually diminishes. In these cases, a bone transport can be performed over a free fibular graft acting as an intramedullary nail, pushed into the medulla of both the fragments.

ROLE OF METATARSL AND CALCANEAL HALF RINGS IN TIBIAL FRAMES

Equinous of foot is a common occurrence during the course of management of tibial fractures with Ilizarov. The calf muscles and triceps apparatus is stronger than the anterior tibial musculature. The muscular architecture and biomechanics of the foot allow it to plantar flex to a greater extent than dorsiflexion. During distraction of the corticotomy site, there is a tendency for the Tendo Achilles to tighten up and the foot to gradually slip into equinous. Sometimes, the patient may be left with a united fracture and equal limb length post treatment, but a fixed equinous foot. To avoid this, a foot frame is applied. This can be in the form of external splints and elastic bands, or by incorporation of the foot in the assembly itself.

A half ring with wires across the metatarsal heads, with or without a calcaneal ring is attached to the tibial assembly to keep the foot plantigrade during proximal distraction. The following are the indications for a foot assembly:
1. Preexisting equinous or other foot deformities
2. Non-unions in the lower third of the shaft
3. Direct docking with corticotomy
4. Transports longer than 5 cm

Two olive wires in opposite direction tightened over a half ring provide enough stability to the foot. If the equinous is fully correctable under anaesthesia, a metatarsal half ring will suffice. This is attached by hinges and plate to the upper ring to keep the foot plantigrade and allow the patient easy walking during the course of treatment. On the other hand, if the equinous is not correctable on the table, both calcaneal and tibial half rings need to be used. The calcaneal half ring will be distracted from the lower tibial ring to stretch the Tendo Achilles, while the metatarsal half ring will bring the foot plantigrade.

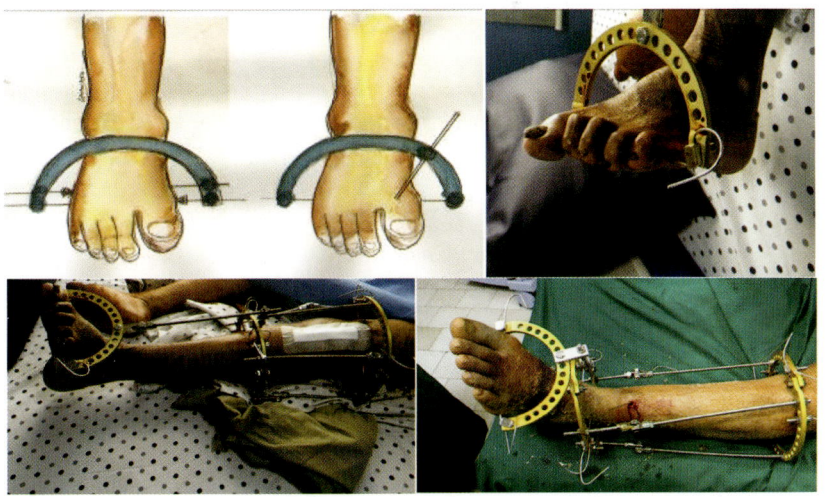

Picture 158: Foot rings to prevent equinus

REMOVAL OF THE APPARATUS:

The following criteria are to be followed before one decides to remove apparatus:

1. The new bone has filled the entire gap end-to-end in the corticotomy site and radiologically good bone is visible in both AP and lateral views.
2. Radiological union of the fracture, with bone in both cortices in both views.
3. The dynamization test is positive.

Dynamization test: Once we have achieved a radiological union, we have to decide upon the time of removal. Ilizarov is a prolonged procedure. Hence even the most enthusiastic and compliant patient becomes weary after some time and insists on removal. Premature removal will defeat the very purpose of surgery, because if the regenerate is in a plastic stage, it will deform and if the fracture is not fully united, it will displace. Some surgeons use a plaster or splint for a few weeks of additional protection. However, I conduct a dynamization test which will convince both surgeon and patient that the time for removal is correct. The following are the steps:

1. On day one, all nuts over the threaded rods are loosened by two full turns. This leaves the frame collapsible, without angular or shear stresses. The patient is allowed full weight bearing.
2. Within 24 to 48 hours we can get the test result, which is both subjective and objective. The subjective part is the patient's experience. If he feels that the limb is stable and experiences no pain either at the fracture site or corticotomy junction, the time for removal has come.
3. If loosening of the nuts suddenly produces pain anywhere except near the wires, then they are all tightened again, and we wait for the fracture to consolidate a little more.
4. In all cases, it is preferable to dynamize the frame by loosening the nuts on the index threaded rods (those which actually bind bone discontinuity), and ask the patient to weight bear for two weeks, towards the end of treatment and just prior to removal.
5. When in doubt, protection in the form of a plaster, fibre cast or splint can be given until full consolidation.

CONCLUSION:

For perfect results, the stability of the assembly is very important and the following parameters are useful:

1. Smaller the diameter of the ring, greater the stability. Likewise, greater the number of rings, more the stability.
2. Greater the tension in wires, more the stability. A perfect placement of wires in relation to the long axis of the bone increases the stability.
3. Greater number of rods and secondary elements provide added stability.

CLINICAL EXAMPLES: (courtesy Dr. Jishnu Baruah)

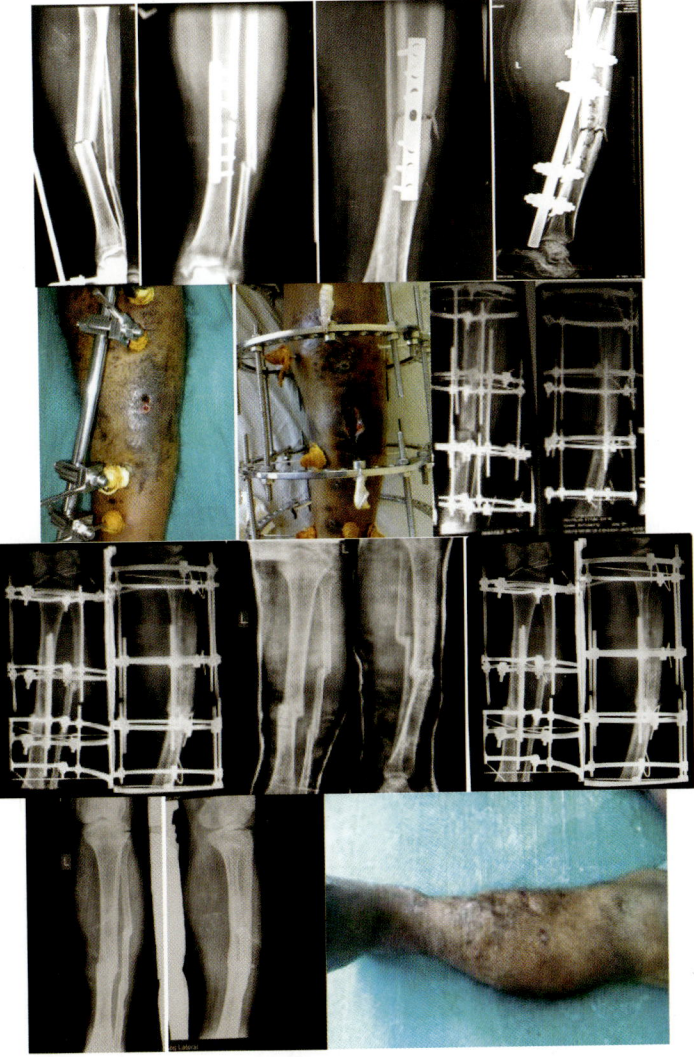

Picture 159: Compound fracture tibia treated by piano accordion compression/ distraction/ compression method.

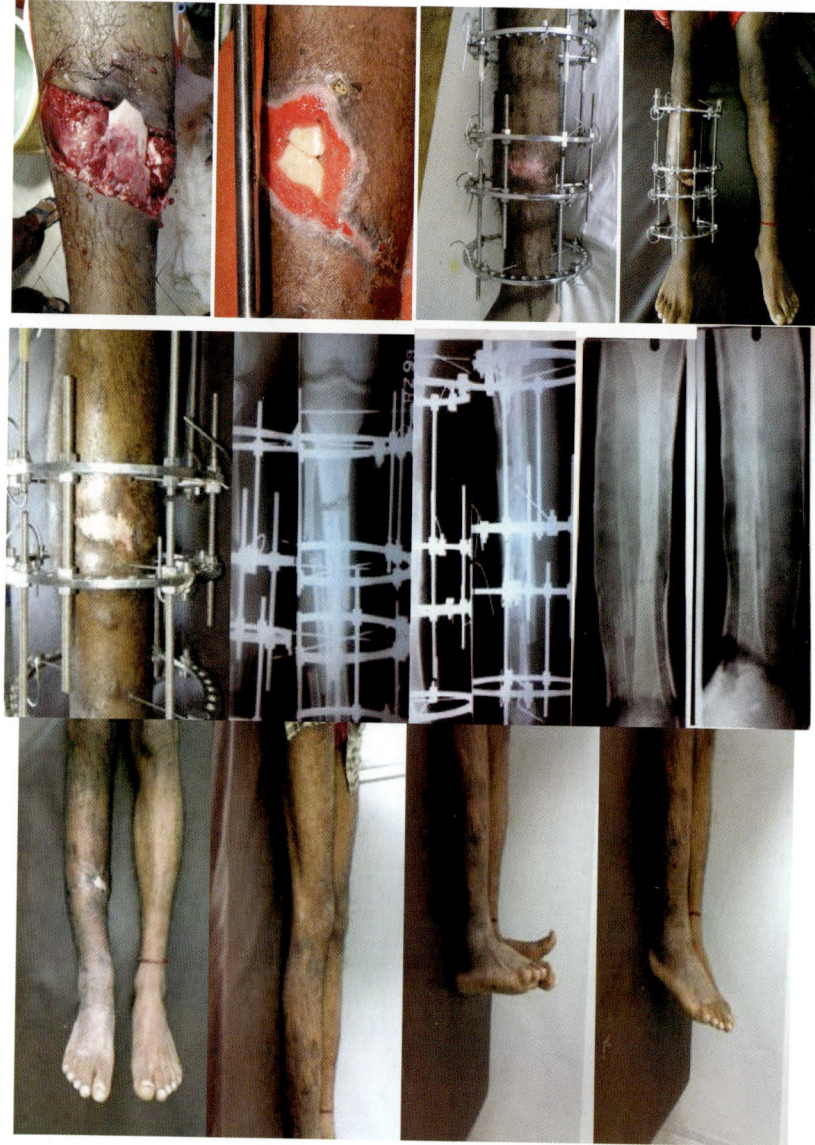

Picture 160: A case of compound fracture of tibia treated by bone transport.

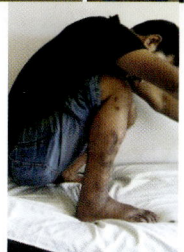

Picture 161: Bone transport for a compound fracture tibia

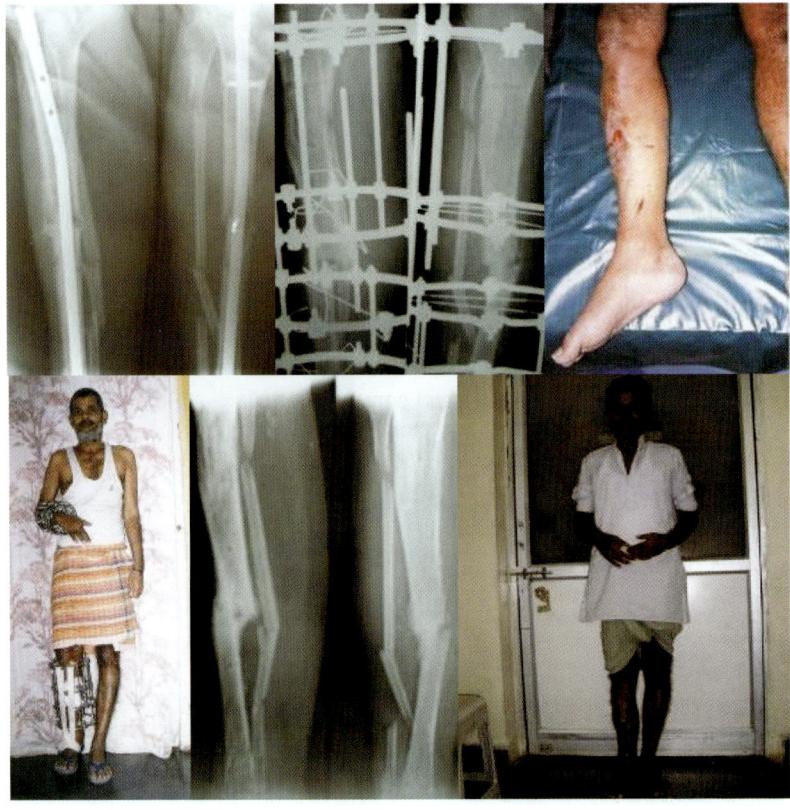

Picture 162: A case of compound fracture tibia treated by bone transport.

The aim of treatment is to allow a gradual expansion at the corticotomy site leading to abundant formation of regenerate and callus. This simultaneously allows a gradual reduction of the fracture gap, followed by compression of the fracture site. The frame assembly will result in minimizing angular and rotatory stresses while encouraging linear micromotion which acts as a stimulus for new bone formation.

Non-Union of Femur

The fundamental principles for treating femoral non-unions are very similar to that of tibia. The use of proximal femoral arch and half rings for the upper part of femur have greatly improved the patient's acceptance and tolerance of the system. Here it may not be possible (except for a highly experienced surgeon) to use all wire constructs, especially in the proximal femur, and a couple of Shanz screws make both the procedure and compliance easy. A brief description of various types of non-unions and the assemblies needed to correct them are:

Type A1 Non-unions: Corticotomy, compression and distraction. If the gap is big after resection, a bone transport is needed.

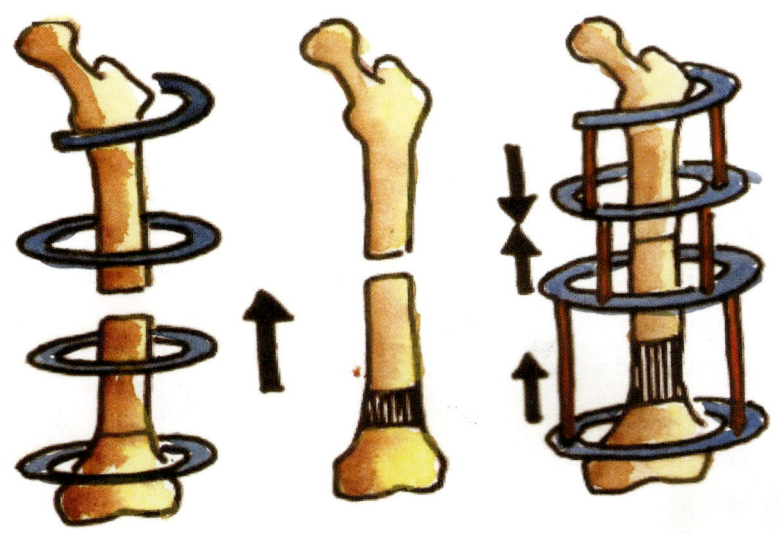

Picture 163: Frame assembly for A1 non-unions of femur

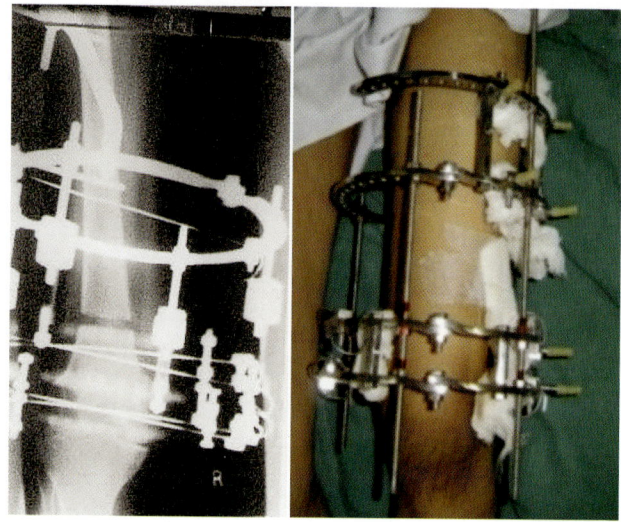

Picture 164: Treatment of A1 non-unions of femur

Type A2 Non-unions: These are treated by compression, distraction and then compression.

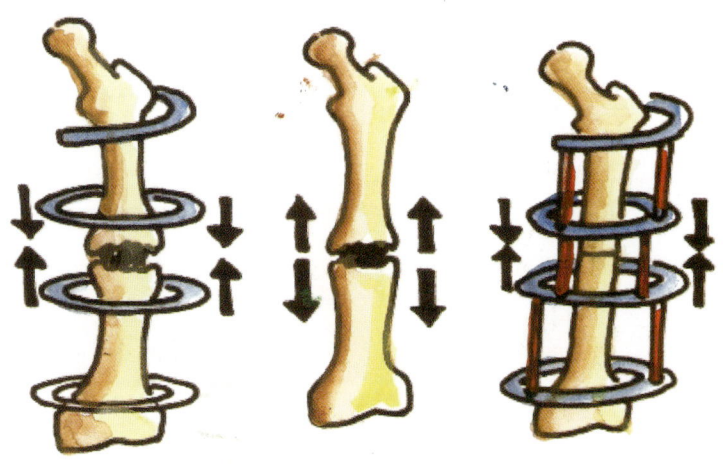

Picture 165: Assembly for A2 non-unions of femur

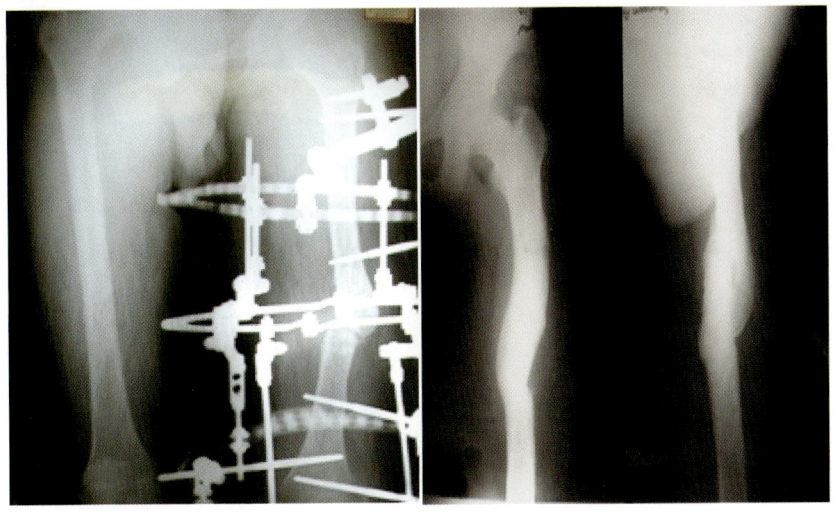

Picture 166: A2 non-unions of femur

Type A3 Non-unions: Compression with deformity correction with hinges, olive wires, or threaded rods.

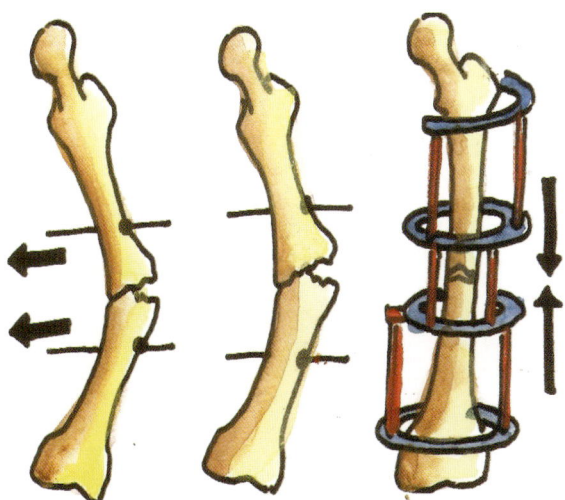

Picture 167: Schematics for an olive wire correction of A3 femoral non union.

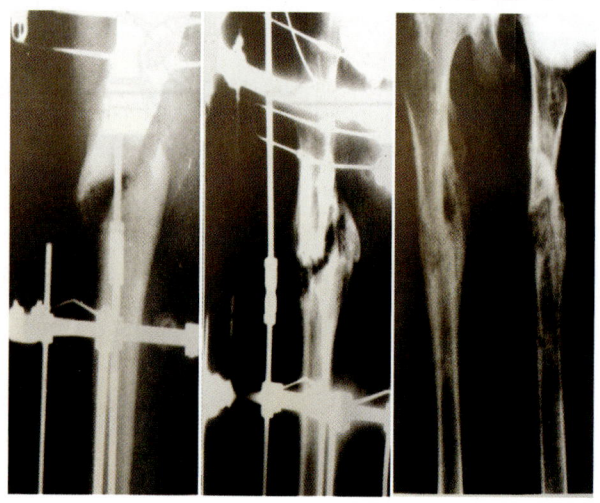

Picture 168: Clinical example of management of A3 non-unions

Type A4 Non-unions: Corticotomy, bone transport and compression.

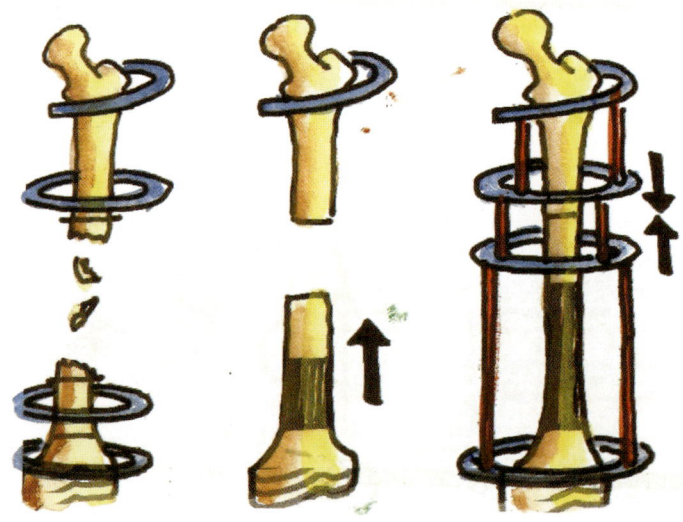

Picture 169: Frame scheme for A4 non union.

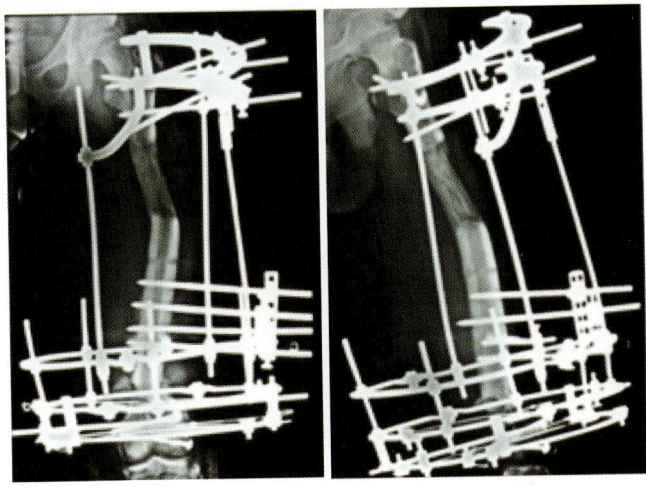

Picture 170: Management of A4 non-unions of femur

Type A5 Non-unions: Two level corticotomy, bifocal expansion and bone transport for the gap. Here this is between 5 to 10 cm. These are pretty difficult problems and tax the ingenuity and engineering skills of the surgeon.

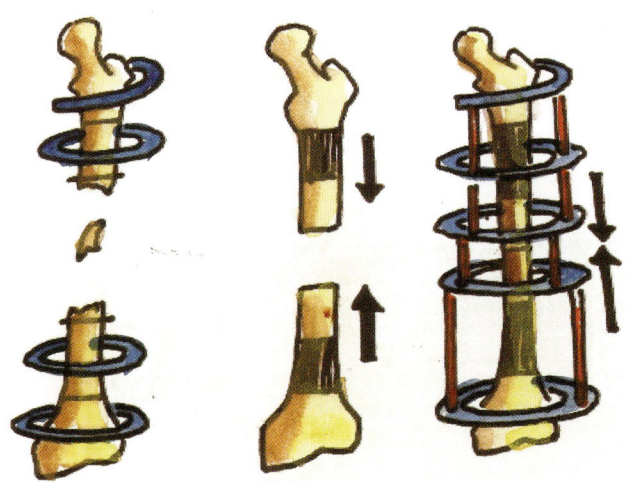

Picture 171: Schematics for bifocal transport in A5 non unions.

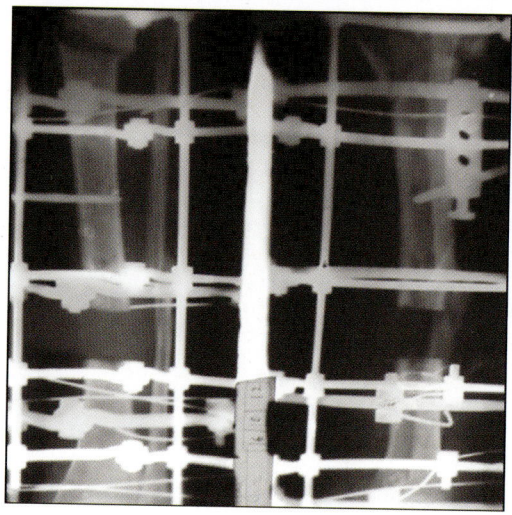

Picture 172: Treatment method for A5 femoral non-union

TypeA6 Non-union: Bone transport using crossed olive wires, followed by compression.

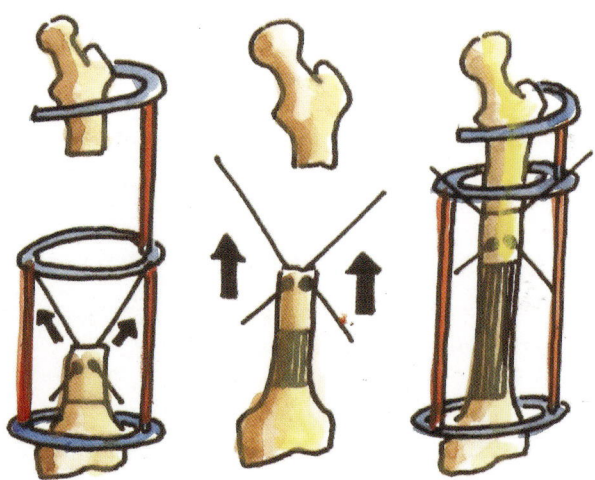

Picture 173: Apologies for absence of radiographs. I could not find them on the Net, nor did I have one in my records.

Type B1 non-unions will need a control of infection followed by corticotomy, compression and distractions, while type B2 non-unions will be amenable to compression, distraction and then compression. The magical telescope/ shock absorber, or piano accordion method, produce dramatic results.

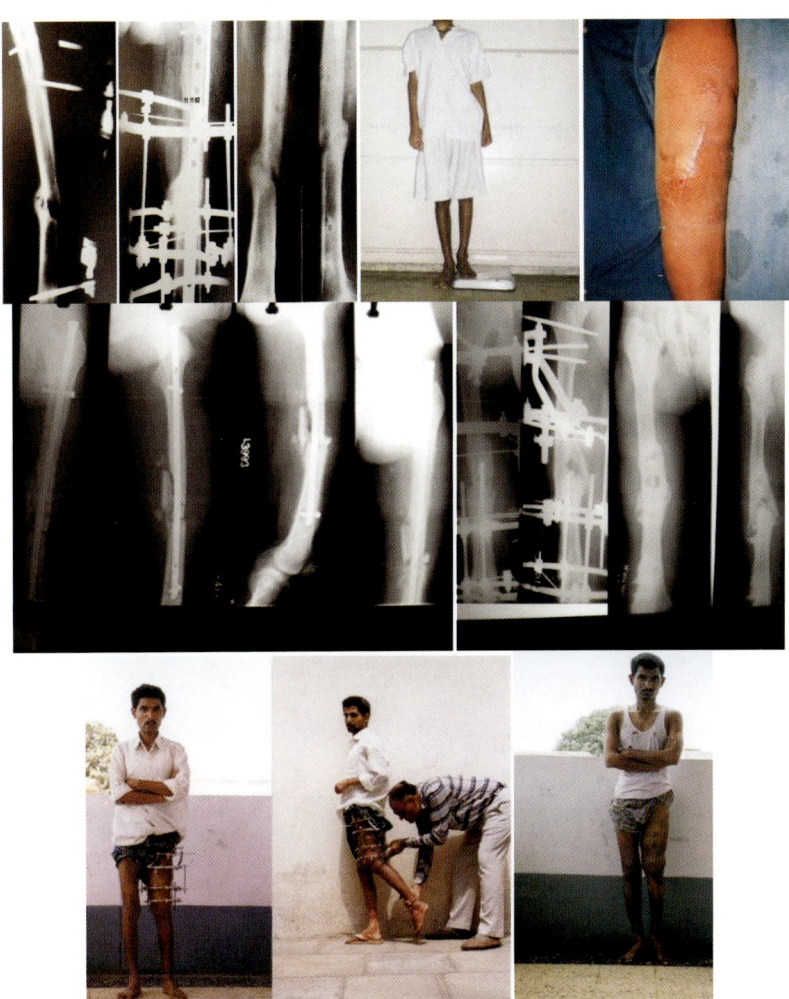

Picture 174: This case from Dr. Adke shows the modalities of managing a femoral B2 femoral non-union in a young patient. See the simple elegant frame!

Type B3 Non-unions: Infection control, sequestrectomy, followed by compression. with deformity correction using hinges, olive wires or threaded rods.

Type B4 Non-unions: Infection control, corticotomy, bone transport and compression.

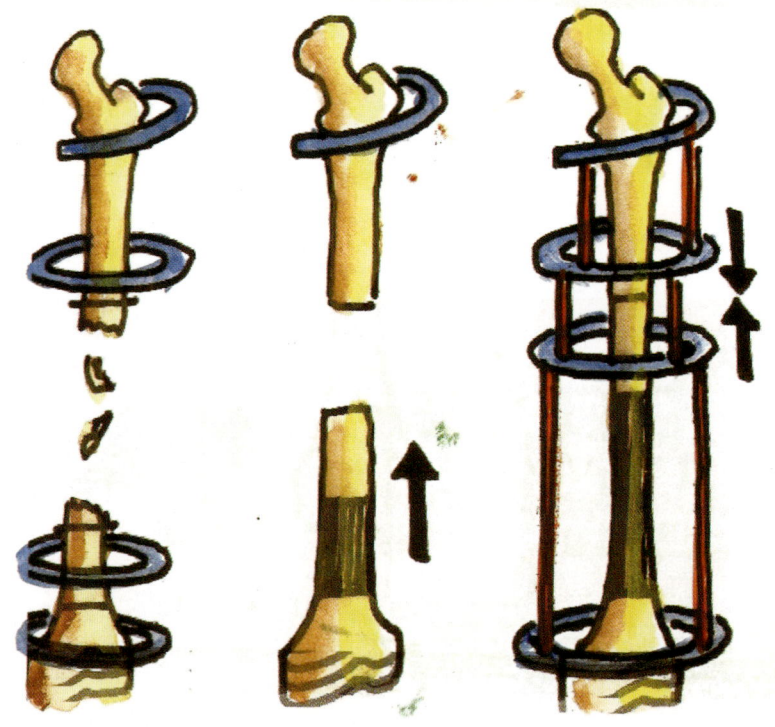

Picture 175: Treatment modalities for B3 and B4 femoral non-unions

Type B5 Non-unions: Infection control, sequestrectomy, bone end re-fashioning, two level corticotomy, bifocal expansion and bone transport for the gap (5 to 10 cm).

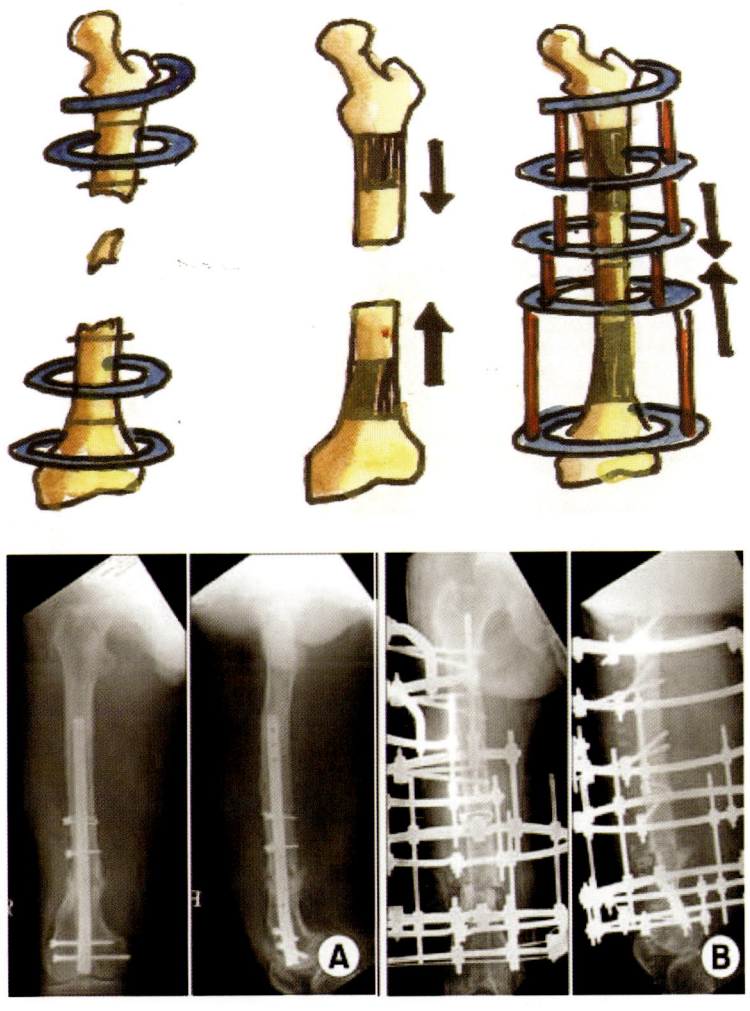

Picture 176: Bifocal transport for a B5 non-union

Type B6 Non-unions: Infection control, followed by bone transport using crossed olive wires, followed by compression. Alternatively a bifocal transport achieves the same results.

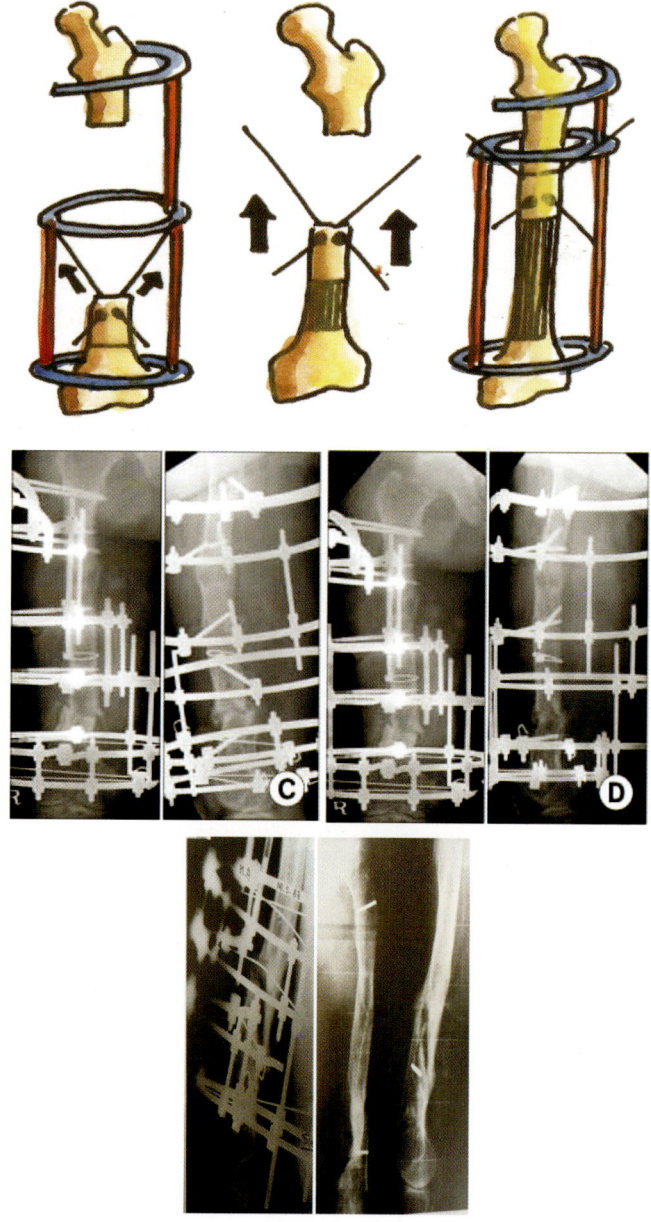

Picture 177: A B6 non-union treated bifocal transport.

Non-Union of Humerus

Because the upper limb is not used for locomotion and is not weight bearing, and because it hangs to the site, rotatory-malalignment is very common in non-unions of the humerus. It is best to use an Omega or five-eighth or arch type of ring proximally, a five-eighth ring distally, and full rings in the central portion. The fundamental principles are the same as described previously and summarized below:

Type A1: Non-unions: Corticotomy, compression and distraction. An arch or omega ring is needed at the uppermost level.

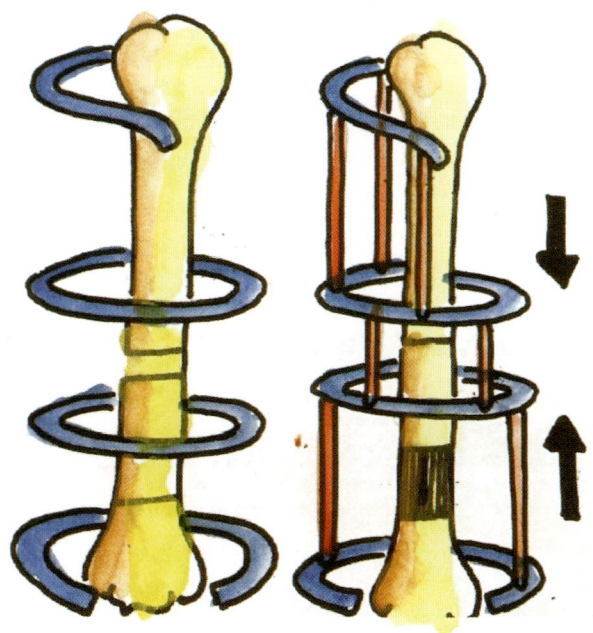

Picture 178: A1 non union and the frame construct.

197

Type A2: Non-unions: Compression, distraction and then compression.

Type A3: Non-unions: Compression with deformity, correction with hinges, olive wires or threaded rods.

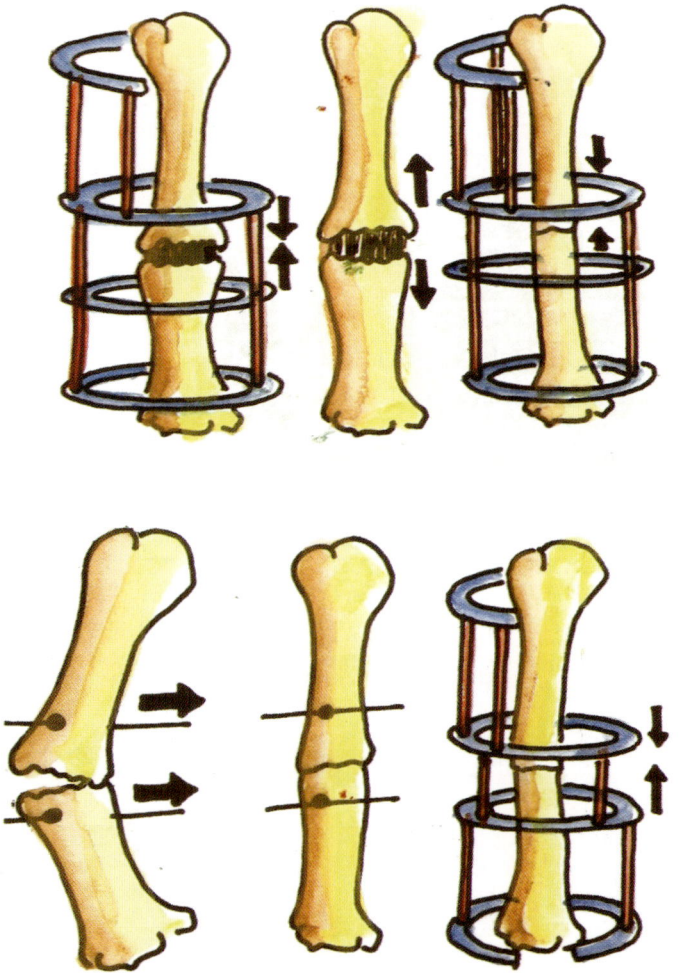

Picture 179: Frames for A2, and A3 non-unions of humerus

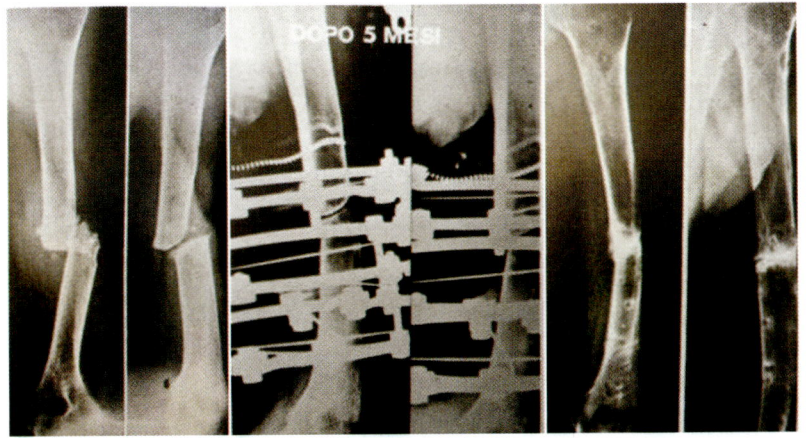

Picture 180: Clinical example of an A3 non union corrected with olive wires.

TYPE A4: Non-unions: Corticotomy, bone transport and compression..

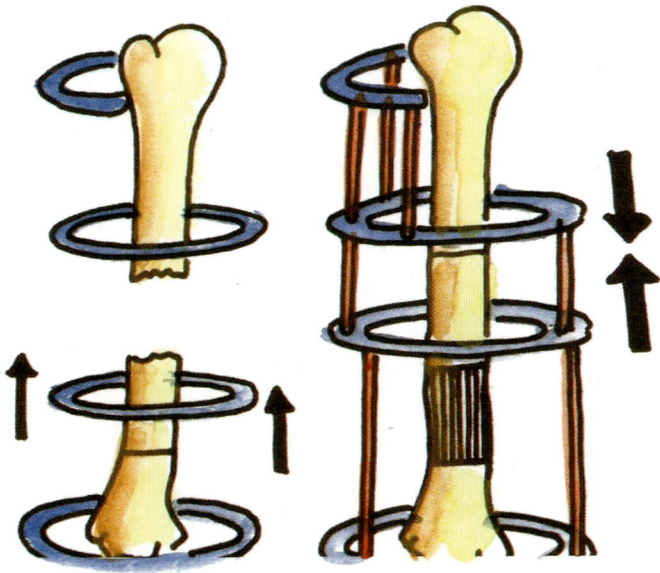

Picture 181: A frame construct for A4 Non union of humerus

Type A5: Non-unions: Two level corticotomy, bifocal expansion and bone transport for the gap (5 to 10 cm).

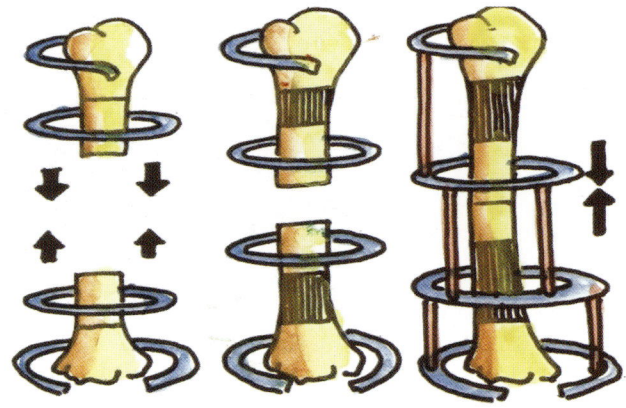

Picture 182: A frame construct for A5 Non union of humerus

Type A6: Non-unions: Bone transport using crossed olive wires, followed by compression

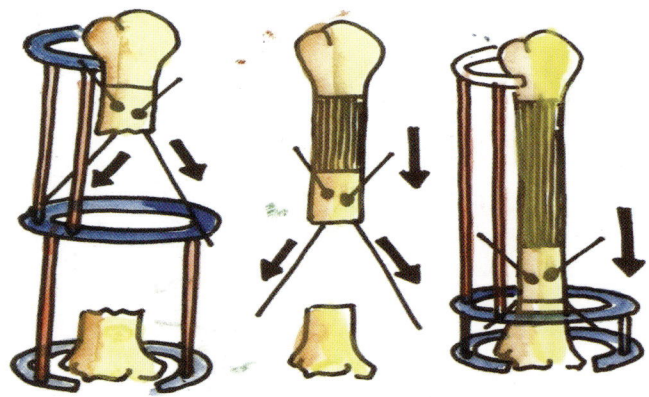

Picture 183: A frame construct for A6 Non union of humerus

Type B1 Non-unions: Control of infection, followed by corticotomy, compression and distraction.

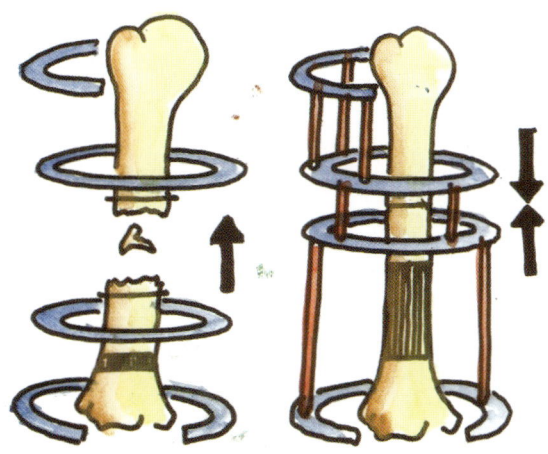

Picture 184: B1 non-union of humerus and its treatment procedure

Type B2 Non-unions: Compression, distraction and then compression

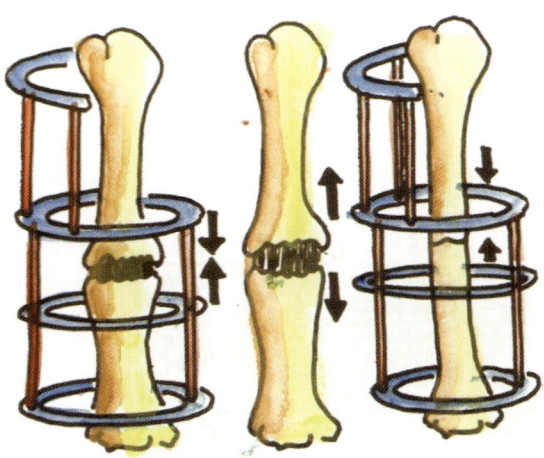

Picture 185: B2 non-union of humerus and the appropriate frame construct.

Type B3 Non-unions: Infection control, sequestrectomy, followed by compression with deformity correction using hinges, olive wires or threaded rods.

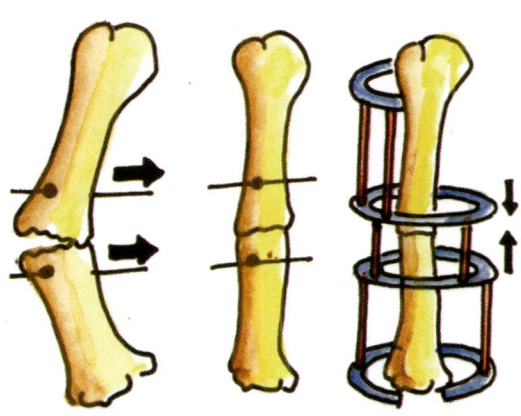

Picture 186: B3 non-union of humerus and its treatment procedure

Type B4 Non-unions: Infection control, corticotomy, and compression.

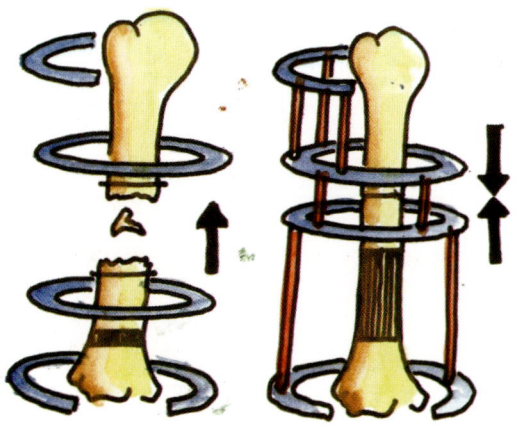

Picture 187: B4 non-union of humerus and its frame construct.

Type B5 Non-unions: These have a gap between 5 to 10 cm. Infection control, sequestrectomy, bone end re-fashioning, two level corticotomy, bifocal expansion and bone transport for the gap.

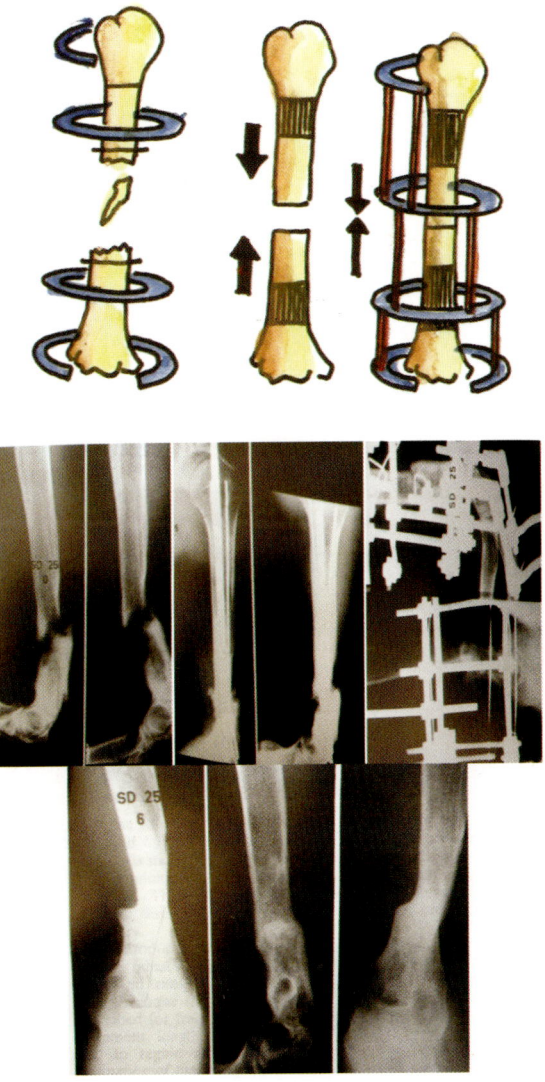

Picture 188: Treatment protocol forB5 non-unions

Type B6 Non-unions: Infection control, followed by bone transport using crossed olive wires, followed by compression.

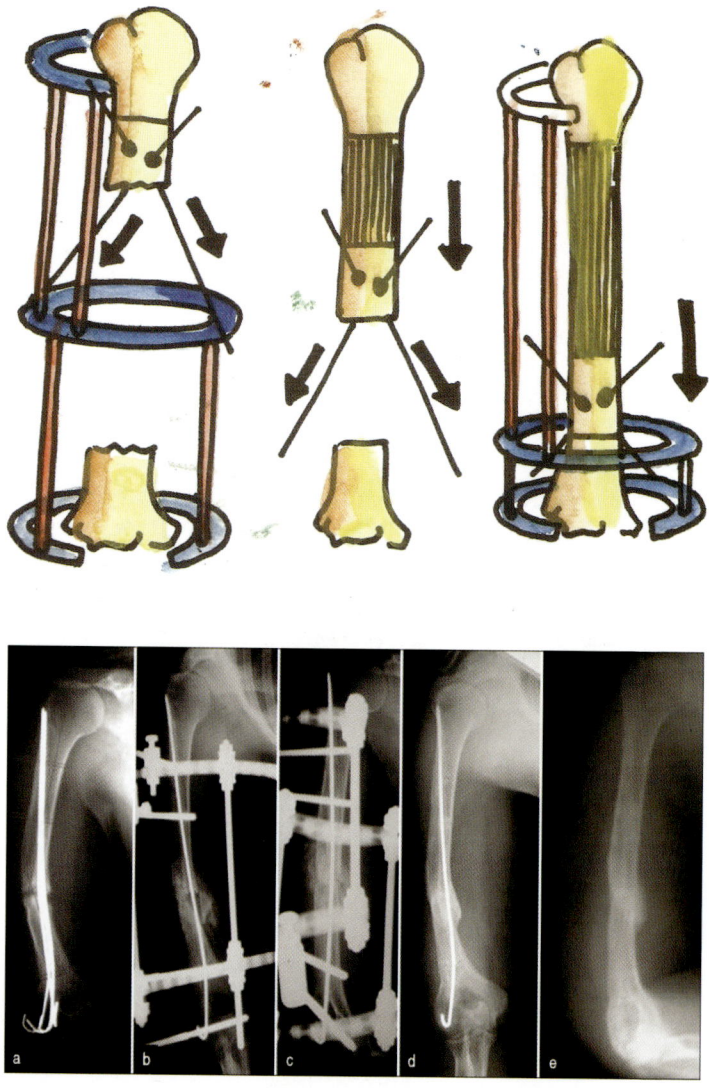

Picture 189: Frame construct and clinical example of a B6 non union of humerus.

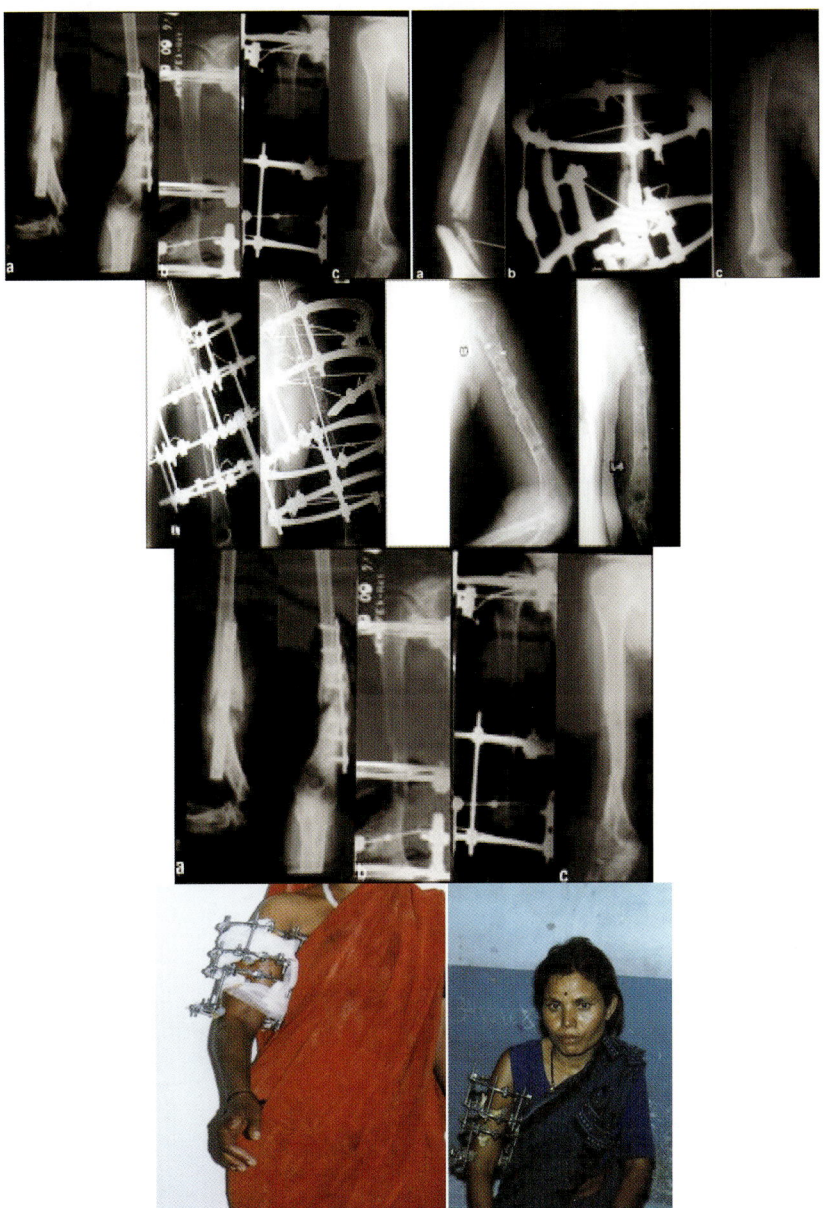

Picture 190: B6 non-union treated by bone transport. Case courtesy Dr. Sandeep Adke

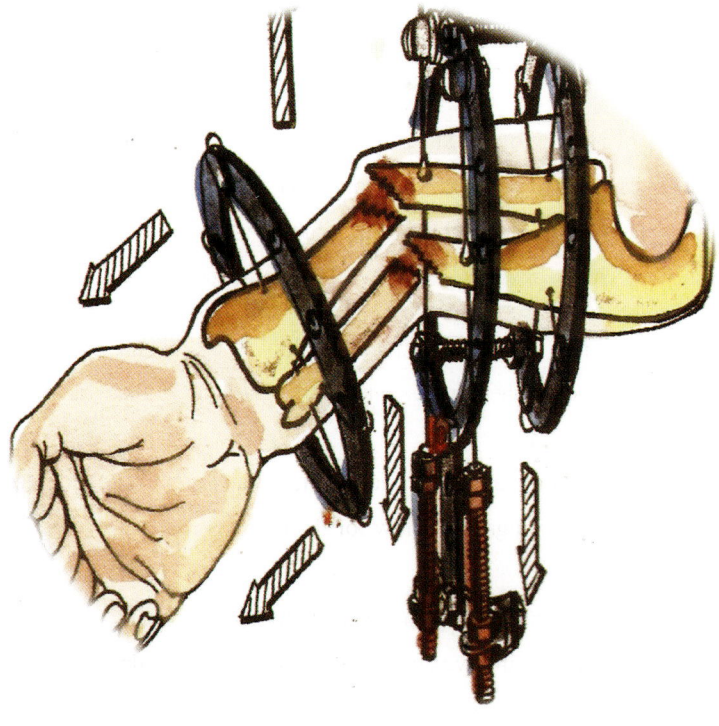

Non-Union of the Forearm Bones

As the forearm has two equal bones which participate in a complex rotatory movement, treatment modalities are addressed towards specific problems as they arise.

NON-UNION OF ONE BONE:

A four ring assembly is employed. The proximal ring applied in the region of elbow, and the distal ring applied in the region of wrist will include both the forearm bones. The two middle rings will be anchored to the bone in which there is non-union. The following are the methods employed:

1. For A1 non-union, a corticotomy distraction followed by compression is done. Area of ulna below the olecranon and the radius above the wrist are good sites for corticotomy.
2. For A2 non-unions, a simple compression distraction compression scheme between the two central rings will allow for the union without interfering with the normal bone.
3. For other types, the fundamental principles and methods remain the same. The following drawings will give an idea of the various procedures needed.

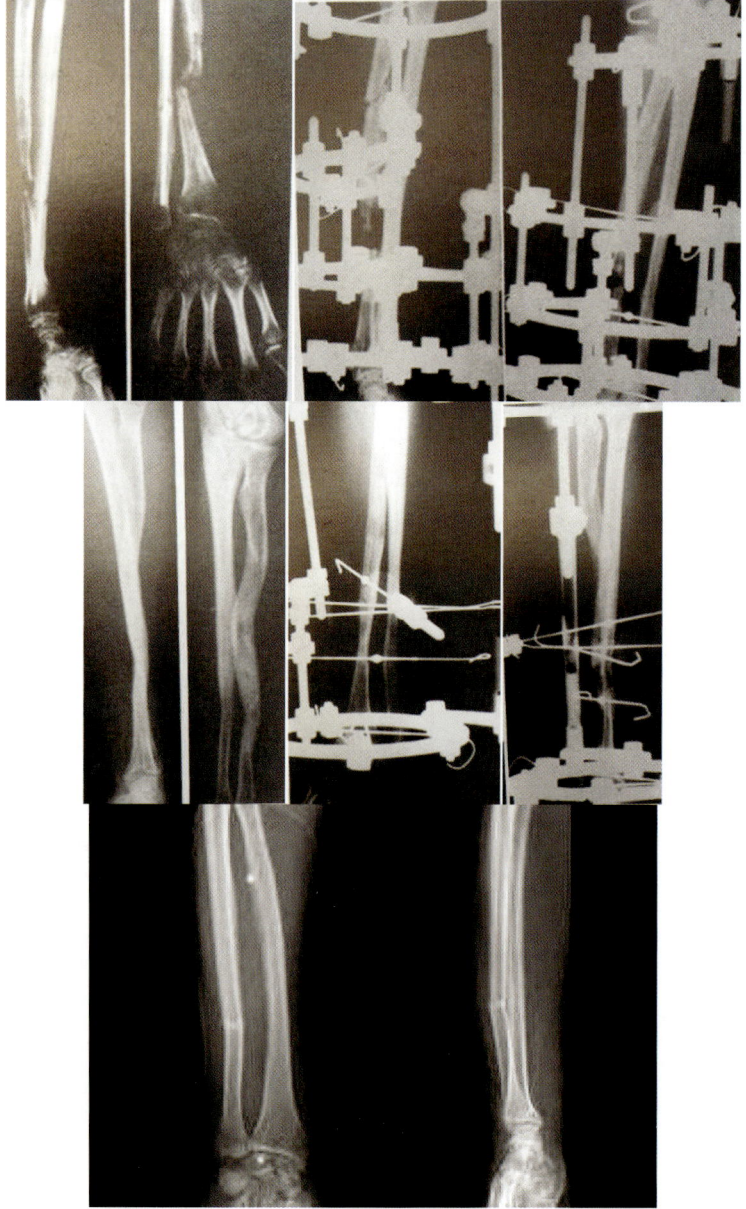

Picture 191: Gap nonunion of forearm treated by bone transport and olive wires

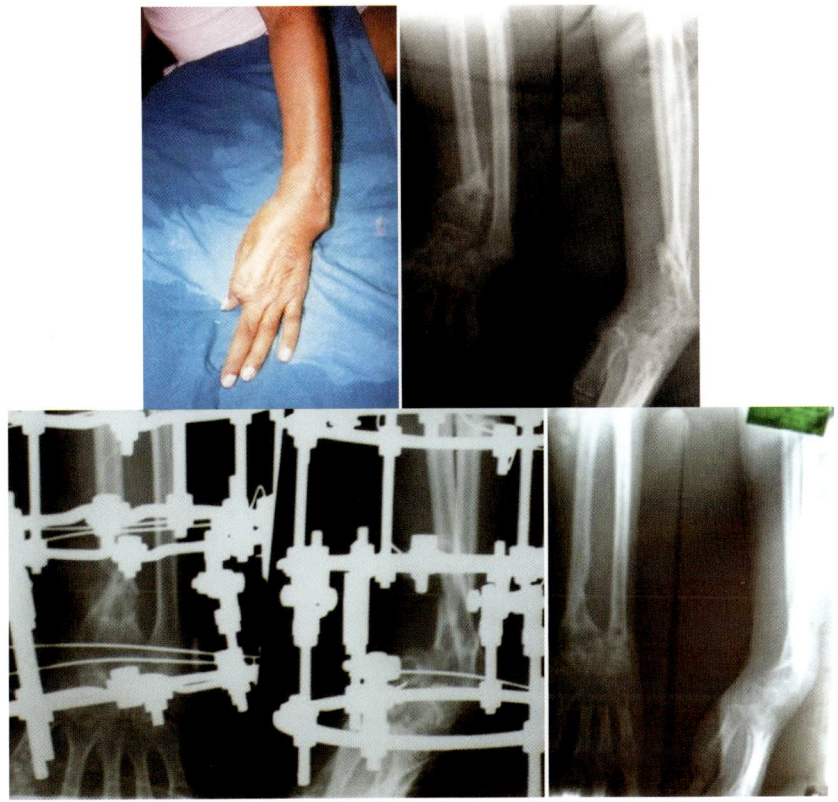

Picture 192: Gap non-union of forearm treated by bone transport and hinges

NON-UNIONS ON BOTH BONES AT MIDDLE THIRD:

Here, a three or four ring assembly is employed with the proximal and distal rings in the region of elbow and wrist. Olive wires are attached proximal and distal to the non-union and connected to the middle rings under tension. The two outer rings can be used to distract the limb and gain length, while the two middle rings with their olive wire configuration will achieve deformity correction and compression at the fracture site.

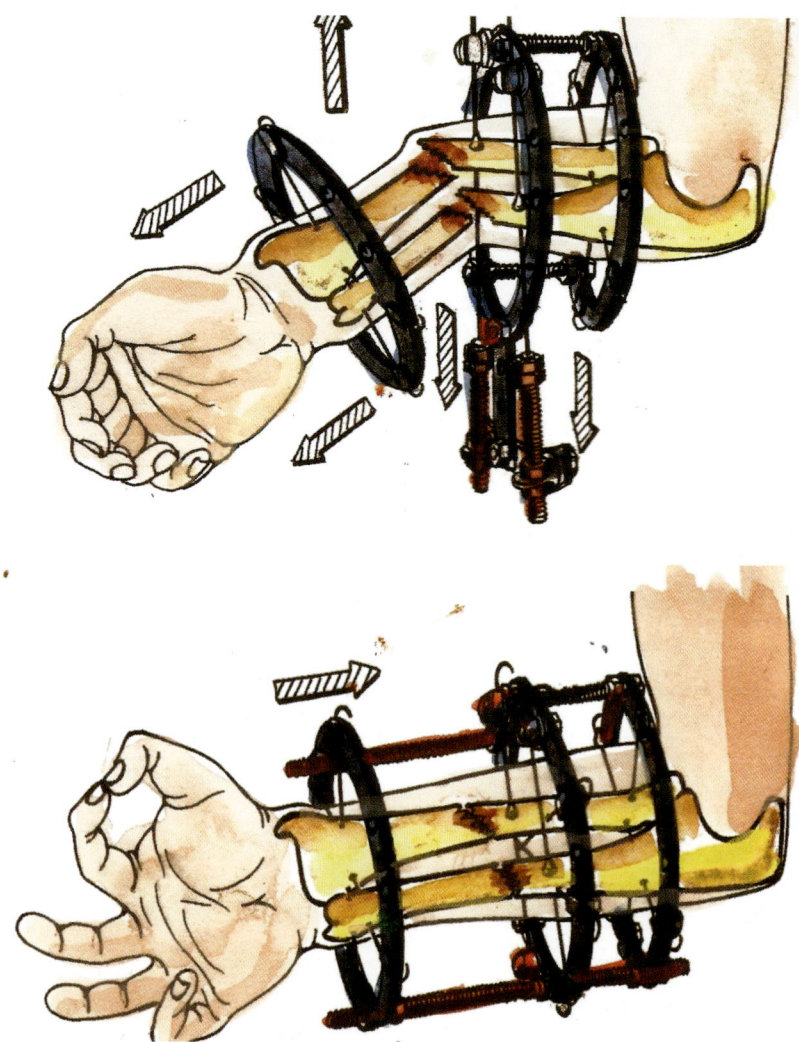

Picture 193: Non unions of mid forearm corrected by a three ring assembly.

Ilizarov in Limb Lengthening

The concepts of management of limb length inequality have undergone a very dramatic change since the introduction of the Ilizarov system. The entire understanding and fundamental principles of bone lengthening is seen with a new eye, thanks to the development of the science of transosseous osteosynthesis. If one consults a standard text book on limb inequality, the following methods are described:

1. The discrepancy be ignored. This would be indicated in discrepancies of less than 2.5 cm.

2. Raised shoes or orthosis. This method would seem to be appropriate for discrepancies between 2.5 to 5 cm.

3. Growth plate arrest and bone shortening procedures. These have to be conventionally indicated in discrepancies between 2.5 and 10 cm.

4. Stimulation surgery to the growth plate by surgical irritation or interposition has been described.

5. Amputation followed by fitting of prosthesis. This has been described in the past as a method of choice in discrepancies in excess of 20 cm. But the entire theory is now being challenged by the advent of Ilizarov Frame Systems.

6. Limb lengthening: Conventionally they have been indicated for discrepancies between 6 and 18 cm, provided the amount of lengthening does not exceed 20% of the pre-existing limb length.

Limb lengthening has always been described as a refractory procedure with great morbidity and a number of complications. This attitude has remained unchanged for many many years. But since the advent of Ilizarov methods, a lot of these pre-existing theories are being challenged. Russian literature mentions expanding amputation stumps to render the use of prostheses altogether unnecessary, and elongation of complex congenital deficiencies, including limb bud failures to give a useful limb.

PRINCIPLES OF ILIZAROV WITH REGARDS TO BONE LENGTHENING:

The following are the principles propounded by Ilizarov and the ASAMI group:

1. Discontinuity of a skeleton segment stimulates the repair processes.
2. The repair process continues as long as the stimulus to the bone and the blood supply is maintained.
3. With the application of a distraction force, new bone forms in the direction of the line of the force.
4. The site of bone regeneration is the centre from which a multi-dimensional regeneration occurs in the muscles, fascia, nerves, blood vessels, subcutaneous tissue and skin.
5. At the end point of stimulation, the regenerated bone undergoes a maturation phase to make the new bone identical to the normal bone.
6. 1 mm per day is the critical rate and 0.25 mm every 6 hours is the critical rhythm.
7. Quality of the new bone is directly dependant on the stability and tensioning of the expansion apparatus.
8. Metaphysis of long bone with a high vascularity is ideal site for corticotomy.
9. Discrepancies of more than 4 cm in the lower limb and 5 cm in humerus are indications for lengthening.

LENGTHENING OF THE TIBIA

There are slight differences in the frame construction for lengthening procedures of tibia in children and adults; hence these shall be described separately.

PROCEDURE FOR ADULTS:

A four ring assembly is used. Here the two proximal rings and two distal rings are close to each other with long threaded rods separating the two units of the rings. We normally prefabricate the assembly one day before the procedure and autoclave is as one unit. The following points are important:

1. The 2 proximal rings and the 2 distal rings are connected to each other with 5 cm threaded rods.
2. The second ring should lie at the length of the middle of the fibular head and the first ring should lie below the knee joint, both exactly parallel to the adjacent joint.
3. The third ring should lie about 4 cm above the ankle and the last one about 2 cm above the ankle.
4. The lengths of the 2 long threaded rods used to attach these 2 units together will depend on the accurate anatomical placement of the rings as mentioned above.
5. The limb is draped in the standard manner and the first ring to be transfixed is ring 1. Using an olive wire passing from lateral to medial side, the first ring is anchored to the upper tibia.
6. A smooth wire is passed parallel to the first wire on the distal surface of ring 4. This wire rests about 2 cm above the ankle.

7. At this stage, one can shift the assembly from side-to-side and make sure that it is central. It is also ensured that a uniform skin clearance is available on all sides.

8. Another transverse olive wire is passed from medial to lateral on ring 2 and tensioned.

9. Additional wires are inserted into all 4 rings proceeding from proximal to distal.

10. All wires are tightened and tensioned.

11. A fibular osteotomy is performed about 8 cm above the ankle joint.

12. A corticotomy is now performed just below ring 2.

13. Closure and post-operative procedures are performed as usual.

14. The 2 threaded rods are now replaced by 2 telescopic rods.

15. The rate and rhythm of distraction depends upon the patient's pain tolerance and the distraction is started after a latency of 2 to 7 days, with a rhythm of 0.25 mm every 6 hours resulting in a rate of 1 mm per day.

TIBIAL LENGTHENING IN CHILDREN

In small children, lengthening can be done using two rings. The proximal ring is placed about 3 cm below the upper tibial epiphysis and the distal ring about 4 cm above the ankle joint. The following parameters are used:

1. Olive wires can be used in the proximal ring to increase stability.

2. For a larger child, additional stability may be achieved by inserting extra wires with posts.

3. For larger children and adolescents, additional half rings can be bolted to the existing rings and the number of wires passed are increased, thereby increasing the stability.

4. A fibular osteotomy is performed.

5. Corticotomy is performed distal to the tibial tubercle.

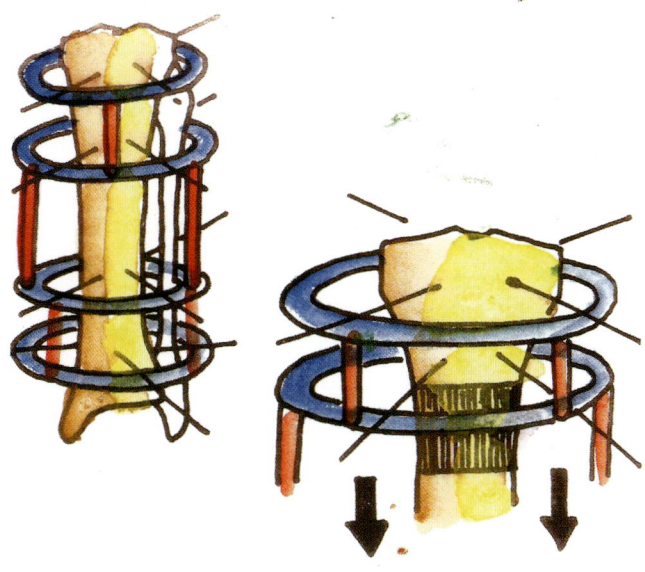

Picture 194: The lengthening frame for the adult.

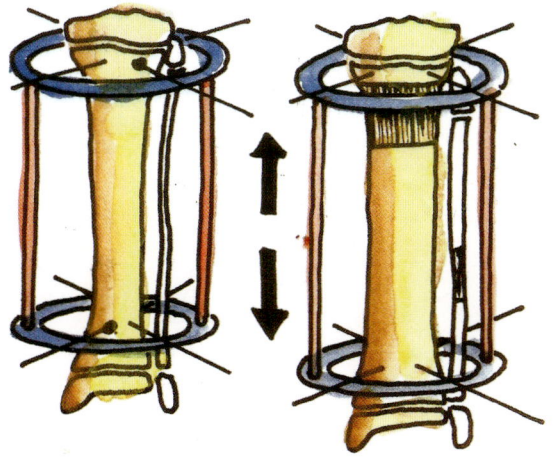

Picture 195: The lengthening frame for the child

TECHNIQUE OF CORTICOTOMY:

This requires a special fish mouth shaped chisel, called the corticotomy chisel. Corticotomy is in fact a low velocity minimum trauma osteotomy without apparently damaging the medullary blood vessels. This is performed through 2 evenly spaced 6 mm incisions. The bone is reached through each incision and the periosteum cut longitudinally in line with the skin incision. Subsequently, using the corticotomy chisel, the cortex is broken in both directions transversely as far as the limited skin incision will allow. The same steps are repeated through other incisions until a complete section of the cortex is achieved. In some cases, one may have to gently rock or twist the bone to complete the break. This is the most important step of lengthening. The premise is that only the circumferential cortex is broken, leaving the periosteal sleeve and the inside medulla intact.

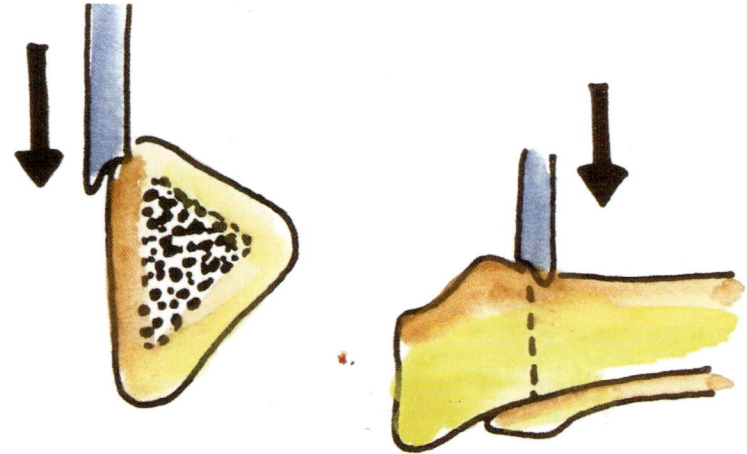

Picture 196: Technique of corticotomy

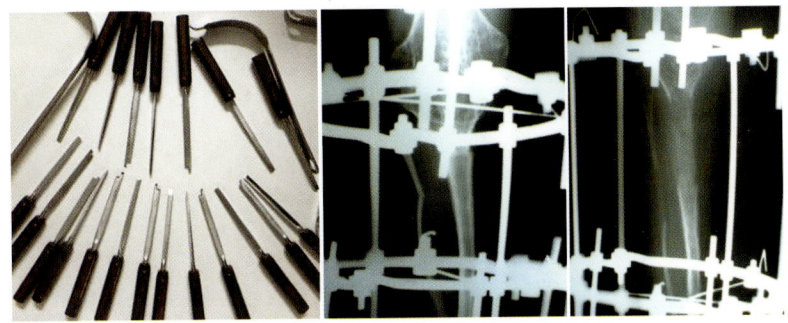

Picture 197: Special corticotomy chisels and bone regenerate

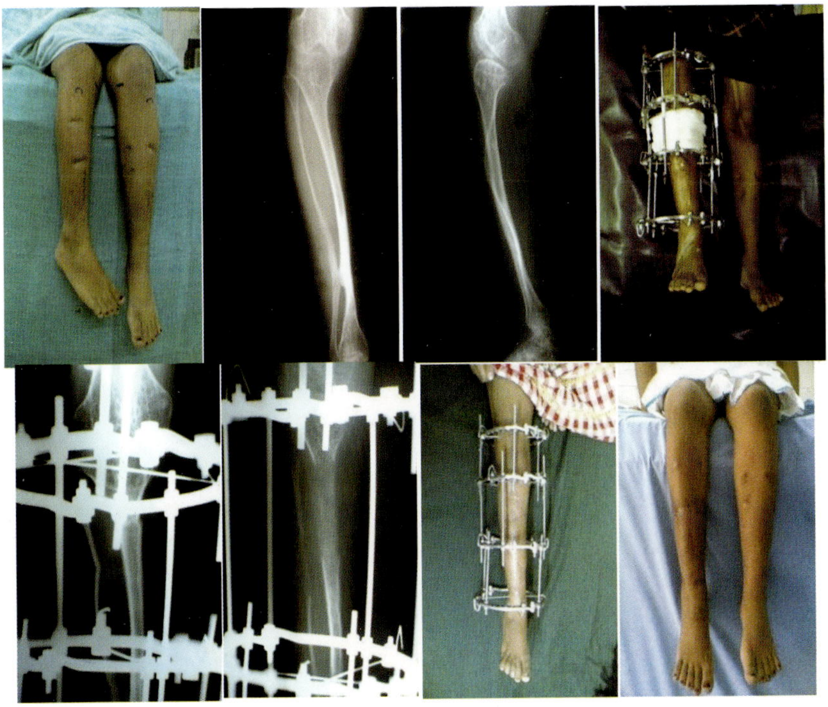

Picture 198: Sequence of limb lengthening in a young adult. (Case Courtesy Dr. Jishnu Baruah)

PROBLEMS ENCOUNTERED DURING LENGTHENING AND THEIR SOLUTIONS

A. ANTERIOR ANGULATION OF THE PROXIMAL SEGMENT:

As the postero-lateral structures are very strong, tension forces generated by these structures can produce an anterior angulation during the process of lengthening.

This can be avoided by placing the proximal 2 rings in 7 to 10 degrees recurvatum in relation to the distal ring. This placement will automatically correct the angulation as it occurs during the process of lengthening. If anterior angulation develops during the course of treatment, it can be corrected by the following method. The support wire is detached from its support plate and attached to a tensioned half ring placed below. This half ring is now attached to the parent ring with 2 or 3 short threaded rods.

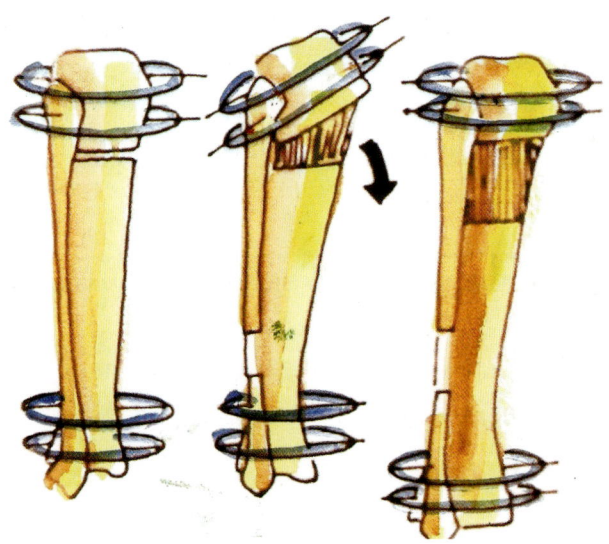

Picture 199: Correction of anterior angulation during lengthening

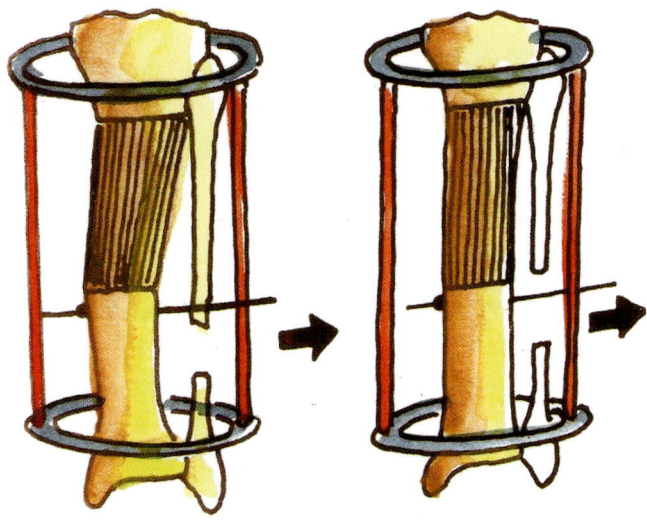

Picture 200: Correction of valgus during lengthening

B. VALGUS OF THE LIMB:

Occasionally, while the lengthening is in process, a valgus deformity can occur. This can be corrected either with traction or with hinge.

1. For the hinge method of correction, the long threaded rods are replaced with shorter rods with hinges at the apex of the deformity. By shifting the focus to the correction of the deformity 0.25 mm every 6 hours, the deformity is corrected. After correction of the deformity, the lengthening process is re-started.

2. In the traction method of deformity correction, an olive wire is inserted from the convex side of the deformity with the olive wire inserted at the apex of the deformity. A long connection plate is attached between the two terminal rings on the concave side of the deformity. The olive wire is anchored to this long threaded rod using a slotted thread rod. Accordingly, traction on this will correct the deformity after which the lengthening process can continue.

219

C. EQUINOUS OF THE FOOT:

Equinous of the foot may occur during lengthening and can be avoided by using rigid orthosis to keep the foot in dorsiflexion during nights. During the day, the patient is subjected to extensive physiotherapy and stretching movements to attain maximum dorsiflexion. If equinous appears during the course of treatment, an additional metatarsal ring can easily be added across all the metatarsal necks to anchor the half ring and enable to allow for a direct lineal pull in the direction of dosriflexion. Gradual turnings of the nut will cause dorsiflexion. The Italian group now routinely uses a metatarsal ring in all cases to avoid foot equinous.

D. FLEXION DEFORMITY OF THE KNEE:

A flexion deformity of the knee occasionally occurs during the course of lengthening. This is corrected by the use of a rigid extension brace worn along with the frame, supplemented by physiotherapy and stretching. If the deformity remains uncorrected with brace, or progresses during the course of treatment, it is an easy job to add an additional femoral ring across the femoral shaft to anchor a full ring, and with the help of hinges to allow for a direct lineal pull in the direction opposite to flexion. Gradual turnings of the nut will cause an extension of the knee.

LENGTHENING OF THE FEMUR:

Femoral lengthening is more difficult than tibial lengthening using the ring fixator. The main reasons are:

1. It is not possible to have a full ring in the upper femur.
2. The thigh girth tapers from the buttock to the knee.
3. If the femur is lengthened along its anatomic axis, medialisation of the knee and ankle results.
4. The critical method of lengthening the femur in relation to the mechanical axis of the hip, knee and the ankle is difficult to achieve.

5. Strong posterior musculature tends to produce an anterior bowing in the femur during lengthening.

FRAME ASSEMBLY:

1. The 4 ring assembly is employed with 3 full rings in the thigh and 1 half ring in the trochanteric region.

2. The 2 distal rings are pulled close to each other with 5 cm rods and the lowermost ring lies 6 cm above the knee joint.

3. Telescopic rods are employed between rings 2 and 3.

4. Half ring 1 and ring 2 are joined to each other using threaded rods. Occasionally one will have to use hinges or bent plates for an uniform transmission of forces from the half ring to the full ring.

5. On certain occasions, ring 2 is left without wires and the entire access of transmission is borne by ring 1.

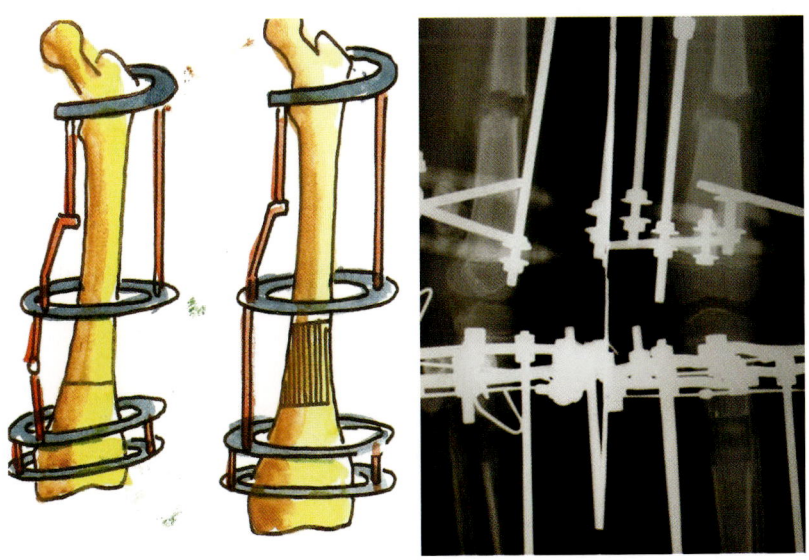

Picture 201: A femoral assembly for lengthening

CORTICOTOMY:

The site of corticotomy is the distal femoral metaphysis just above ring 3. The bone is exposed through a small linear incision in the anterio-lateral aspect of the thigh. The periosteum is split longitudinally. Using a corticotomy chisel a corticotomy is performed as described previously.

LENGTHENING SCHEDULE:

A standard latency, interval and rhythm are followed:

1. Distraction is started after a latent interval of 1 to 7 days. This depends on the problems faced during corticotomy. If the corticotomy is performed with no damage to medullary vessels, the elongation can be started almost immediately. On the other hand, if there has been damage to the medullary vessels, it is best to wait for some time.
2. Rate of elongation is 1 to 1.25 mm per day. If there is very severe pain during the course of the treatment, the rate can be reduced to 0.5 mm per day till the acute crisis is over.
3. A quarter turn of the screw every 6 hours will give an optimum rhythm.

LENGTHENING OF THE HUMERUS

Before the arrival of the Ilizarov system, humeral lengthening was a very uncommon procedure. The advent of Ilizarov frames has demonstrated that lengthening by this method is very easy and practical. Shortening of 5 cm or more is considered a reasonable indication.

In Achondroplastic dwarfs, simultaneous successful lengthening of 8 to 10 cm on both arms have been reported.

FRAME ASSEMBLY:

1. A two ring assembly (an omega ring proximally and a five-eighth ring distally) is employed.
2. These two rings are connected using two telescopic rods.

In case a bifocal lengthening is envisaged, an additional ring is placed midway between the omega and five-eighth rings. This ring is connected proximally and distally using telescopic rods.

CORTICOTOMY:

For a single level corticotomy, the area recommended lies distal to the deltoid tubercle and the insertion of pectorals.

For a bifocal lengthening, the site of second corticotomy is above the distal humeral metaphysis.

LENGTHENING SCHEDULE:

1. Lengthening is started after a latency of 2 to 7 days.
2. Thus, one has to achieve a compromise between the possibility of a good primary fit of the resected surfaces with the promise of lengthening at a later date at the cost of kinking the vessels and other structures or the patience of resection, followed by the maintenance of the gap and a corticotomy with a subsequent elongation. A rhythm of 0.25 mm every 6 hours gives a rate of 1 mm per day.
3. If neurological complications in the form of paresis develop, the speed is reduced to 0.5 mm per day.

Due to good blood circulation in humerus there is a possibility of premature consolidation and this must be avoided by careful attention to the lengthening schedule.

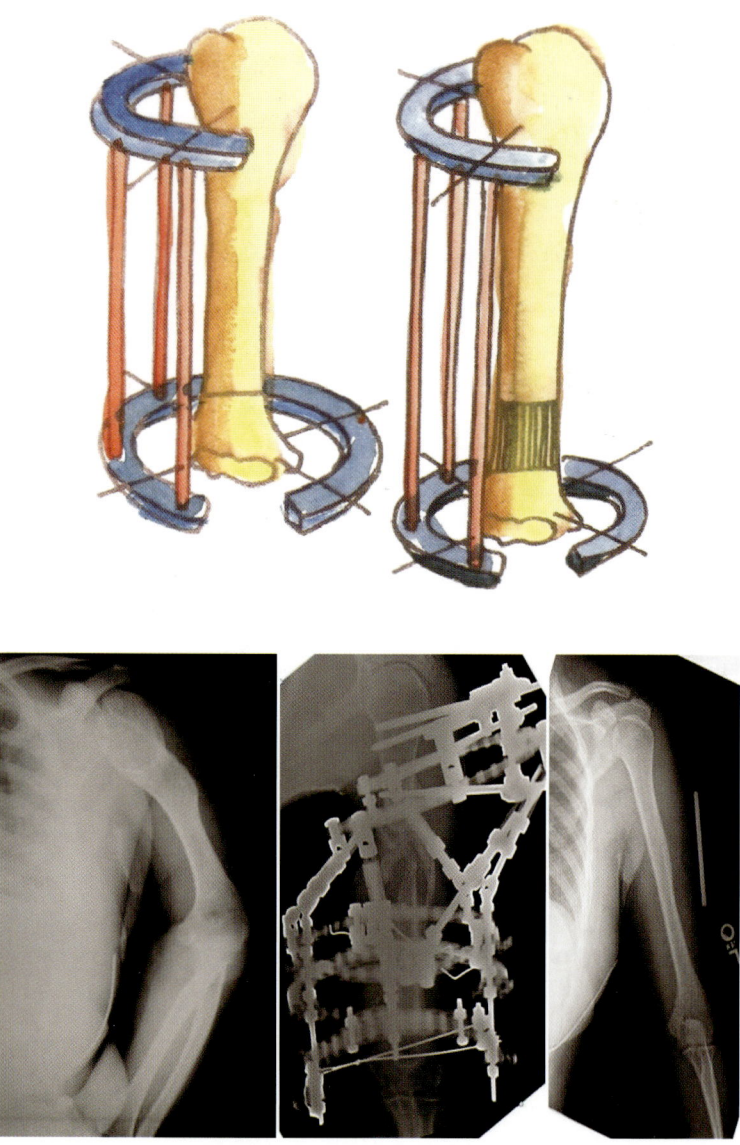

Picture 202: Frame for lengthening of humerus.

Ilizarov in Congenital Pseudarthrosis of the Tibia

This was one of the refractory conditions in the past where most surgical operations failed to produce results. Good results were achieved with the advent of micro surgical procedures, but these facilities are not available in most centres. From Boyd to Sir Peterson and Poh there have been no less than two dozen unsuccessful methods reported in literature. Until the advent of micro vascular surgery, this refractory problem was considered insoluble. The amount of unhealthy bone that needed to be removed was phenomenal. While attempting surgery, one was always worried that the amount of bone resected was not enough. But then the available grafts and implants were *finite* and bone removal had to correspond to the volumes that were *expandable*. Allografts, parental bone, auto grafts, bank bone (frozen), bone substitutes, one fibula, two fibulae, etc. have all been tried. But it was left to the genius of Ilizarov to understand the potential of the human body. The *regenerate* as he called it was a much more superior substance than grafts. Natural patient-produced bone was available. One just had to have the knowledge, patience and courage to harness it. The rest is history!

For the treatment of this condition, the course of management depends on the following factors:

1. The type of pseudoarthrosis
2. The number of operations that the patient has undergone previously
3. The amount of scarring present
4. The presence or absence of neurofibromatosis

5. The amount of bone that has to be resected to allow for a comfortable apposition of the bone ends

6. The age of the patient at the first presentation

As described earlier, the act of getting the ends of the bone together is called docking. The process of docking the freshened bone ends together and compressing them will allow for union of pseudoarthrosis. However, one has to make absolutely sure that all the diseased bone ends are removed prior to docking to allow for a solid union. The procedure could be either be an acute docking accompanied with compensatory lengthening, or generous resection, maintenance of limb length, corticotomy and bone transport.

It is essential to note that bone transports over long segments are prone to develop deformities. These have to be anticipated and their correction planned well in advance.

Acute docking will allow an exact fit of the fragments under direct vision, while bone transport will guarantee a precise limb alignment and length. The former has a disadvantage of the possibility of bunching and soft tissue compromise; the latter has one of deviation of the fragments during transport, needing additional olive wires or hinges!

As a rule of thumb, acute docking should not be done unless the gap after resection is anticipated to be less than 50 mm. Two inches (50 mm to be precise) is the upper limit with which one can get away. For resections beyond this, one has to take up the demerits of slow delayed secondary docking and allow for the deformities to occur during the course of management and plan for the correction of these as they appear during the course of treatment.

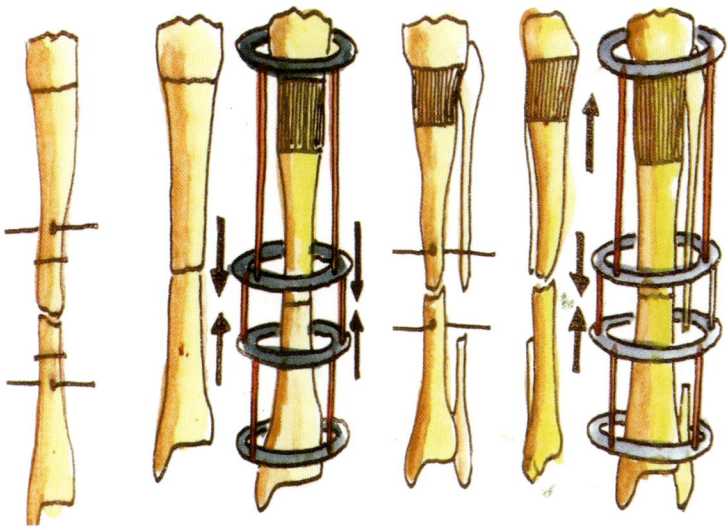

Picture 203: These two approaches are called acute and delayed docking. Both have their advantages though!

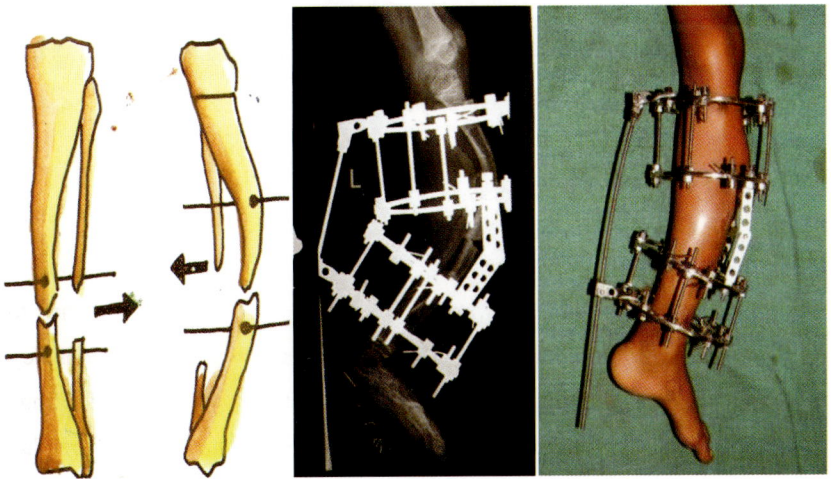

Picture 204: An example of acute docking

227

Younger the patient, better the healing and faster the process. I have operated in children as young as three months (using bangles instead of rings) with excellent results.

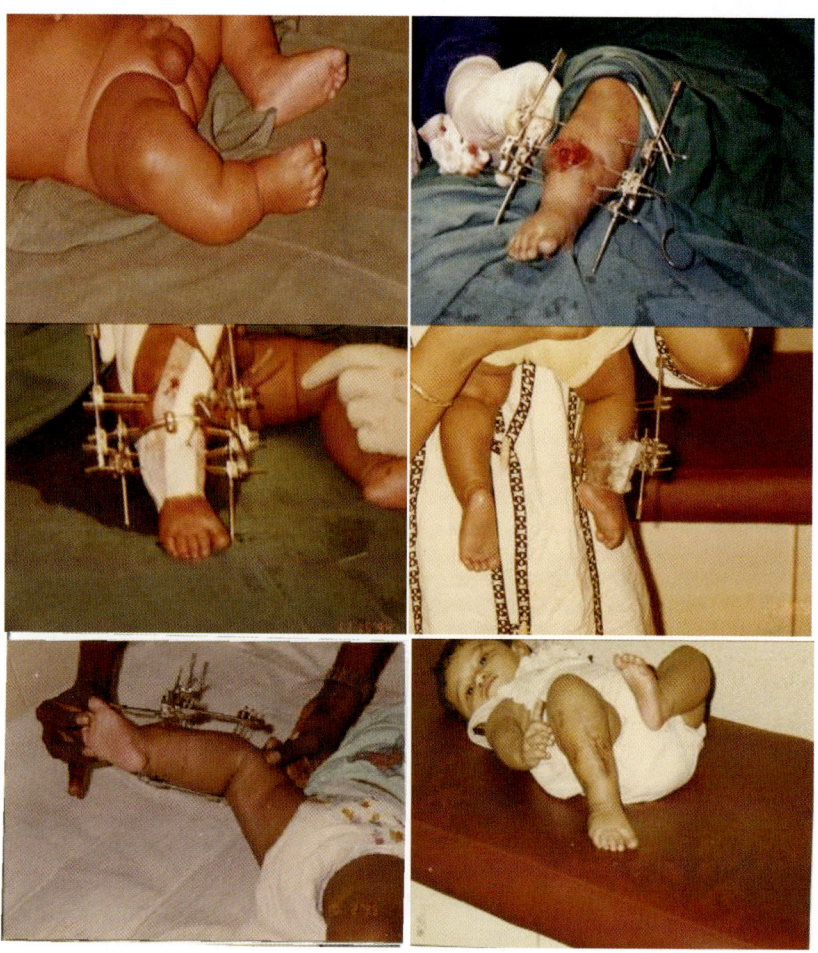

Picture 205: A very young child (70 days) operated for CPT with excellent results

Classification of deformities and their correction with Ilizarov Fixator

The Ilizarov fixation system is a very precise scientific tool for correction of deformities around most joints. Before the advent of this method, deformities were normally corrected by various methods: periodic manipulations, stretching, plaster applications or soft tissue releases. In a skeletally mature individual, osteotomies and arthrodesis were employed. However with the advent of Ilizarov, a wonderful new world has opened and numerous patients with really stubborn or complex deformities have benefitted.

The Ilizarov fixations have the following advantages:

1. Accurate forces can be applied to specific parts of bone or joint.

2. Combination of compression and distraction forces correct most deformities.

3. Direct distraction stimulates expansion of muscles tendons and fibrous tissues.

4. Wire placement dissipates forces across multiple joints simultaneously.

5. A gradual three dimensional correction is possible.

6. Associated lengthening can be done.

7. Open wedge osteotomies can be done with gradual distraction to allow deformity correction without shortening.

But with these advantages, one must also consider the disadvantages of the high technical skill needed in the use of this device. In addition, the patient has to be really motivated and the surgeon dedicated. This is not a *simple fix and forget* approach like a plate to a total joint. Here a constant monitoring and readjustment is needed.

When a surgeon starts with deformity correction, in his initial studies, he invariably reads about the osteotomy rules, encounters many terms describing the different angles propounded by numerous workers: lines, axes, indices, and other formulae and can easily get confused. I find that the literature is definitely written in a user unfriendly language, and appears really complex. If the purported rules and corollaries are not understood in their true context or if multiple philosophies are mixed up, as beginners usually do, deformity correction becomes an ogre which scares the surgeon.

A study of the literature shows that there are two divergent and opposite schools of thought in the field of deformity correction. Surgeons with a vernier in hand, calipers, set squares, multiple X-rays, CORA, angles, index, rules and corollaries at one end, and surgeons with a keen observation, three dimensional visualization, and the patience for regular frequent supervision of deformity correction at the other end. Though I personally belong to the second group, I have just listed and summarized the literature in a simpler and more understandable language for clarity and readers' convenience.

Radiographs show deformities in two planes, while CT scans show them in all three planes. Clinical examination and measurements show the exact 3D extent of the physical deformity. I personally don't think a CT is needed in most cases. Looking at the X-ray, we must imagine the bones inside, and looking at the limb, it is not too difficult to imagine the position of the skeleton beneath.

It is also frequently noticed that what can sometimes be very easy to understand on a piece of paper with a geometry tool box, isn't always easy to apply on a real patient on the OT table. On one hand, we have the mathematical osteotomy rules described by Dror Paley, while on the other end is the original Ilizarov philosophy, to identify the deformity in three planes and correct them in the right order. The middle path is followed by JESS workers who adopt differential compression distractions and the iconic Ponsetti method of manipulation and serial casting. Joshi's fixator is decidedly more scientific and yields better results than Ponsetti for the obvious reason that four small corrections a day are far superior to weekly corrections.

What is CORA?

The theory propounded by Dr. Dror Paley and religiously followed by ASAMI is given below. I have copied their exact language, which the reader will find distinctly different from my laidback style of narration.

Limb Alignment

Assessment of the frontal plane mechanical axis of the entire limb is done rather than single bones. Mechanical axis is the line that passes through the joint centres of the proximal and distal joints. The hip joint centre is located at the centre of the femoral head. The knee joint centre is half the distance from the nadir between the tibial spines to the apex of the intercondylar notch on the femur. The ankle joint centre is the centre of the tibial plafond. Mechanical axis deviation (MAD) is measured as the distance from the knee joint centre to the line connecting the joint centres of the hip and ankle.

Normally, the MAD is 1 mm to 15 mm medial to the knee joint centre. If MAD is greater than 15 mm medial to the knee midpoint it is called *varus* malalignment, and if it is medial to the knee midpoint it is referred to as *valgus* malalignment

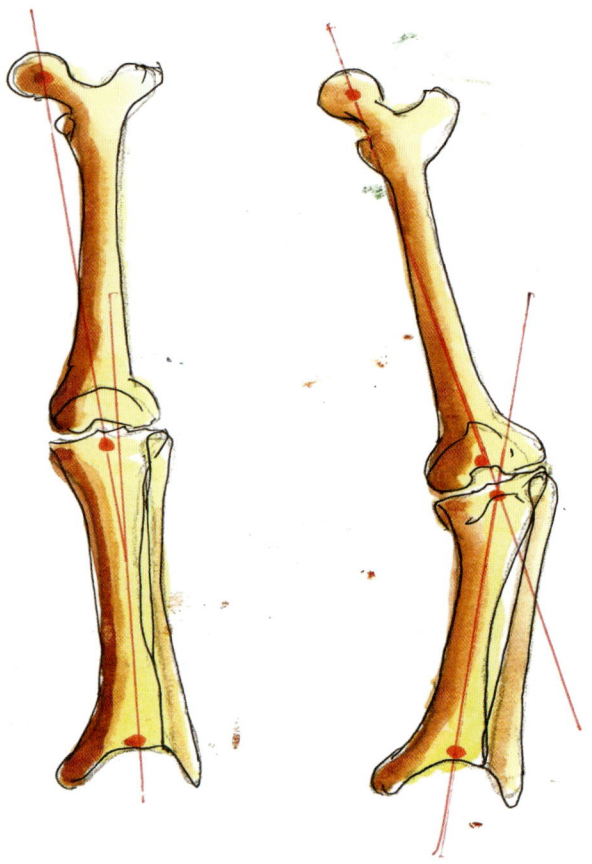

Picture 206: The MAD or mechanical axis deviation

Anatomic Axes

The line that passes through the centre of the diaphysis along the length of the bone is called the anatomic axis. In a normal bone, the anatomic axis is a single straight line, while with deformities or in a malunited bone with angulation, each bony segment can be defined by its own anatomic axis.Figure 153. Anatomic axis

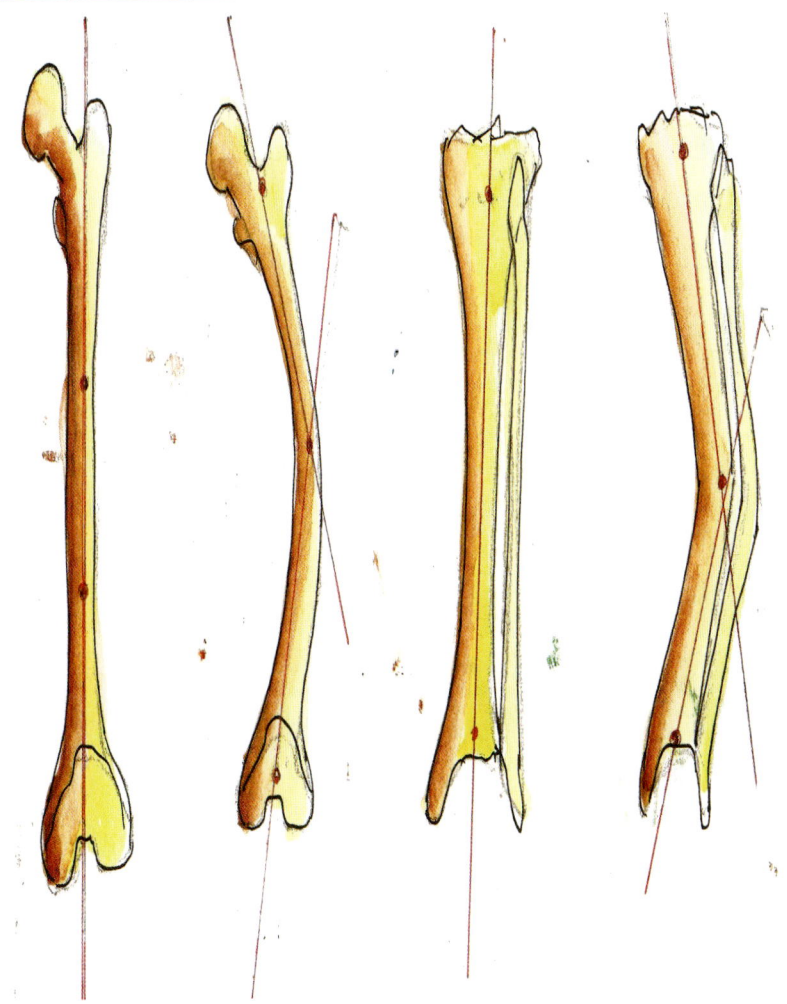

Picture 207: Anatomic axis. In normal bones it is a straight line. In deformities, two or more lines will bisect each other.

Joint Orientation Lines

Joint orientation describes the relation of a joint to the respective anatomic and mechanical axes of a long bone.

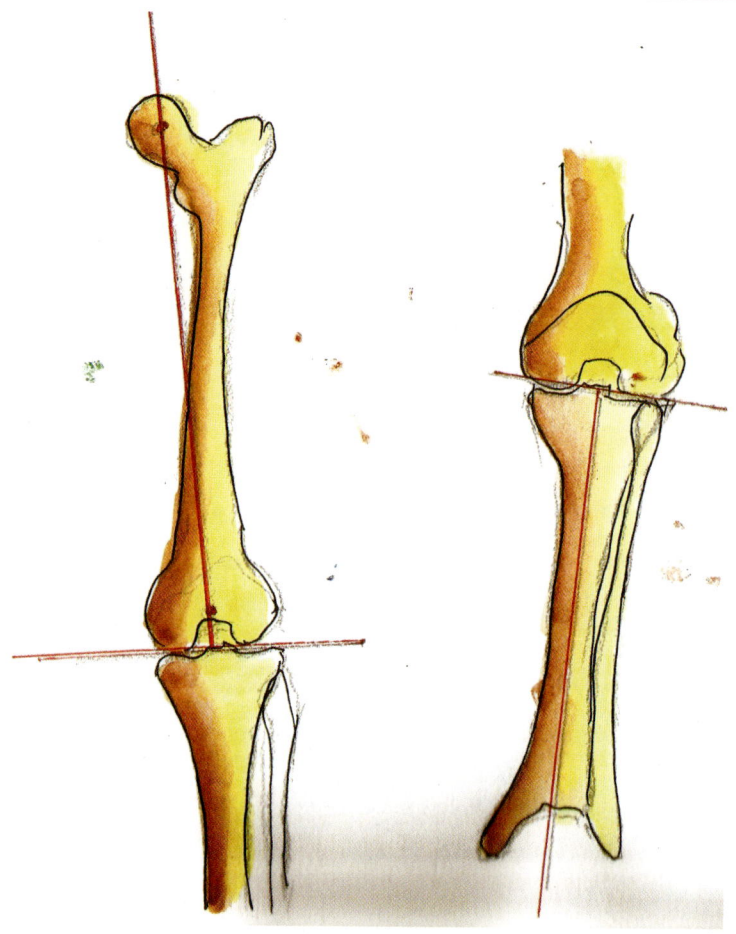

Picture 208: Joint orientation lines

Centre of Rotation of Angulation

The intersection of the proximal axis and distal axis of a deformed bone is called the CORA. It is the point about which a deformity may be rotated to achieve correction. The angle formed by the two axes at the CORA is a measure of angular deformity in that plane.

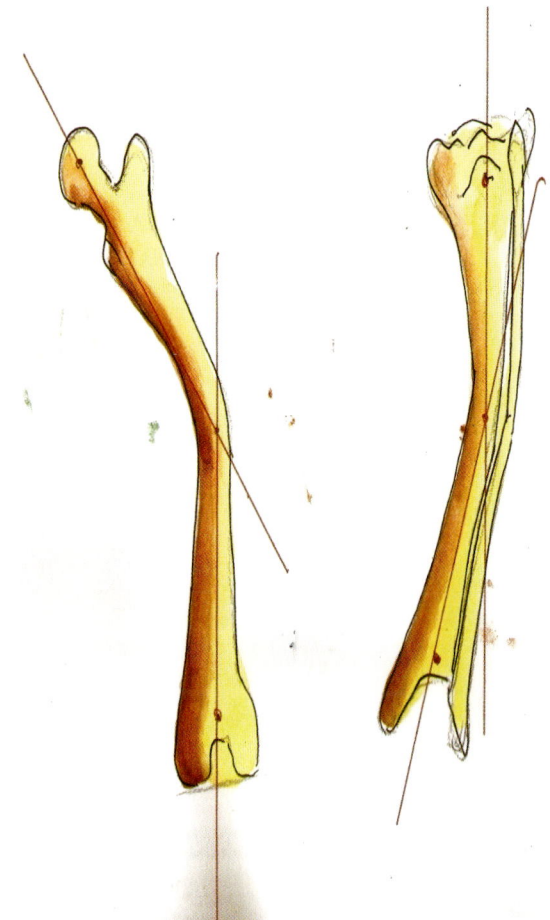

Picture 209: Cora or centre of angle of rotation.

According to Paley theories, which not all Ilizarov surgeons agree with, if CORA lies at the point of obvious deformity in the bone and the joint orientations are normal, the deformity is uniapical (in the respective plane).

If CORA lies outside the point of obvious deformity, or either joint orientation is abnormal, either a second CORA exists in that plane and the deformity is multi-apical, or a translational deformity exists in that plane.

When the CORA lies outside the boundaries of the involved bone, a multi-apical deformity is likely to be present.

Bisector

The bisector is a line that passes through the CORA and bisects the angle formed by the proximal and distal axes. Angular correction along the bisector results in complete deformity correction without the introduction of a translational deformity.

In addition, there are rules of osteotomy which I feel add to confusions, rather than give the surgeon clear proven guidelines. I'm refraining from confusing the reader further with rules of osteotomies and their corollaries, because I am not too convinced of their practical usefulness. You can get the rules, etc. from the literature if you need more theory. Here I will stick to an extremely practical work book manner with clarity and reproducibility.

In my view, indications of deformity correction by Ilizarov can be summarized in two words, *large* degree of deformity and those associated with *shortening*.

A. Deformities that are mild, probably below 15 degrees, and which can be predictably corrected in one stage, may be easily done with the various osteotomies described in the texts. This is a lot easier for both surgeon and patient.

B. With greater degrees of deformities, where soft tissue elements have to be taken care of, or where gradual correction is essential to achieve proper balance (e.g. a high tibial osteotomy), then Ilizarov will give predictable reproducible results.

C. Where there are associated limb length discrepancies, this method provides versatility and is the best solution.

The first step is to assess the deformity thoroughly, both clinically and radiologically, for a proper preoperative planning. A classification is needed that suggests the mode of the treatment according to the type of the deformity. (A classification of deformities, rather!)

An angular deformity may be present in one plane or more. It's not absolutely essential to determine how this plane is angled to the frontal or the sagittal planes (as some methods suggest) because even in the simplest of cases, there is no application of the deformity correcting techniques in either the frontal or the sagittal planes; all the correction has to be done in the original plane of the deformity only.

The Paley or ASAMI type of complicated mapping for deformity correction may have its applications in computer assisted automatic devices where such input has to be made, but in the case of surgeons using the basic Ilizarov frame, it is a confusing and unnecessary exercise. Because in a situation with multiple deformities, correction in one plane most certainly messes up with the original plane of the other deformity and one has to reassess that plane for the subsequent stage of correction. This also applies to shifts and rotations that are invariably associated with angular deformities. These can get revealed for the first time after one component gets gradually corrected, or they can get better or worse.

It is doubtful if all the individual components can be predicted, mapped and hinged with one universal hinge in the first instance on the operating table to get complete correction in one go. So one has to wait, observe and make suitable adjustments to the frame at suitable times. Experience and skilled approximations contribute to the art component of orthopaedic surgery! This is where the osteotomy rules don't throw enough light. Osteotomy rule 1 gives adequate guidance for uniplanar angular deformities and how they can be compressed or distracted at the same time, but things get tricky when the CORA or the needed osteotomy gets into the level of the joints, in cases where the deformity is metaphyseal. Osteotomy rule 2 and its corollary address part of this problem by predicting shifts that creep in and advising appropriate adjustments to get these shifts to the desired direction and extent, but still doesn't allow us to deal with the original hinge or any new deformity that might have crept in during the process. Invariably some frame readjustments will be required depending on the nature of this new deformity, mostly changing the plane and the level of the hinges.

Osteotomy rule 3 (and corollary) simplifies complex deformities by allowing us to find a resolution CORA for the correction. However, dividing a big deformity into multiple CORA might not be practical, if one takes into account the constraint of space for putting in the smaller, angulated individual parts of bone into a fixator. Besides, it still deals with deformities in one plane.

Therefore one can have a relook at our classification and deformity correction principles to see if some unnecessary elements can be ignored partly just to avoid confusing a beginner, while the practical principles retained and simplified.

Dr. Jishnu Baruah of Assam has proposed the following classification of deformities, which I have found extremely practical, useful and logical. He has classified deformities into five types, based on a 3D visualization of both the deformity and the radiographs. It is easy to learn and fully reproducible.

TYPE ONE: Uniplanar Angular diaphyseal deformity

TYPE TWO: Uniplanar Angular metaphyseal deformity

TYPE THREE: Multiplanar Angular deformity

TYPE FOUR: Angular deformities with rotation.

TYPE FIVE: Complex Multi joint deformity including joint contractures

If any rules of deformity corrections have to be proposed, in my view they are these!

1. Rotation has to be corrected on the table, no matter what! It helps patients to mobilize and rehabilitate faster, and avoids other plane translations if

attempted at a later stage. In addition, I believe that delayed correction of rotation causes a kinking or hour glassing of the regenerate, delaying the treatment process.

2. There has to be a proper corticotomy, which has to be precisely performed. Periosteal slitting, special chisels, cutting the cortex alone circumferentially, and break the last third. The X-rays may look ghastly, but regenerate is lovely. I have seen radiographs with clean oscillating saw-like corticotomies, and I shudder! Pity the poor patient.

3. Deformity correction is essentially more of a soft tissue procedure, stretching the skin, sub cutaneous tissue, fat, muscles, ligaments, nerves, vessels, etc. on the concave side. Any rule that disregards this essential step is wrong. As Sir John Charnley has stated in his historical book *Closed Treatment Of Common Fractures,* the orthopaedic surgeon's job is more of a gardener than a carpenter.

4. Angular metaphyseal deformities need an open wedge. Angular diaphyseal deformities need an additional metaphyseal corticotomy. The *hinges are never placed in the precise coronal or sagittal planes; they have to exactly mirror the plane of deformity.*

5. The final rule is that there is no rule!! Each deformity is evaluated individually and corrected. Frequent regular follow-up, and a combination of surgeon's patience and patient compliance is the key to success. You don't correct deformities by the *fit and forget* technology of internal fixations or joint replacements. You work hard patiently to get results.

Approach in individual types:

1. Uniplanar angular diaphyseal deformity

This the basic, common deformity and the outline to manage these uses the Joint Referencing Method. The joint referencing proximal and the distal rings are the foundation on which the frame can be progressively constructed towards the apex of the deformity, leaving adequate space for distracting components on the concave side. With experience, these frames can also be preconstructed. Care must be taken to maintain the axis of the bone segments and the axis of the frame in the same line when fixing the middle rings. Slight errors in this step are forgivable, because the frames can always be under corrected or over corrected depending on the follow-up X-rays after achieving clinical correction. It only leaves a skewed frame with hinges during the consolidation phase and not the perfectly parallel fixator where the hinges can be exchanged with straight connecting rods for better frame stability and dynamics.

If a simple open wedge correction is desired, the hinge is placed close to the convex cortex; if some lengthening is desired, it is placed further out towards the convexity. The length which will be achieved can be calculated by the difference in the length of the arms of the hinges compared to another identical hinge temporarily placed in the neutral axis of the bone at the centre.

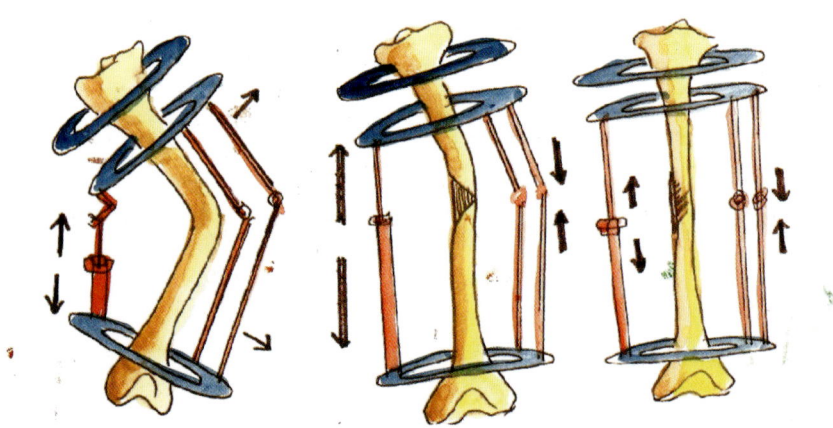

Picture 210: Frame for type 1 deformity correction

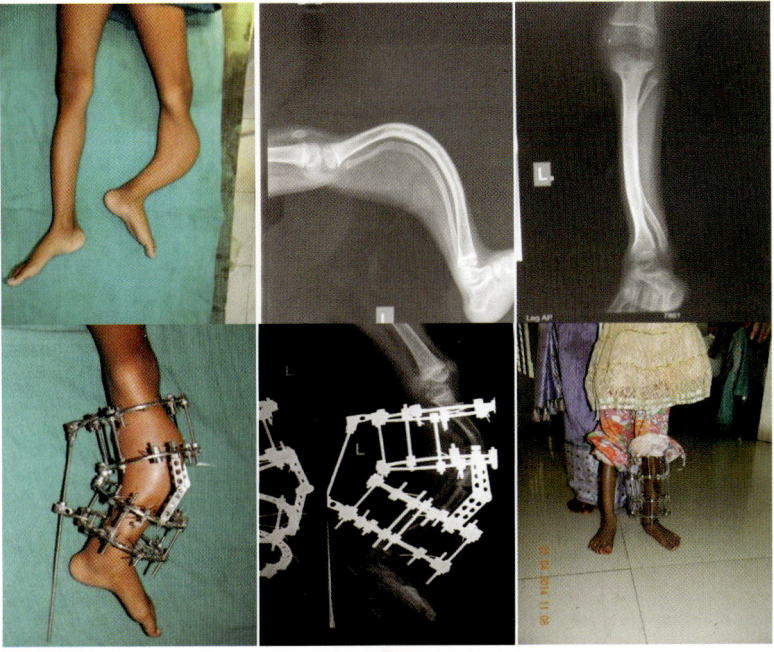

Picture 211: Correction in a type one deformity

The rate of distraction needed at the distractor at the convex side can be assessed by the rule of similar triangles. This distractor is turned in the amount given by the ratio (distance of the hinge from the distractor) divided by (distance of the hinge from the neutral axis). That amount of distraction at the distractor calculates to one unit at the neutral axis. However, it must be understood that there is a cone of soft tissue that is distracting at different rates, more towards the distractor and less towards the hinge, and this has to be factored in to decide upon an optimum rate.

2. Uniplanar Angular metaphyseal deformity

This is a common deformity in adult osteoarthritis of the knee. Other examples would be malunions, congenital or metabolic deformities. As the deformity is in the metaphyseal bone, it is an easy matter to do an open wedge, and distract the concave side till the desired correction is achieved.

Occasionally, the apex of the deformity lies close to a joint or even partly within a joint. Wire fixation and/ or osteotomy in such a constrained space becomes taxing and complex. A correction in any level other than the apex of the deformity will lead to a shift in the mechanical axis. So if one is forced to do an osteotomy at a level other than desired, one has to plan the hinges between the middle two rings in such a way that they correct rather than aggravate the shift in the mechanical axis after correction of angular deformity. This can be done by changing the level of the hinges to place them either more proximal or more distal to the normal bisector line.

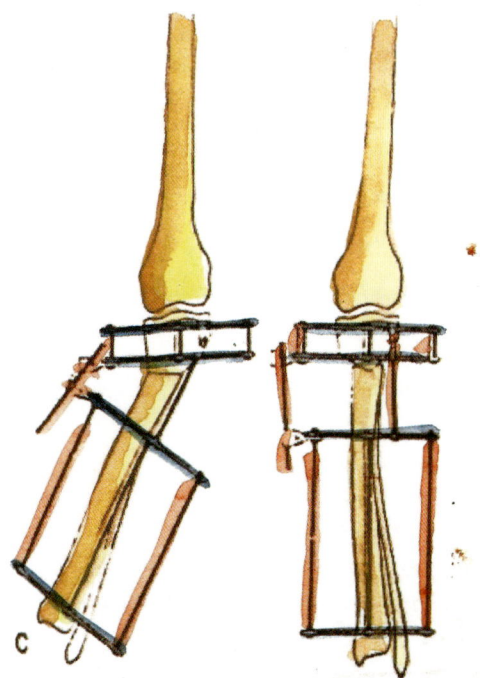

Picture 212: Schematics for a type two deformity

A varus knee with medial compartment arthritis, bow legs and a practically normal lateral half of the joint is an ideal indication for a high tibial osteotomy by an open wedge distraction as shown in the following case. Other examples would be Coxa Vara, or Genu Valgum, in which the deformity will be in either the proximal or distal femoral metaphyseal area.

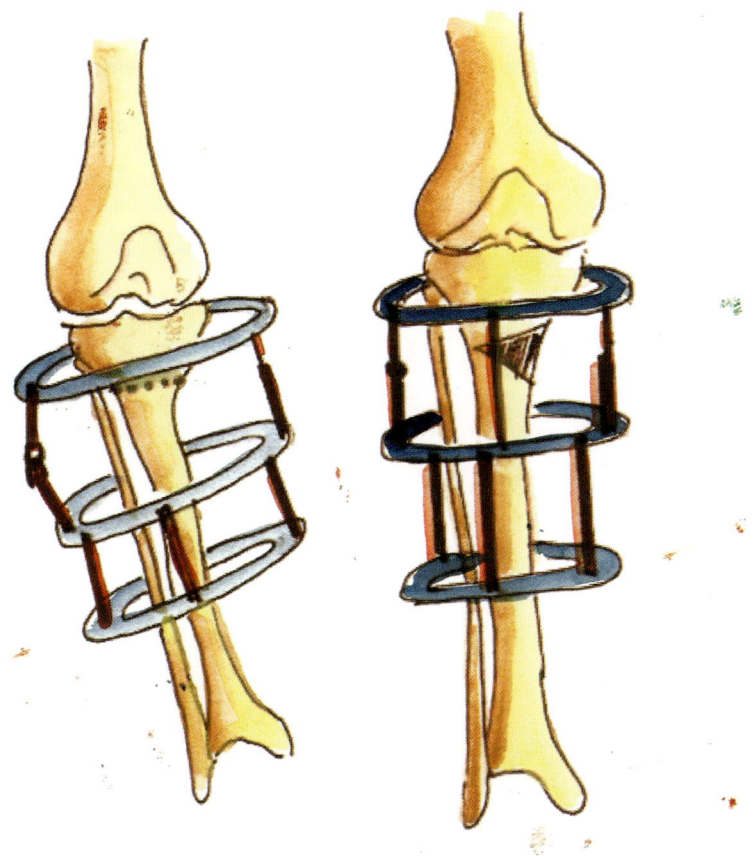

Picture 213: simple three ring frame is enough for most metaphyseal deformities in a single plane. The most important trick is the appropriate placement of the hinge and the positioning of the distracters or extension rods exactly at 180 degrees to that plane to ensure that the wedge is opened in the correct axis without deviation.

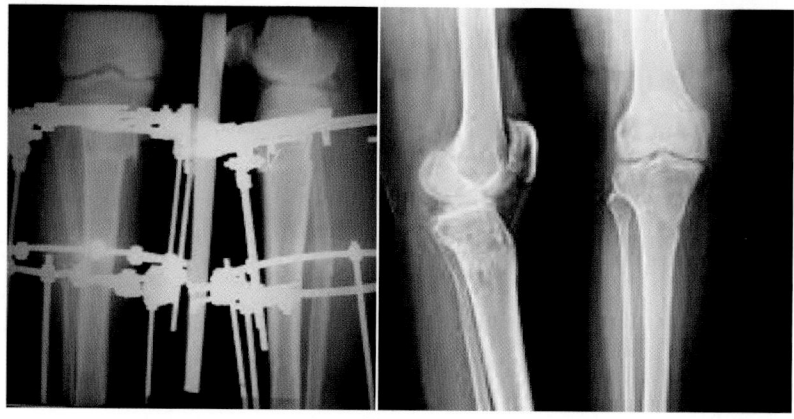

Picture 214: A precise hinge placement is the essential trick

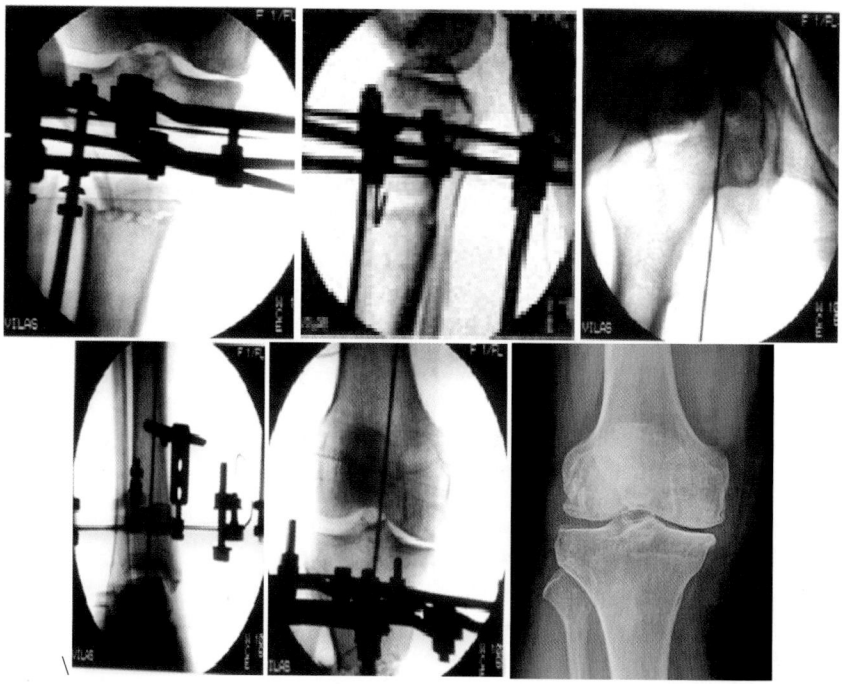

Picture 215: A properly executed correction will produce a medial joint space and align the limb

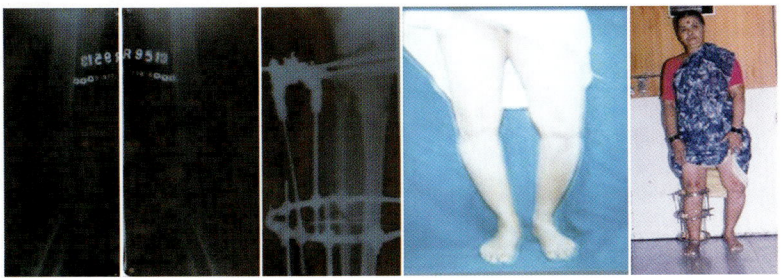

Picture 216: This patient underwent an osteotomy only on her right side

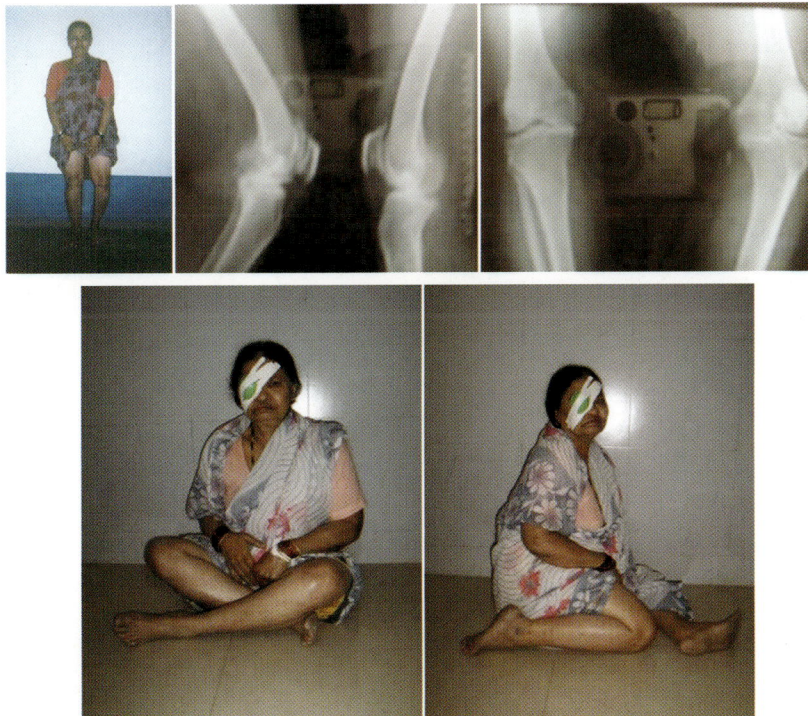

Picture 217: Follow-up after 19 years shows a pain-free knee with excellent range of motion.

Case courtesy Dr. Adke

3. Multiplanar Angular deformity

These can be either diaphyseal, metaphyseal or involving the entire length of the bone. In a lower limb around the knee we can expect the deformity to be either varus/ valgus or procurvatum/ recurvation. If the limb has a combination of both, it becomes a type three deformity.

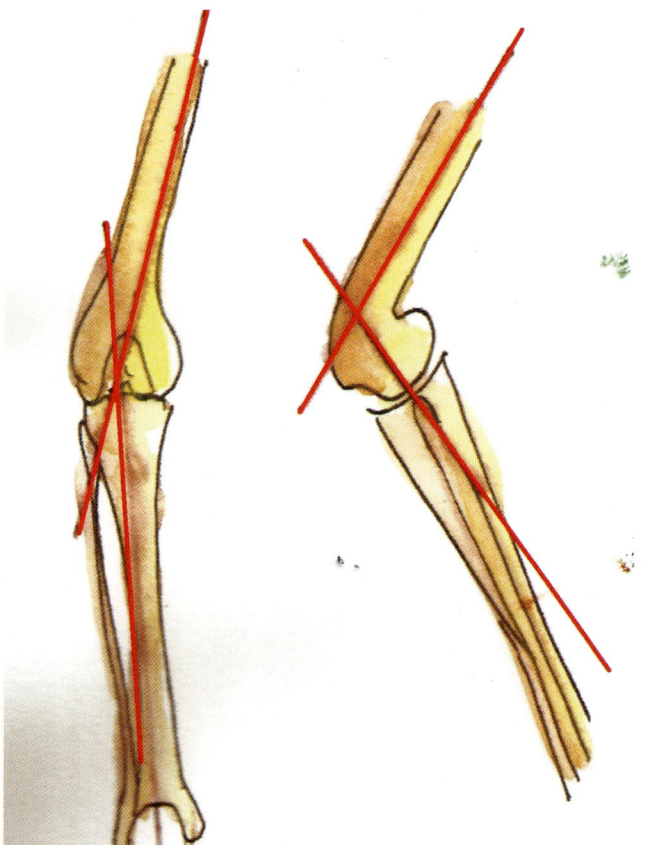

Picture 218: It is essential to remember that a type three deformity exists in two planes and hence a correction is planned keeping both these in mind.

Lesser of the two can be corrected acutely at the osteotomy site to convert it into a uniplanar deformity that can sometimes lie in between the two planes. But the plane of maximum deformity after such a correction should be chosen to apply the axis of the hinge; the remaining steps can follow. If both deformities are so excessive that the proximal and distal rings cannot be brought perpendicular to the plane of deformity on the OT table, a gradual correction of both deformities can be done later by completely reapplying the hinges as indicated in that situation. A second osteotomy can also be done for the second plane in its own apex of deformity, provided there is space for it.

Here it is essential to use hinges or olive wires in both planes to achieve a correction at the osteotomy site. If this leads to shortening, a metaphyseal corticotomy should be done. In case the deformity is in the metaphyseal area, the same corticotomy site can be used both as the correction axis and distraction point for regenerate.

It is important to point out that though we imagine and discuss radiographs in the AP and lateral views, and thus imagine only the sagittal and coronal planes, but actual deformities are seldom present in these exact planes. The hinges and wires should thus be placed on the appropriate points to exert a three dimensional force to correct deformities in both planes.

In the subsequent drawings, I have shown the rings in different colors in relation to each axis of the deformity, and it is easy to see that both planes are in oblique views in reference to our standard AP and lateral radiographs. In my opinion teaching the use of an X-ray, and geometry box with set squares and protractors, over the Radiographic Lobby, seldom conveys what is actually done in the operating room.

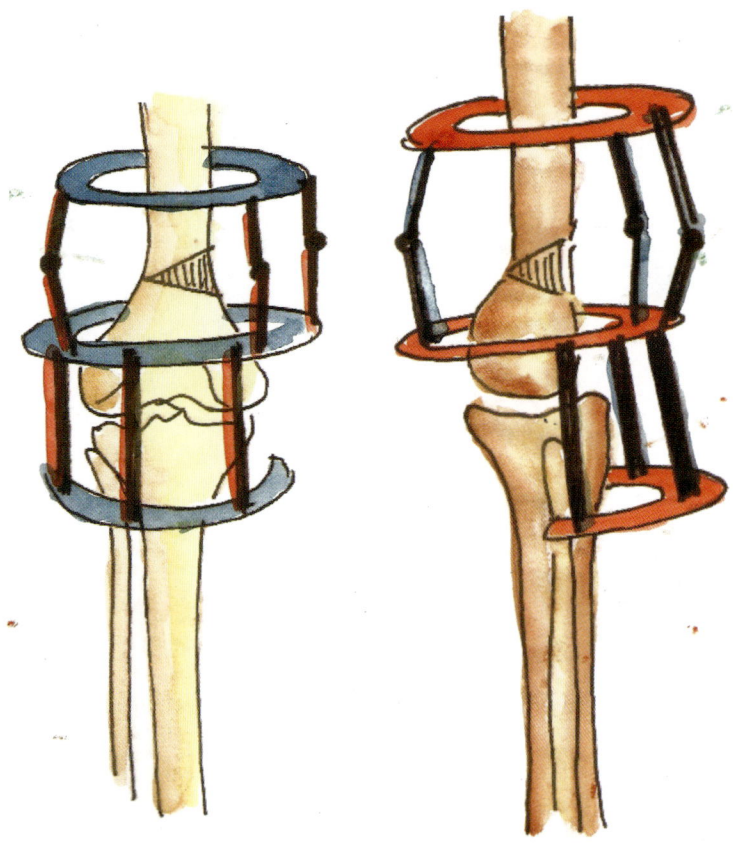

Picture 219: A type three deformity and the construct needed for its correction. Note that neither deformity is in the strict AP or Lat plane.

The following clinical examples will explain this point further.

This patient shown below, has a combination of varus and procurvatum, both arising in femoral metaphyseal area. The stages of correction show how the line of forces, precisely applied, produce expected results.

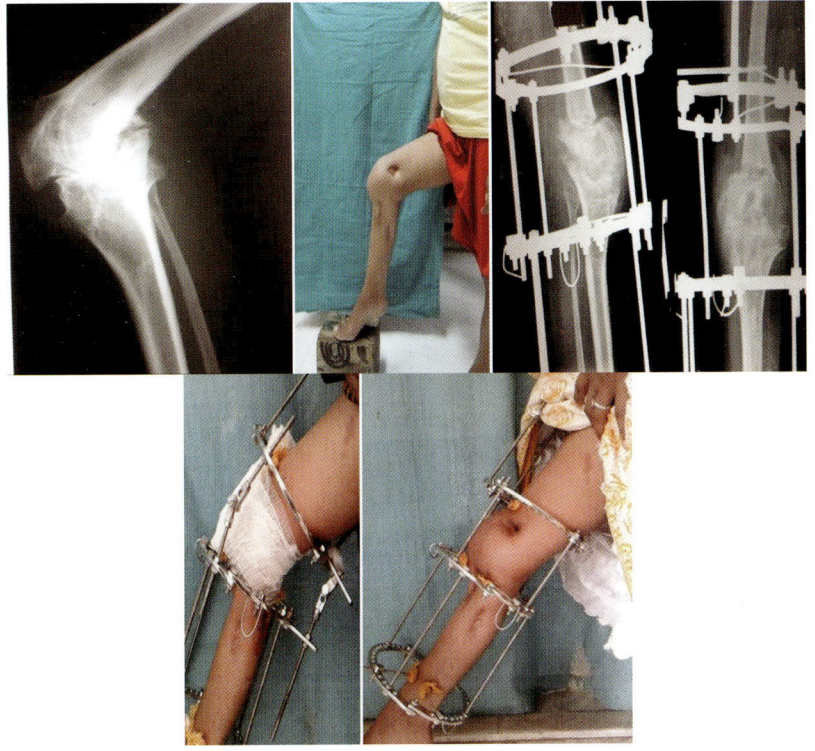

Picture 220: Type three deformity and its correction

4. Angular deformities with rotation

A rotational malpositioning of a limb causes serious functional deficit during locomotion. The most important point here is to completely correct the rotation during the primary surgery. Many surgeons state that because the frame is Ilizarov, rotation can be corrected at any stage. This is not correct. Once elongating the corticotomy has begun, the regenerate forms as a sleeve of highly enriched vasculature. The intactness of this tube is essential for healthy regenerate and sound callus formation. Rotation of the two segments in opposite directions during the course of treatment causes an *hourglass* effect or even kinking of the regenerate tube. This will suddenly cause cessation of regenerate formation. The other reason why correction of rotational deformity in a single shot is advisable is because it facilitates walking post operatively.

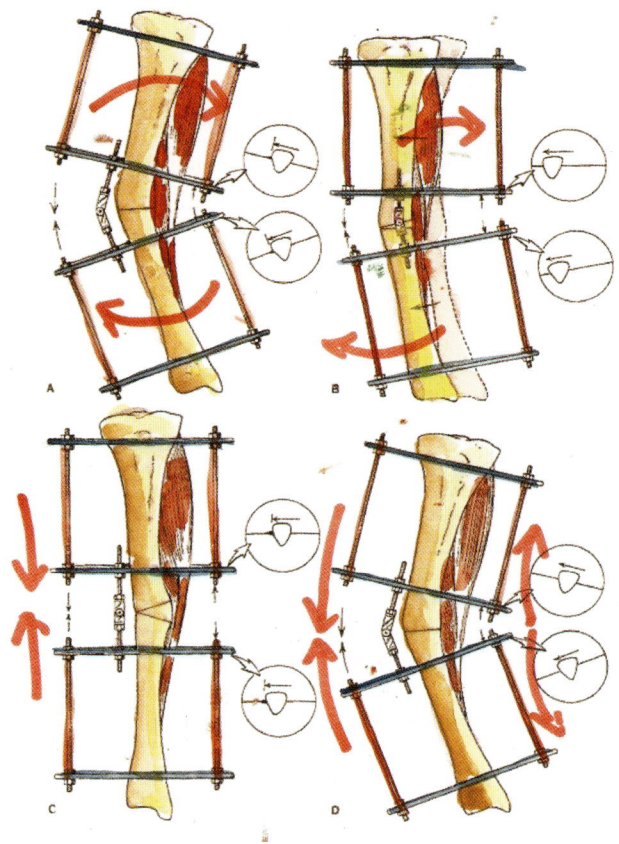

Picture 221: It is essential to imagine the type four deformities with their rotational elements and appropriate corrections planned.

The following observations by Dr. Jishnu Baruah shed more light on this important aspect:

Literature suggests that rotation is the last element to be corrected when it is present along with other deformities. The suggested sequence has been,

Angulation-Lengthening-Shifts followed by Rotation. It has been explained that, this is easily done only between parallel rings. However at the same time it is mentioned that a significant de-rotation can induce shifts between the bone ends. It is obvious because we cannot guarantee concentric bone ends within the rings being de-rotated. And shifts thus appear. Also, leaving the rotations to be dealt with at the last means we are told to de-rotate a newly formed regenerate! This might not be a very physiological way to manipulate a regenerate, particularly when it is obvious that rotation can induce shifts; no one welcomes a shift within a regenerate. The fitment of cumbersome perimounting de-rotation components is also not an easy job, even if the limited space can be managed. Too many components also lead to heavy frames, mechanical issues and sometimes difficulty for the patients to follow the distraction protocol.

It gets significantly easier if the rotation element is the first to be corrected, particularly as we will be doing a osteotomy in every case and the ends can be acutely de-rotated at that site itself, converting the complex picture to a simpler Type 1 or Type 2 deformity. It can then be managed as such with a simpler angular correction frame. This acute correction is in fact a restoration of the otherwise deranged local anatomy and so should be better tolerated than a rotation of a freshly formed regenerate. If the soft tissues allow the remaining angular deformity to be corrected with a couple of weeks, theoretically at least the ends can be distracted to correct any small residual limb length discrepancies following the principles of callotasis-distraction at half the rate after a 2 weeks latency. However in the case of inability to get angular correction fast enough or any doubt about regenerate potential in the corrected gap, the situation can be managed by bifocal osteosynthesis with another corticotomy while the osteotomy site is compressed to union.

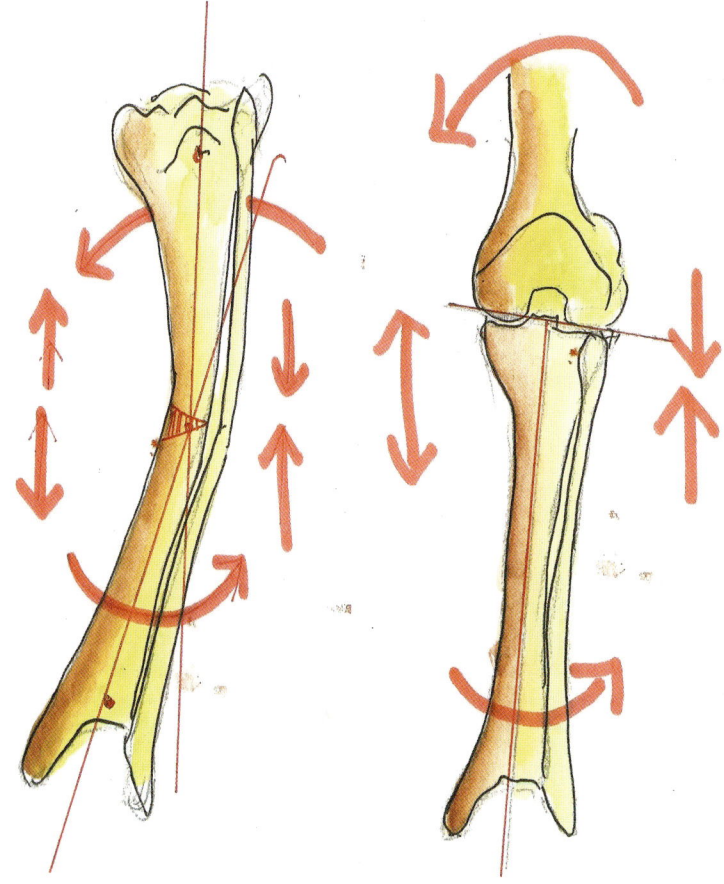

Picture 222: Correction of a type 4 deformity involves rotational correction as the first and most important step.

The following clinical example illustrates this more clearly.

This is a tibial procurvatum deformity due to amniotic band. The child was operated at one month of age; within four weeks, deformity correction and union of osteotomy were achieved.

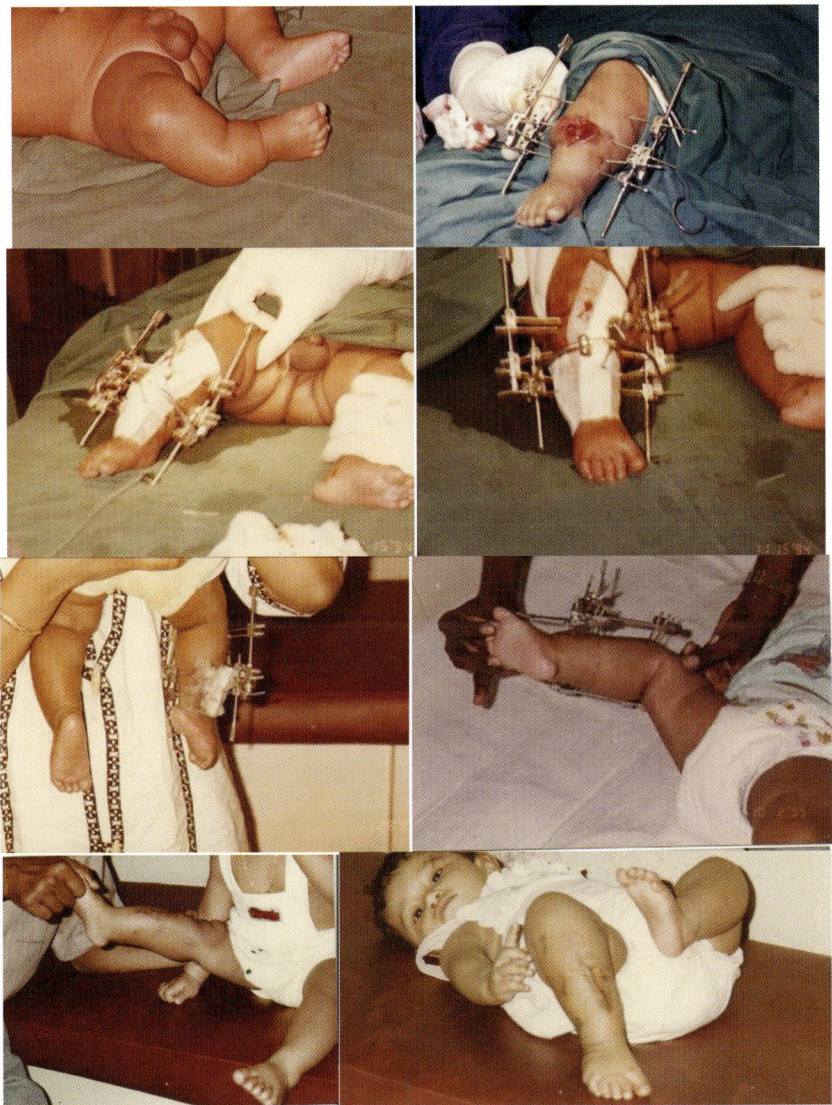

Picture 223: Procurvatum of tibia with internal rotation, treated in a very young child

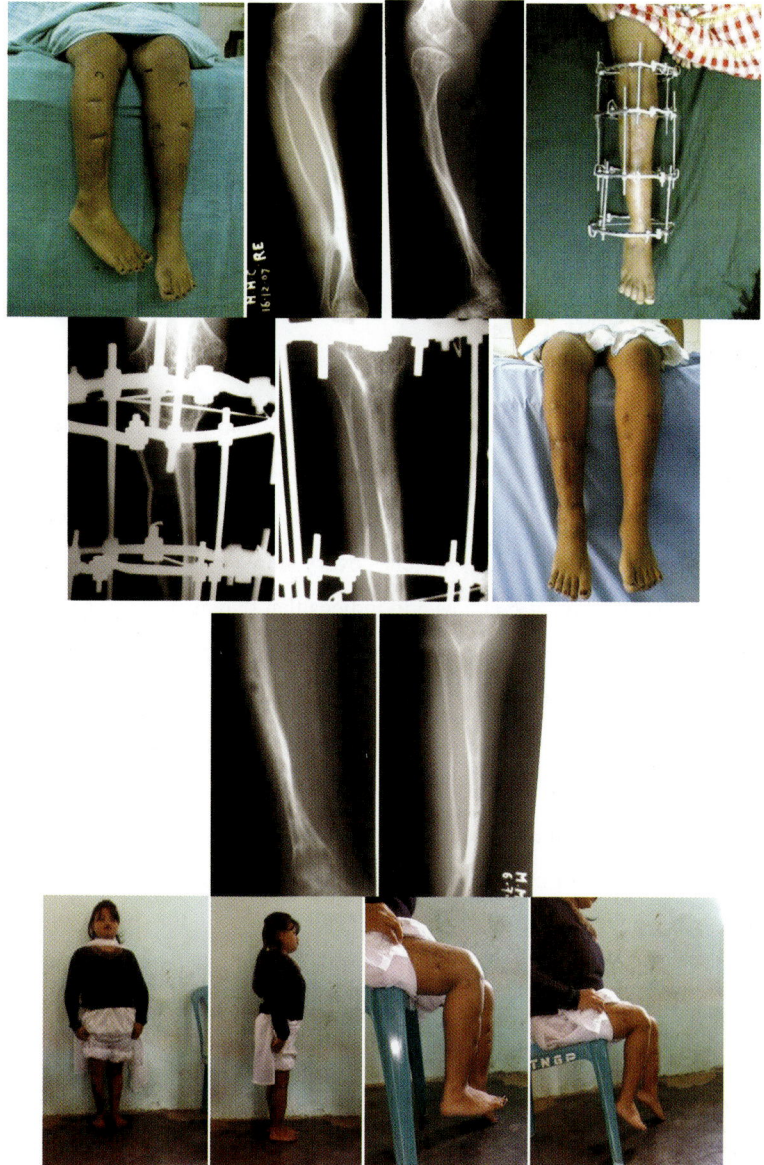

Picture 224: In type four deformities, it is essential to correct the rotation element first

5. Complex multi joint deformity including joint contractures

Type five deformities include those with a greater soft tissue component than bony deformities alone. It spans across many joints and is mostly due to congenital anomalies or neglected or complicated trauma. Foot with multiple joints usually presents with deformities like club foot, rocker bottom, hemimelias or other defects. I have excluded club foot from this chapter as it will be covered separately. In type five deformities, the following points have to be considered for management.

1. We must treat the limb as a whole and not X-rays alone. Deformities are seldom corrected on X-ray lobbies.
2. Ilizarov is magical in the sense that gradual distraction elongates not only the corticotomised bone, but also stretches every single soft tissue. The beginner gets so carried away with angles and indices that they usually forget about the gardening part. The tiny releases and the constant adjustments make the difference between success and failure,
3. For these deformities, no rules can be laid down. Each patient and limb has to be evaluated on the table and appropriate frame applied to correct all deformities in all planes, including regaining of lost limb length.
4. Unlike total joints or internal fixations, we simply cannot have a fit and forget approach. This is a continuous ongoing process of management, requiring a lot of patience from both surgeon and patient.
5. Many times, when bony or soft tissue problems appear in mid-treatment, we must follow a gentle reverse, pause and then forward approach. This means if a corticotomy site does not throw expected callus, or if transient neuropraxia develops, we have to slowly loosen back the frame, wait for a few days, and do a compression-distraction-compression manoeuvre, to get things back into shape, before resuming further distraction.

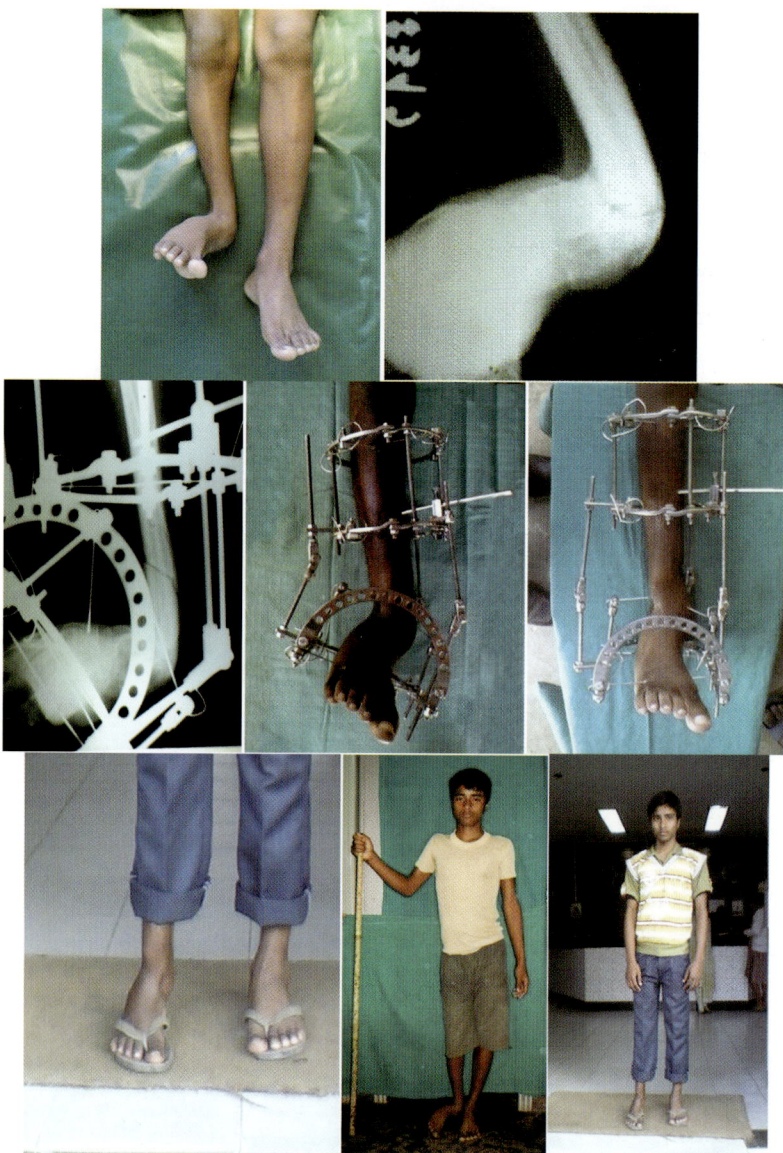

Picture 225: Correction of a type five deformity

6. The satisfaction felt by both surgeon and patient when the foot is plantigrade for the first time and the patient feels the ground, is impossible to describe in words.

7. More than rules and drawings, the accompanying pictures show how these problems are dealt with.

The following interesting case illustrates this further. This female teenager with Ollier's disease had an ulnar elbow and a radial wrist.

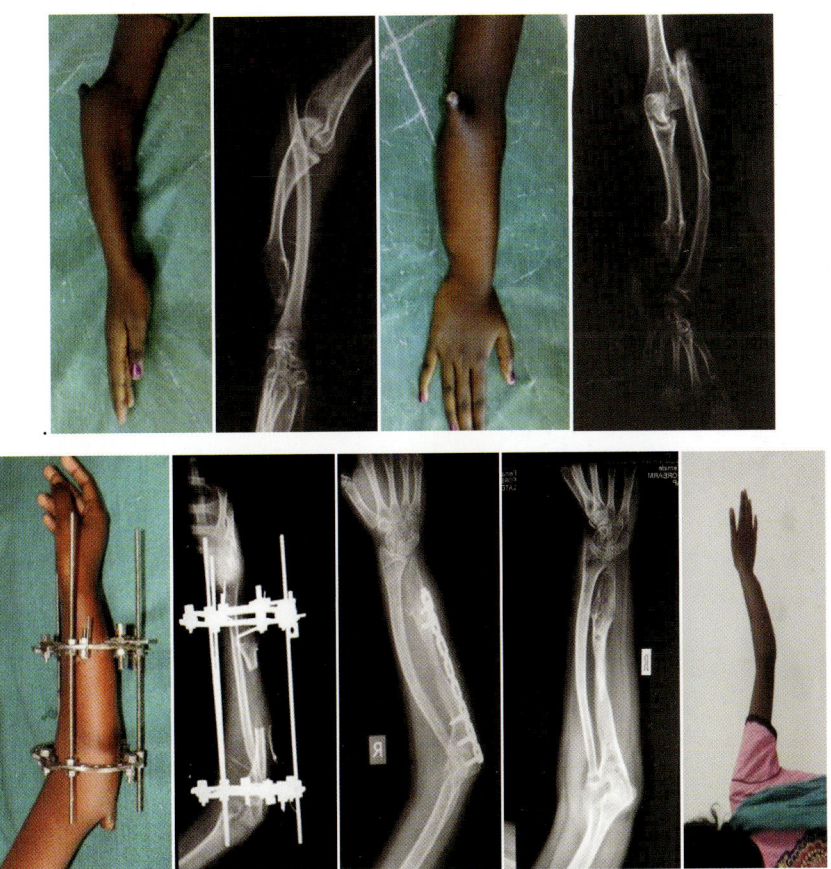

Picture 226: Correction of a complex type five deformity with shortening

257

The intelligent use of plate at the correct time hastened return to function.

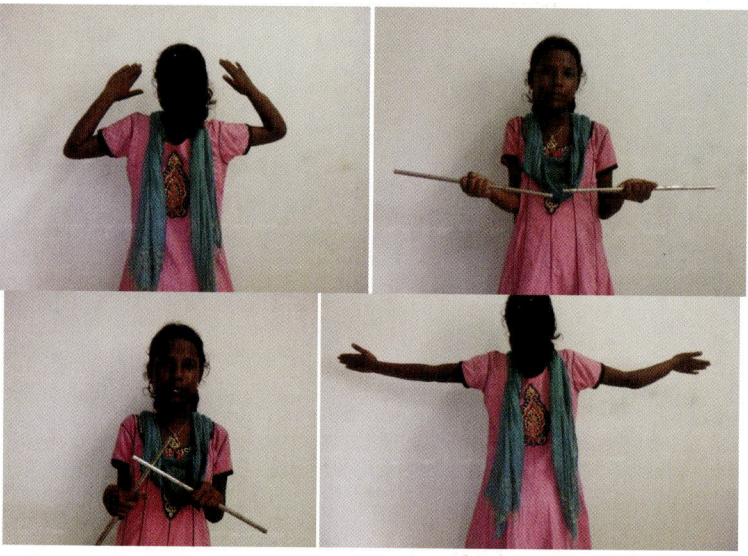

Picture 227: See the excellent range of function and excellent cosmetic results

The next case illustrated here is a neuropathic-equino-cavo-varus foot with a fungating ulcer. This thirteen year old girl had two problems: she had not walked on her foot for two years, and the fungating non-healing ulcer was obnoxious. She was advised amputation by many surgeons, but Ilizarov magic prevailed again and these pictures show the extent of corrections that could be achieved.

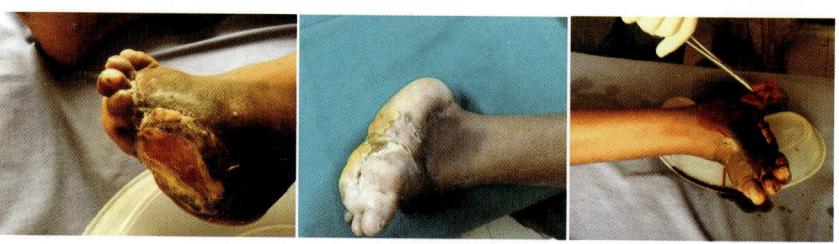

Picture 228: Neuropathic equino-cavo-varus deformity

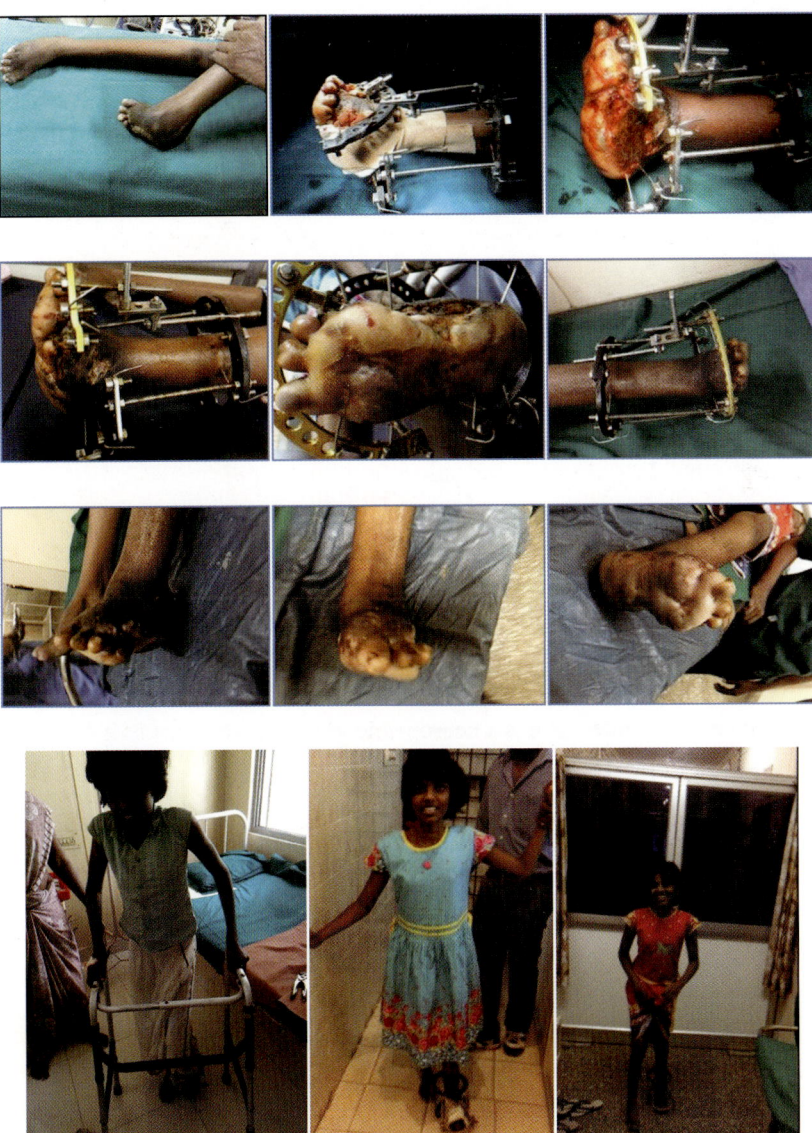

Picture 229: Ulcers healing during the course of correction and full weight bearing mobilization from day one

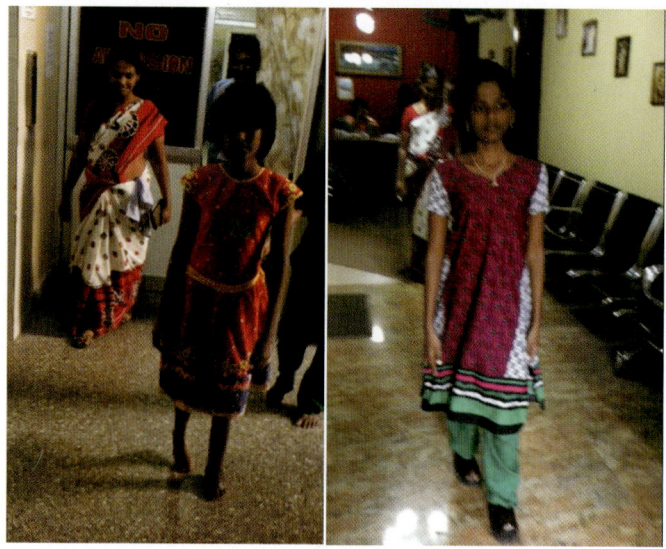

Picture 230: Excellent final results

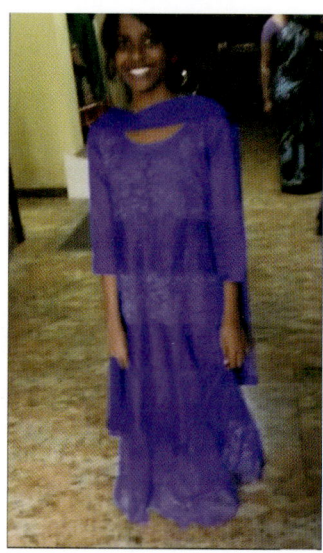

Picture 231: The Smile on her face tells it all!

Flexion Contracture of the knee

Flexion contracture of the knee may be either because of developmental disorders, poliomyelitis, or due to scarring and tethering of the tissues due to trauma, burns or infection and is treated by the following method.

1. The distance between the buttock and the heel is measured; this will be expanded at the rate of 1 mm a day.
2. A standard 4 ring assembly is used with 2 rings in the thigh and 2 in the leg.
3. Judicious placement of olive wires will allow increase of stability and possibility of correction of associated deformities.
4. The posterior aspect of the thigh and the calf are taken as the concave component, and anterior aspect of the thigh and the shin are taken as the convex component of the deformity.
5. Threaded rods with hinges or telescopic rods are anchored to the rings.
6. A gradual distraction of 1 mm per day is well tolerated by the soft tissues.
7. Transient neuropraxia may be encountered during rapid distraction; this can be avoided by slowing the speed of distraction or stopping the distraction temporarily.
8. If there is an associated varus or valgus deformity, placement of additional hinges and threaded rods will ensure correction of the same simultaneously.

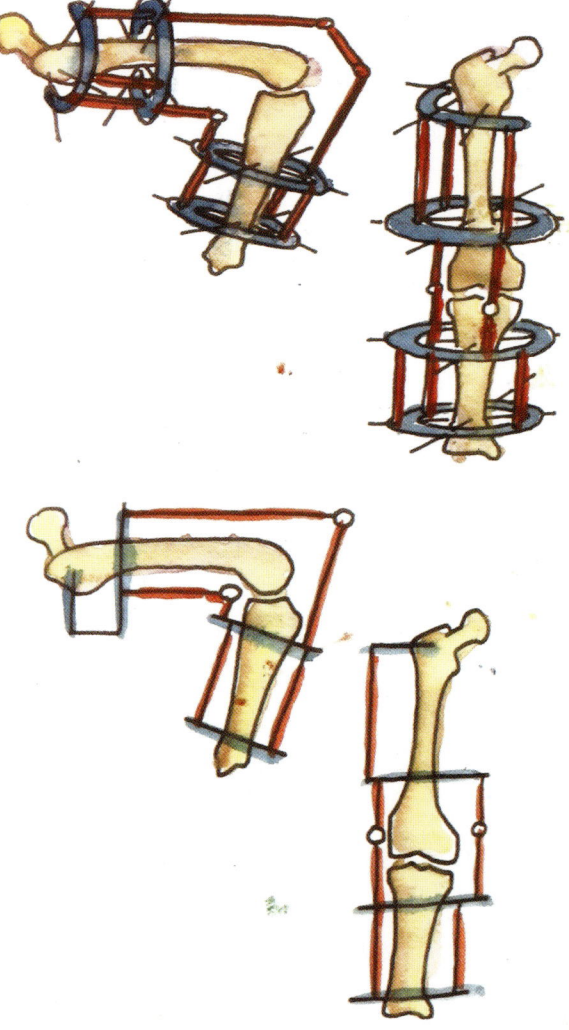

Picture 232: Correction of flexion deformity of the knee

Congenital Club Foot and other foot deformities

Club feet have been traditionally treated by either manipulative correction or by open soft tissue releases. Ponsetti method of serial castings at weekly intervals is still the gold standard for club feet treatment. The result from these procedures seems to be extremely satisfactory. Nevertheless, the ring fixation system can be used in the following conditions:

1. Children above the age of three years.
2. Recurrent or relapsed club feet.
3. Feet that have had multiple surgical operations with a lot of fibrosis and scarring.
4. Arthrogryphotic feet or those with bony deformities in the foot.

Dr. B. B Joshi of Mumbai has devised a simple method using L and V rods instead of rings and arches to achieve the same result. Good results have been reported using his system, but I feel that the Joshi method misses out the important Ilizarov principle of tensioning. The wires act as a biaxial transfixions, similar to Shanz pins and not as tensioned wires. In addition, one has to wait for the child to be a little older before attempting this procedure. On the contrary, the original Ilizarov system is a little more stable biomechanically and less traumatic on the bones and soft tissues, especially in a young child. I had devised a bangle fixator in 1991 which was in extensive use for some time, and then fell out of fancy, purely due to the unavailability of the device. I have devoted a whole chapter to this (The Prakash CTEV fixation). The following are the principles of treating CTEV:

1. A transverse ring is fixed to the middle of the leg.

2. The calcaneum is fixed by a half ring or a five-eighth ring.

3. The metatarsals are fixed with one or two half rings. The transverse wire passes through all the metatarsals just below the neck. One or two olive wires through the second and third metatarsals at right angles to the transverse wires will stabilize the rings in both axes.

4. The rings are joined to each other using posts, hinges and threaded or telescopic rods on the basis of three dimensional foot visualization. There is only one rule: Stretch the concave structures and compress the convex side. A representative assembly is shown in the drawings.

5. By increasing the length between the tibial and calcaneal rings, an elongation of the heel chord is achieved with the correction of calcaneal equinus.

6. By bringing the metatarsal rings closer to the leg rings, the forefoot equinus is corrected.

7. By moving the calcaneal rings away from the metatarsal rings, the cavus deformity is corrected.

8. By expanding the medial threaded rod between the calcaneum and the metatarsals and compressing the lateral threaded rods, one achieves correction of the varus of the foot.

9. All deformities can be corrected under vision, and suitable modifications can be introduced during the treatment to tackle fresh problems as they arise.

10. The secret of a successful, pain-free assembly is a *stable frame*. All wires should be properly tensioned, and all nuts fully tight at all times. A tight, tensioned stable frame is absolutely pain-free and well tolerated by most patients.

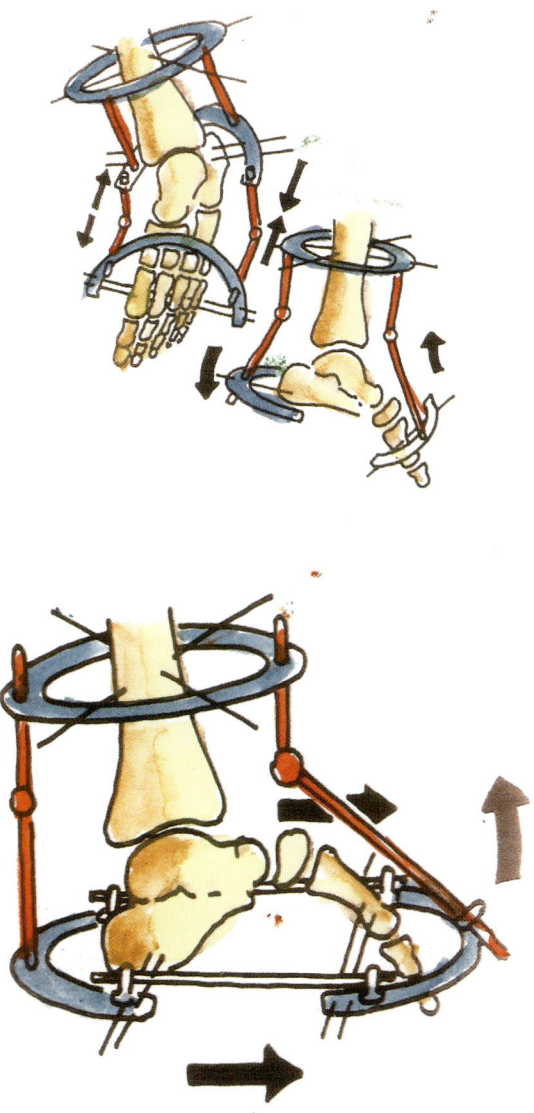

Picture 233: Frame application for foot deformities

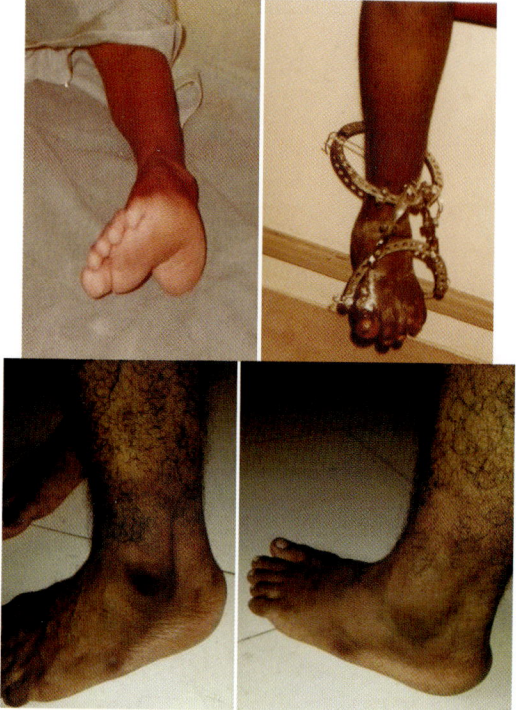

Picture 234: A fourteen year follow-up of a grossly deformed club foot treated by Ilizarov method.

MISCELLANEOUS FOOT DEFORMITIES

The Ilizarov method can be used to correct practically all the deformities of the foot.

The following parameters must be kept in mind:

1. Child must be at least three to four years of age. There have been reports in literature about corrections in younger children, but this requires very great co-operation of the parents.
2. The foot is divided into four components: the leg component, the hind foot component, mid foot component and forefoot component.

266

3. One ring fixed to the middle of the thigh will participate in correction of deformities of the ankle.

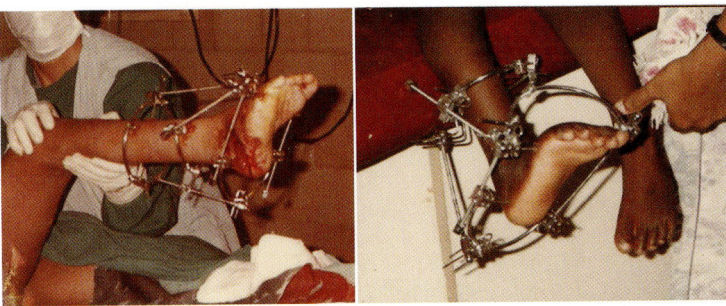

Picture 235: Most foot deformities will need metatarsal, calcaneal and tibial rings

4. A half or a five-eighth ring is fixed to the calcaneum; this will control the hind foot. From the middle of this ring, threaded or telescopic rods are connected to the proximal ring for tackling ankle deformities.

5. The forefoot is fixed to the 2 rings across the metatarsal shafts. Additional stability can be achieved by olive wires perpendicular to this.

6. These metatarsal rings are connected to the calcaneal rings with posts and telescopic rods. By expanding or contracting either the medial or the lateral threaded rods, a correction of varus or valgus of the foot is achieved.

7. By simultaneously expanding both the medial and flip lateral threaded rods, correction of the cavus foot is achieved.

8. By compressing both the medial and the lateral threaded rods, a correction of a planus or rocker bottom foot is achieved.

9. During the course of correction, a radiological evaluation of all the concerned joints is done. If it is found that any joint is subluxating, additional corrections are done by pulling specific bones using olive wires.

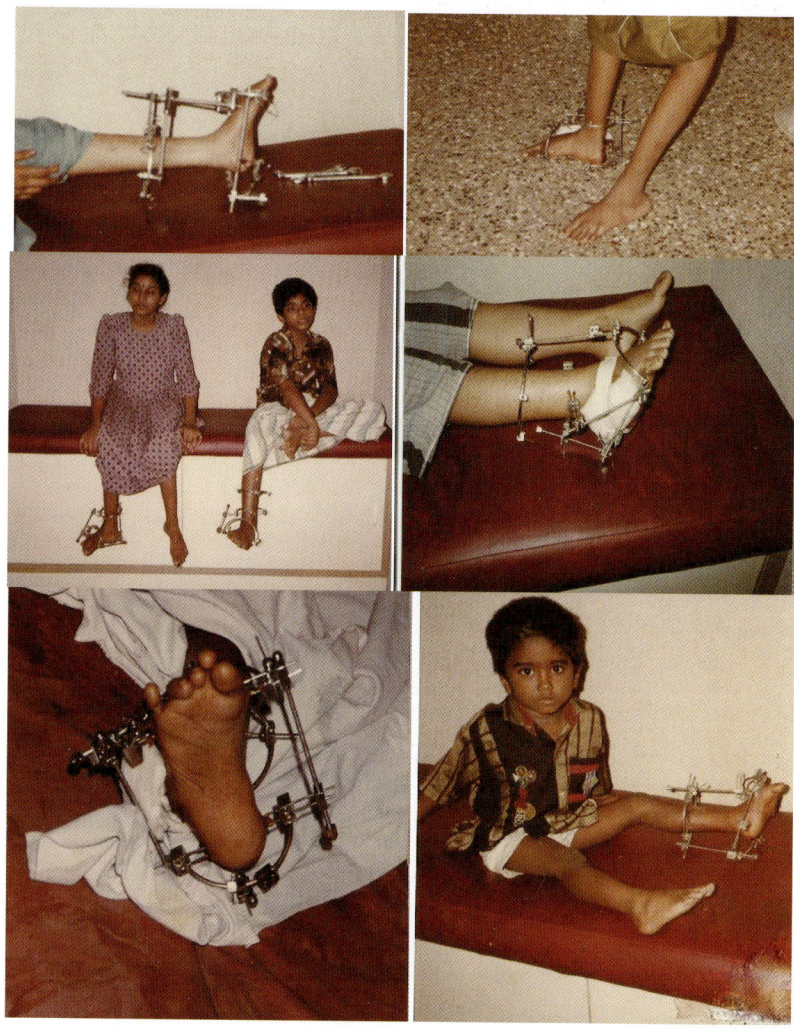

Picture 236: A properly applied frame is extremely well tolerated

The Prakash CTEV Fixation

One of the major advances that have happened in the treatment of club feet has occurred after the advent of the Ilizarov frames. Irrespective of the system employed, methods that rely on the principles of thin wire transfixation and gradual periodic distraction have resulted in a tremendous boon for treating these conditions. Rigid and resistant feet that have suffered many surgical assaults resulting in small scarred feet are the most benefited.

Dr. B. B. Joshi was the first to pioneer a fixator assembly using small cubes to transfix the K-wires and introduced his version in India. (Rancho cubes are the American version.) Of course, one can very well use the original Ilizarov apparatus for the same purpose. However, each system has its own advantages and disadvantages.

ADVANTAGES OF THE ILIZAROV SYSTEM:

1. Accurate forces can be applied in a three dimensional axis.

2. Wires can be tensioned; thus thinner wires can be used.

DISADVANTAGES OF THE ILIZAROV SYSTEM:

1. The apparatus becomes very cumbersome and bulky to apply.
2. The weight of the system is by far too much.
3. Due to the tremendous amount of forces generated, it is quite easy for the pins to tear off the soft bones making this system inadvisable in very young children.
4. While the Joshi system tries to eliminate a few of these disadvantages by making the system lighter and less cumbersome, it loses out on the important advantage of tensioning, as no full rings are employed. Thus the wires act

merely as stiff pins anchored at both ends and consequently have to be a little thicker.

I have attempted to take the advantages of the Joshi system in creating an extremely light system, at the same time retaining the advantages of the ring fixation system by designing a simple set specially for treating foot deformities. This is called the Prakash CTEV set, and I think that it would not be out of place to describe this system here.

This system employs the cubes as used by Joshi, but they are threaded on rings. Unlike Ilizarov rings that are flat, Prakash rings are stainless steel bangles with loose cubes threaded on them. These cubes can be locked at any level depending on the placement of the K-wires. And as the wires are anchored at both ends, it is possible to give them a certain amount of tension. In addition, due to the availability of half and full rings, it is possible to anchor the tensioning and distracting rods at the essential and critical points to provide a better dissipation of forces.

The Prakash CTEV set consists of the following components:

The metatarsal bangle

The calcaneal bangle

The tibial full ring

Small distracters

Large distracters

Straight and L rods

Hairpins

K-wires

The metatarsal bangle: This is a rod bent to a semicircle with permanently welded K-wire fixation blocks at both ends, These blocks are welded perpendicular to the long axis of the bangle, which helps to distinguish them from calcaneal bangles which otherwise look identical. Freely sliding over the bangle are four Joshi-like cubes, which can be locked anywhere along the bangle's perimeter.

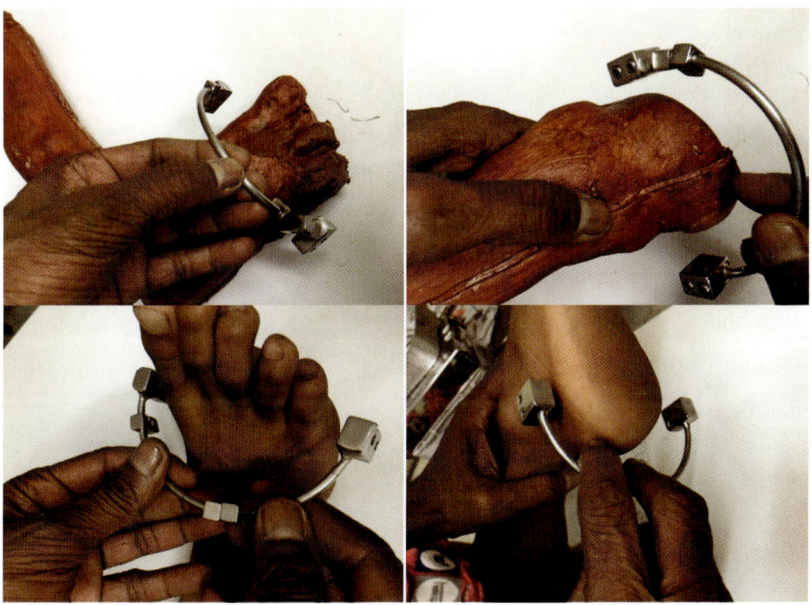

Picture 237: Positioning of the metatarsal and calcaneal bangles shown over a rubber model and a normal foot.

The calcaneal bangle: This is identical to the metatarsal bangle, but the end blocks are welded parallel to the long axis of the bangle. This distinguishes the calcaneal from the metatarsal bangle. Threaded on to the bangle are four free sliding Joshi-like cubes, which can be locked anywhere along the bangle's perimeter.

The tibial full ring: A straight rod is bent into a circle and the ends are welded together to form a round bangle, the dimension and thickness of which depends upon the size of the set and the age of the child on whom the set is being used. Threaded on to this ring are eight cubes of Joshi type which are free sliding and rolling on the ring.

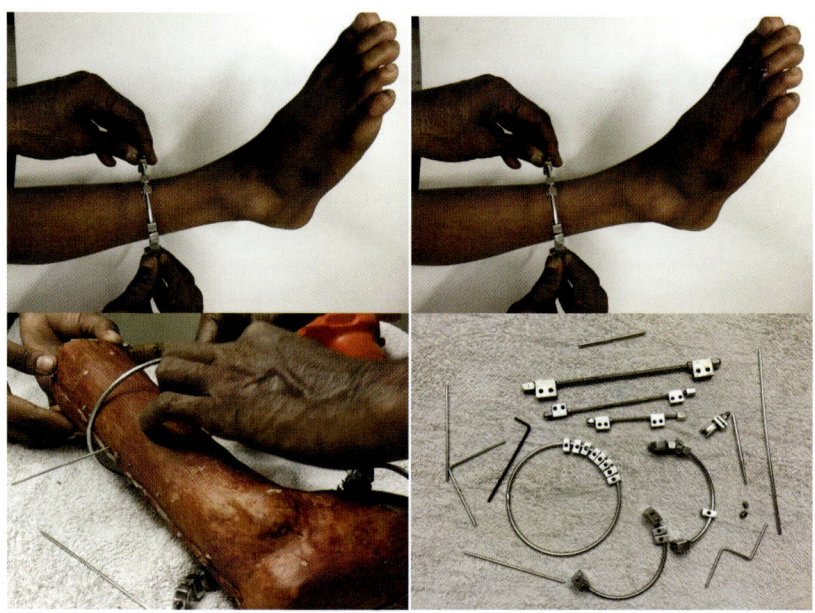

Picture 238: Position of the tibial bangle, and the other components of the system

The distracters and compressors: These are the standard Joshi type compressors and distraction assemblies, consisting of a threaded rod with wire fixation blocks at both ends. One block slides freely on the threaded rod and its propulsion is inhibited by a locked nut beyond the block. The other wire fixation block is threaded on to the threaded rod. One end of the threaded rod is anchored to a standard hexagonal head which can be rotated by a spanner. The other end of the rod is fixed to a square nut with numbers 1 to 4 on the sides, which tells the patient what movement has been achieved and also ensure that exactly one quarter turn is made every six hours.

Straight and L rods: These are rods of varying lengths and can be inserted into the cubes. Additional rods are also available which can be bent in any shape (Z, L, U, V or S) to allow anchorage of additional components in whatever manner one decides during the operative procedure.

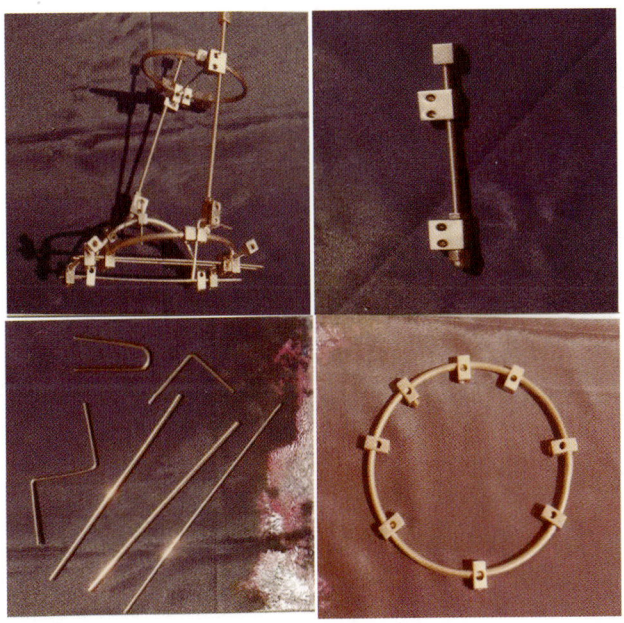

Picture 239: The various components; bangle, L rods, Z rods, distracters etc

Hairpins: These U shaped threaded rods allow for anchorage of two sets of components in which the holes are parallel to each other with the possibility of the holes being at different distances.

K-wires: These are conventional Ilizarov K-wires that are of 1.6 or 1.2 mm diameter depending upon the age and skeletal maturity of the child/ patient.

INDICATIONS OF THE PRAKASH CTEV FIXATOR:

I have personally used this fixator in over 500 children with excellent results, followed up to 25 years. At the end of this chapter, I have given representative examples. I have found my fixator extremely useful in the following conditions:

1. Club feet in children over three years old and who have not received treatment.
2. Club feet that have not responded to conservative treatment in children over two years old.
3. Failed operations on feet for children who are at least three years old.
4. Other foot deformities that are missed, neglected or relapsed after treatment in children over three years of age, including those caused by birth, poliomyelitis, or miscellaneous conditions.
5. Congenital pseudoarthrosis of tibia in a child older than three months or 6 Kg weight.

THE LOWEST AGE AT WHICH THIS FIXATOR CAN BE USED IS THREE MONTHS. THE MAXIMUM AGE AT WHICH IT SHOULD BE USED IS TWELVE YEARS.

After twelve years of age the bones are sufficiently mature and rigid to allow the application of a conventional Ilizarov fixator. Below three years it is better to attempt primary treatment of foot deformities by conservative or surgical releases; if these methods do not work, it may be advisable to go in for the Prakash fixator.

SURGICAL TECHNIQUE:

The actual surgical procedure depends upon the age of the child. The premise on which the system works is identical to the Ilizarov principles. Gradual periodic distraction stimulates formation of new tissues, i.e. the regenerate. This is not only applicable to bones, but also to soft tissues, tendons, nerves, blood vessels, fascia, ligaments and skin.

It is an established fact that when one cuts, then sutures a tissue, the elastic tissue heals by a poor quality fibrous tissue. The premise behind procedures of gradual periodic distraction is to allow for a stretching of all contracted tissues and make them regenerate in the form of the original first class tissue, rather than the second class fibrous tissue that would result if one attempted to cut and elongate them by Z plasty or otherwise.

For a regenerate formation, both the rate and rhythm of distraction are important. Published literature talks of a 1 mm distraction per day at a rhythm of 0.25 mm 4 times each day; this will ensure a smooth and gradual elongation.

During the course of performing many operations, I have found that though the surgical procedure is essentially non-surgical, it makes the treatment process very easy and the results much better if the surgeon combines closed tenotomies and minimal bony procedures along with the fixator application to achieve more predictable and certain results. I shall first describe the operative procedure of the use of the CTEV fixator. Then I shall describe the tips and tricks to make the job quite easy.

FRAME ASSEMBLY:

1. The full ring is slid on to the tibia. This is a very important step as the tibial ring is a solidly welded full ring and once the calcaneal or the metatarsal ring has been anchored, it is virtually impossible to slide the full ring over.

2. The metatarsal ring is now affixed. A thin K-wire, the diameter of which depends upon the skeletal maturity of the patient, is used. Usually 1.2 mm wire is used in children below three years, and 1.6 mm wire for older

children. This wire is drilled from medial to lateral through the metatarsals. The point of entry is just below the head of the first metatarsal; the wire passes through the first metatarsal and thereafter an attempt is made to impale as many of the metatarsals as possible. It would be ideal to fix all five, but one must attempt to transfix at least three including the first and fifth. The wire should pass a little below the epiphyseal line.

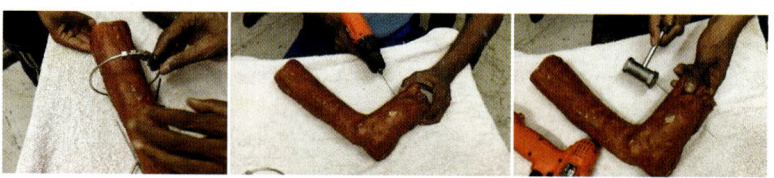

Picture 240: Tibial ring is slid in and the metatarsal wire is passed

3. After transfixing the K-wire, it is hammered from the medial to the lateral side, ensuring that equal lengths of wire are protruding on both sides of the foot. The metatarsal ring is now threaded on to this wire. From the medial side one passes the wire through the fixation block and then passes the other end through the same. In case the wire is too long, one may have to cut a little to allow free passage through both ends. The two ends are now tightened using the Allan key. If the child is older than 6, one may elect to impart tension of 40 to 50 Kg to the wire.

4. The second metatarsal wire is now passed distal and parallel to the first. The important point is that the distance between these two wires is predetermined by the wire fixation block. Thus one has to ensure that the second wire is passed through the distal hole of the wire fixation block. Here, if the second wire gets parallel to the first while passing, we need to tension it. In case the wire gets passed with a slight deflection, one stops immediately as it pierces the skin when it emerges from the opposite side. Thereafter one bends it towards the appropriate hole in the wire fixation block; once it emerges from

the opposite end, it is anchored. The mere act of tightening the Allan key allows tensioning of the wire!

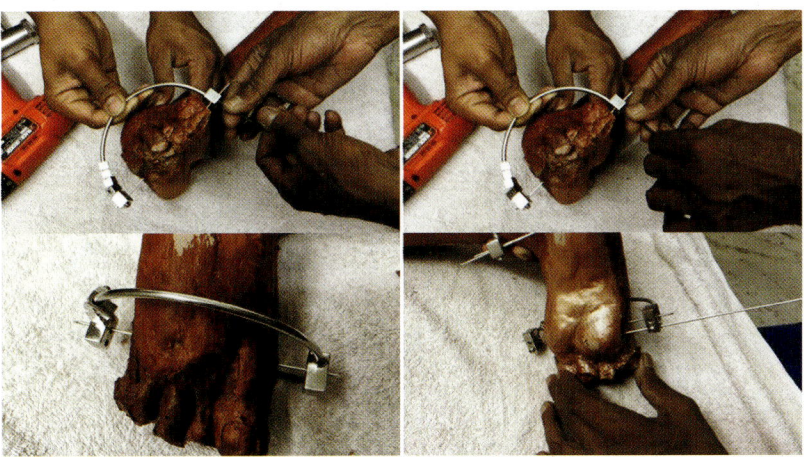

Picture 241: Insertion of the second metatarsal wire

5. The second half ring or bangle to be anchored is the calcaneal bangle. A thin K-wire is passed through the calcaneum, parallel to the axis of the calcaneum in the sagittal plane without relation to any other component of the foot. After transfixing the K-wire, it is hammered from the medial to the lateral side, ensuring that equal lengths of wire are protruding on both sides of the foot. The calcaneal ring is now threaded on to this wire. From the medial side, one passes the wire through the fixation block and then passes the other end through the same. In case the wire is too long, one may have to cut a little of it to allow the free passage through both ends. The two ends are now tightened using the Allan key. If the child is older than 6, one may elect to impart tension of 40 to 50 Kg to the wire.

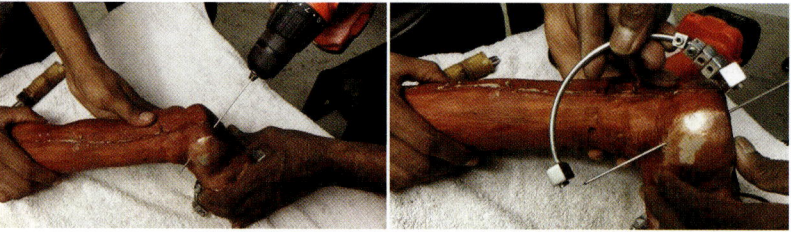

Picture 242: The calcaneal bangle application

6. A parallel K-wire is now inserted to give additional torsional stability to the calcaneal anchorage. Again, the distance from this wire to the previous calcaneal wire is predetermined by the wire fixation block through which the second wire passes. If the wire emerges parallel, one tensions this too. If the wire emerges at an angle, the mere act of tightening the Allan key allows tensioning of the wire!

7. At this stage we have a metatarsal ring anchored by two parallel K-wires and a calcaneal ring anchored by two more wires.

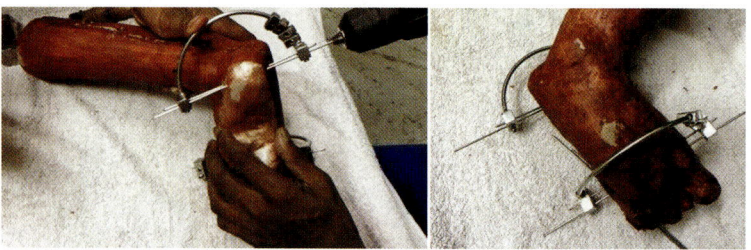

Picture 243: The foot after fixation of calcaneal and metatrsal rings

8. Now we affix the tibial ring. *(Hope we have not forgotten to pass the full ring on to the calf prior to anchoring the calcaneal and metatarsal rings!)* The level of placement is around the middle of the leg. It is advisable to go at least 7.5 cm above the level of the musculo-tendinous junction where the Achilles tendon flares to become triceps. First a K-wire is passed from

lateral to medial, keeping due regard for vital structures. This wire is actually passed first through one cube, then across tibia, and as it emerges from the other side, a cube is slid and placed just opposite the exit point of the wire, and the same wire is passed through the cube on the exit side. Because the cubes are free sliding on the ring, the need for special wire fixation bolts is completely eliminated. While affixing the cubes to the wire, it must be ensured that the same number of free sliding cubes is present on both sides of the wire. The second wire is now passed and can be nearly perpendicular to the first. I have personally not faced any problem with the wire going through the calf muscle. This wire is also anchored in exactly the same manner as the previous wire.

9. An important step to keep in mind is that the wire ends protruding beyond the bangles and the cubes are not cut or trimmed. (They will be used for the anchorage of the secondary components.)

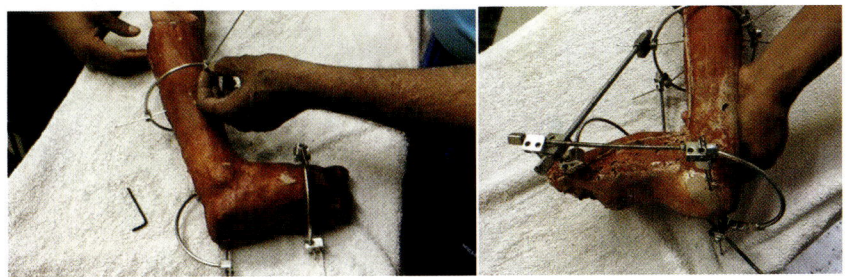

Picture 244: Fixation of tibial ring and distracters

10. Additional procedures like subcutaneous tenotomies, fasciotomies, de cancellations, etc. are now performed. These depend on the age of the patient and the severity of the deformity and are described in detail later.

11. Now we plan to anchor the secondary components and four compression distraction assemblies. The order commonly followed is medial, lateral, posterior and anterior.

12. *The medial support strut*: From the two protruding wires on the medial metatarsal bangle, a distracter is anchored. This distracter is kept with the wire fixation blocks close to each other and the protruding wires from the calcaneum are now anchored to it. The Allan key is used to tighten the wires on to the distracter. Occasionally the wires may not be in the exact parallel plane as the holes in the block of the distraction rod; in these cases it may be a good idea to gently manoeuvre the wire by bending it.

13. The lateral support strut: From the two protruding wires on the lateral metatarsal bangle, a distracter is anchored. This distracter is kept with the wire fixation blocks away from each other and the protruding wires from the calcaneum are now anchored on to this. The Allan key is used to tighten the wires on to the distracter. Occasionally the wires may not be in the exact parallel plane as the holes in the block of the distraction rod; in these cases, it may be a good idea to gently manoeuvre the wire by bending it. Here the distracter is fully expanded at the time of application and will be used as a compression device.

14. The posterior support is now affixed. Here the plan is to allow for pulling down the calcaneum to give space for the talus to relocate as correction is in progress. The distracter is anchored using a hairpin. First a hairpin is inserted through the two link joints in the calcaneal bangle. These link joints are now tightened on the bangle. The protruding end of the hairpin which is perpendicular to the long axis of the calcaneal bangle is affixed to the posterior column distracter and the Allan screw tightened. If it is possible to twist and pass the other end of the hairpin through the second hole of the distracter block, this is done. Else a small straight rod is used to join the cube on the bangle to the distracter.

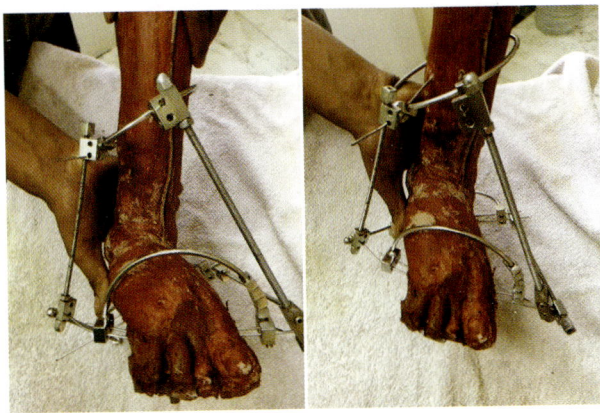

Picture 245: Finalization of the assembly and beginning distraction compression

15. Now the upper end of the distracter should lie at the level of the tibial ring. The protruding end of the anterio posterior K-wire is anchored to one hole of the distracter. A hairpin is used to affix one of the free cubes on the ring and the distracter assembly. An important point to be noted here is that the distracter should have the two wire fixation blocks close to each other to allow for proper length of distraction.

16. The last segment needed for completing the frame is the anterior column support. This is to be anchored anteriorly between the apex of the metatarsal ring and the tibial bangle. The device will achieve gradual compression and hence should be applied in full expansion of both ends. The K-wire protruding anteriorly is first affixed to one hole in the end lock of the distracter. A hairpin is used to fix one of the loose cubes to the other hole. Both nuts are now tightened with appropriate Allan keys. The lower end is now fixed to the metatarsal bangle by anchoring the lower block to the free cubes of the latter with one or two straight rods or bangles.

17. As shown in the diagrams below, the assembly is now complete. By distracting the medial column, the forefoot adduction is gradually corrected. Compression of the lateral side results in a corresponding shortening of the

lateral column. Elongating the posterior column pulls down the calcaneum and compression of the anterior rod corrects the equinous.

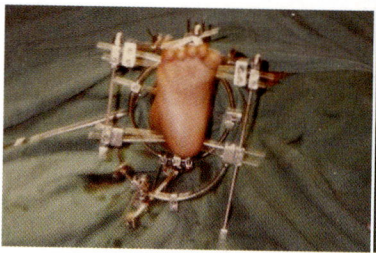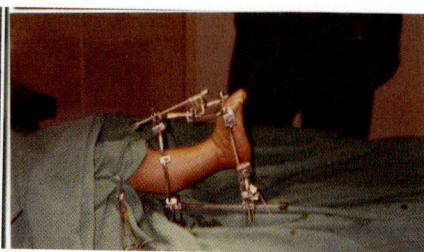

Picture 246: Clinical examples of Prakash bangle fixator

ADDITIONAL PROCEDURES:

A few additional procedures are needed; these depend on each individual patient. The premise for using the fixator is to avoid open surgery that needs cutting of the tissues with resultant repair, resulting in second class fibrous tissue. But fixator and mechanical forces alone may not always be enough to achieve full correction, hence we may need to resort to additional procedures that are minimally invasive.

1. Tendo Achillis elongation: This is performed by a sharp knife percutaneously. As shown in the diagram, through three or four small incisions, fibres of one-third of the diameter are cut in different directions at different levels. Circumferential cut to the paratenon is studiously avoided.

2. Posterior capsulotomy: This is performed from the lateral side just by the side of the TA. The foot is dorsiflexed and a tight capsule is cut using a sharp knife through a pin pointed incision.

3. Plantar fasciotomy: By stretching the sole and using a sharp pointed tenotomy knife with multiple small pointed incisions, the plantar fascia is cut across.

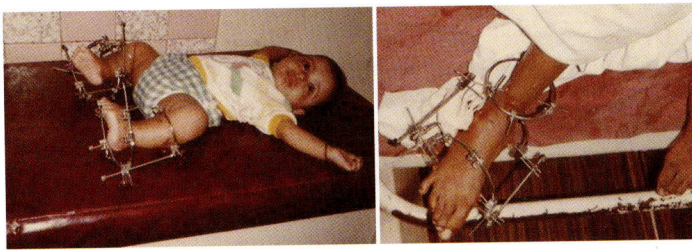

Picture 247: The Prakash bangles can be used in patients of the age group of three months to fourteen years

3. Decancellation of the Cuboid: In children older than four years with a rigid lateral column, this procedure is needed. At the apex of the curvature, the cuboid is palpated. A small incision is made over the bone and the incision goes bone deep. Using a very small curette, the entire interior of the cuboid is curetted out. By a gentle manipulation, one can crust the hollow cuboid, resulting in a good amount of lateral column shortening.

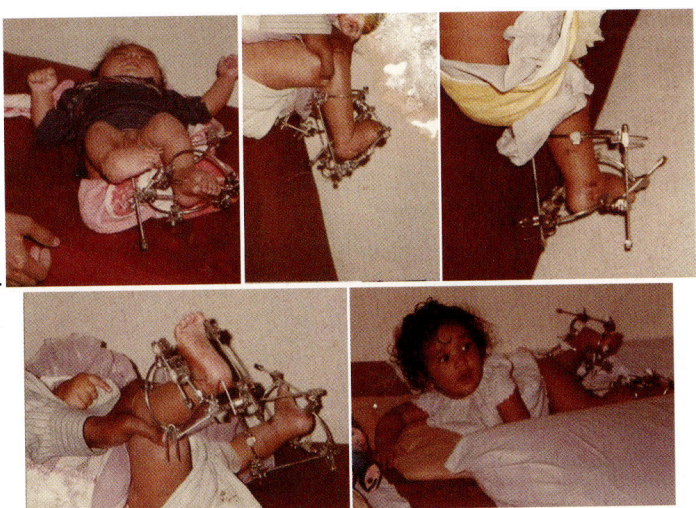

Picture 248: A properly applied frame is well tolerated even by infants as young as three months

4. Bony wedge resections: In children over six years old, the bony changes would have become fixed and it may not be possible to correct the deformity by soft tissue procedures alone. In this case, appropriate wedges are resected prior to application of the distracters.

APPLICATION OF FORCES, AND SCREW TURNINGS: One must not attempt acute correction as it may hamper the blood supply and lead to ischemic changes. Minimal correction is done and all the Allan screws are tightened. While applying the distracters, it is better to retain the twisting end distally and the square nut proximally. Thus in the foot, the two square nuts will be around the metatarsal area and the rotating nuts will be in the calcaneal side. Likewise, the proximal distracter rods will have the square nut at the apex of the metatarsal and calcaneal bangles while the twisting nuts will lie anteriorly and posteriorly across the tibial ring.

COMPLICATIONS AND PITFALLS:

1. As with other ring fixation systems, one must be aware of the anatomy and be careful not impale neurovascular structures.
2. In severely deformed feet, the calcaneum may be tiny and the neurovascular bundle may be too close on the medial side. In these cases, one has to keep one finger on the neurovascular bundle to avoid impaling.
3. Too rapid a distraction causes transient neuropraxia; in these conditions, one must stop the turnings for a few days, then resume.
4. Swelling might occur during the process of treatment; this is overcome by elevation.
5. Claw toes almost always occur; this is prevented by using a plastic foot plate strapped to the toes.
6. Improper frame application leads to a flat foot. This occurs if the equinous alone is corrected without regard to distal translation of the calcaneum and a

squashing of the talus results. One must understand the principle correctly and make sure that the heel is pulled down sufficiently to allow for a space for talar relocation.

DEGREE OF CORRECTION AND TIME OF REMOVAL:

It is better to over correct than to under correct. Once the deformity has been corrected in all planes, and the foot is neutral, one continues until 20 degrees of dorsiflexion is achieved. Medial column is stretched until it is 15 to 20% longer than the lateral column. Radiographs are taken during the course of treatment to look for talar relocation. After removal of the frame, it is advisable to use appropriate footwear for 3 to 6 months to avoid recurrence.

I have illustrated this system with a random collection of clinical photographs from my patient database.

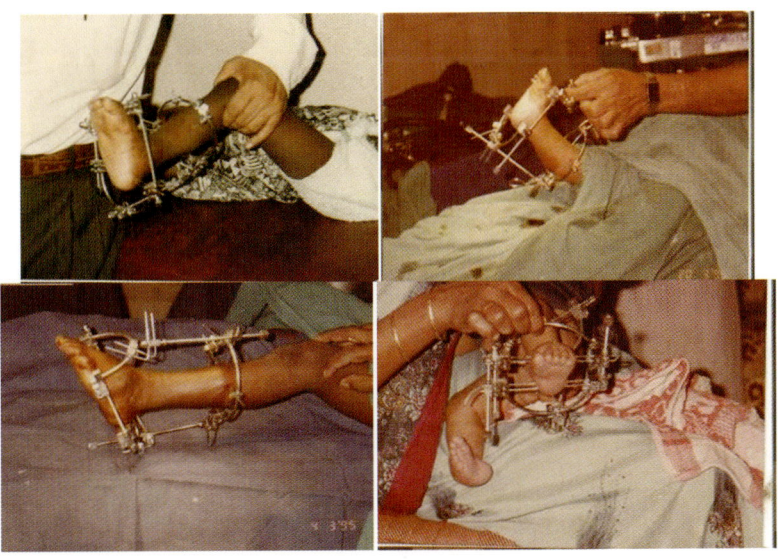

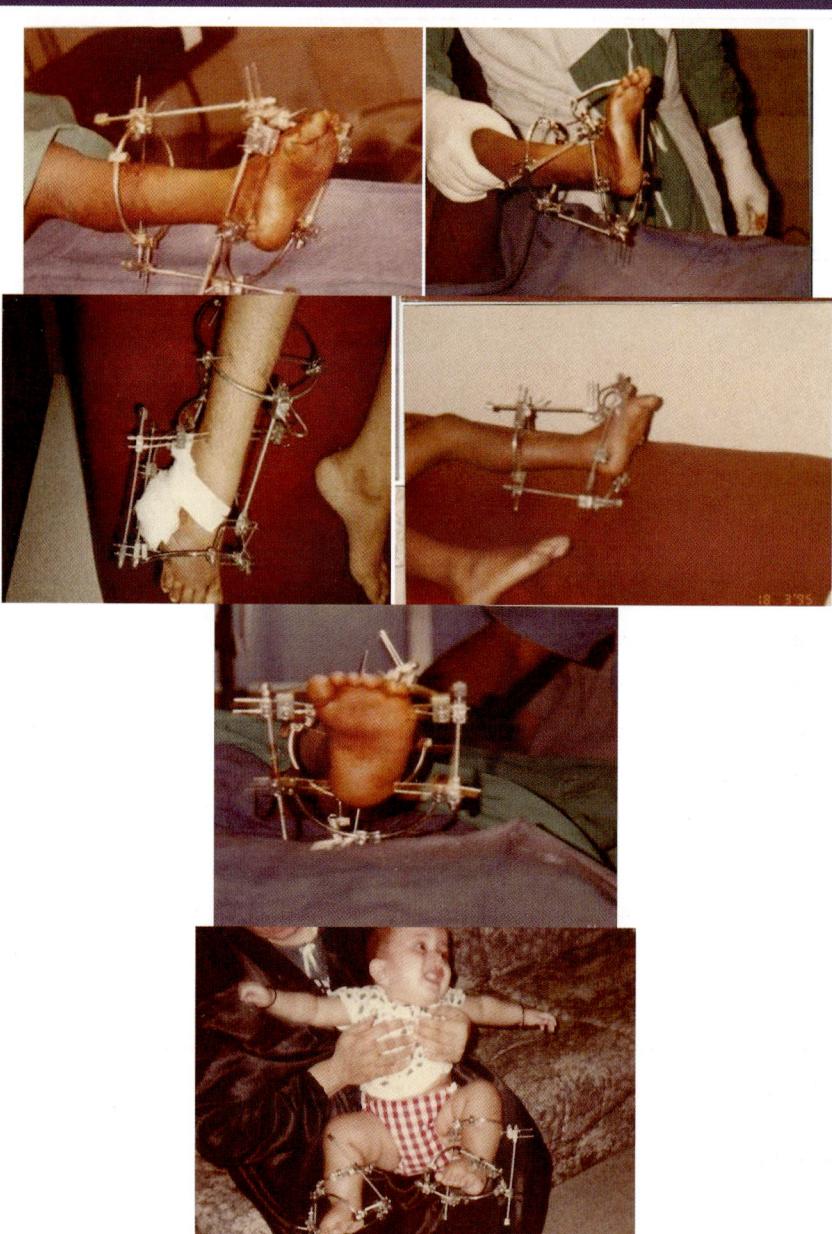

Picture 249: Various clinical applications of the Prakash bangle fixator

Flexion Deformity at the Elbow

These occur either due to congenital or developmental conditions or due to contracture of the anterior structures of the cubital fossa due to scars, burns or infections. The steps for correction of flexion deformities of the elbow are:

1. The distance between the deltoid and the palm is measured; this will be expanded at the rate of 1 mm a day.
2. A standard 4 ring assembly is used with 2 rings in the arm and 2 in the forearm.
3. Judicious placement of olive wires will allow increase of stability and possibility of correction of associated deformities.
4. The anterior aspect of the arm and forearm are taken as the concave component of the deformity and the posterior aspect of the arm and forearm are taken as the convex component of the deformity.
5. Threaded rods with hinges or telescopic rods are anchored to the rings.
6. A gradual distraction of 1 mm per day is well tolerated by the soft tissues.
7. Transient neuropraxia may be encountered during rapid distraction; this can be avoided by slowing the speed of distraction or stopping the distraction temporarily.
8. If there is an associated varus or valgus deformity, placement of additional hinges and threaded rods will ensure correction of the same.

Special precautions to be taken during correction of elbow flexion deformities

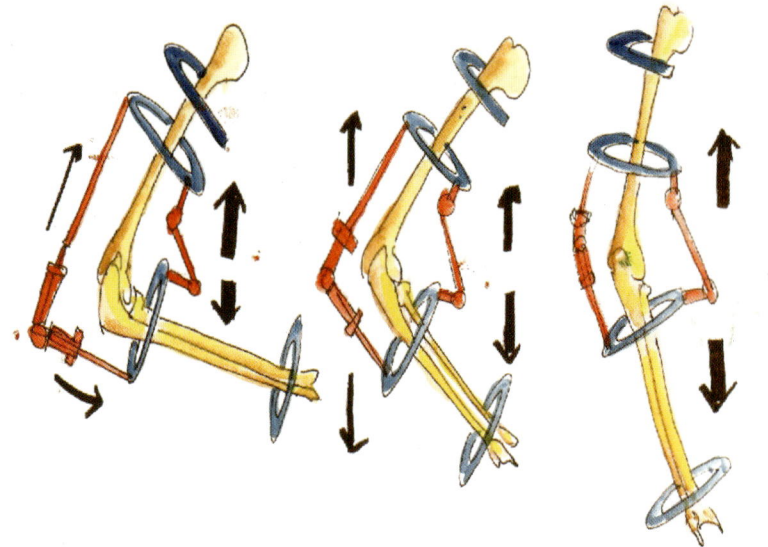

Picture 250: Placements of hinges and rings for correction of flexion deformity of elbow.

1. It is essential to define the cause of elbow stiffness. Pure soft tissue contractures will need percutaneous releases, while bony deformities will need corticotomies and osteoclasis.

2. Transient wrist drop occurs in almost half the cases. One needs to stop distracting for a few days, allow the wrist drop to recover, and then resume distraction.

3. The most important point to remember is that the best position for a fused elbow is right angle for the right hand and extension for the left hand.

4. Stiff elbows are a little tricky and should be attempted only by experienced surgeons.

Ilizarov in Tumours

The role of Ilizarov in tumours can be simply defined as *a better substitute for bone grafts*. Aggressive and malignant tumours should be managed by the standard limb salvage protocol. In benign, well-encapsulated, or moderately aggressive tumours where a resection and bone grafting is planned, Ilizarov can produce more bone and avoid shortening during arthrodesis.

The two situations where Ilizarov frame can be useful are:

A. Diaphyseal tumours, which have to be excised with healthy margins leaving a bone gap. With monofocal or bifocal bone transports, one can bridge the gap while maintaining the limb length.
B. In metaphyseal tumours, where an excision/ arthrodesis is planned with grafting, Ilizarov is an excellent substitute for bone grafts. It will however be a poor substitute to a megaprosthesis, which has the benefit of joint mobility.

The following illustrations shed light on various situations and how they can be appropriately managed. However, it should be clearly understood that though Ilizarov produces distinctly better bone than grafts, the time taken is prolonged and the process is taxing, both for patient and surgeon. Likewise, Ilizarov is the only solution available for poor patients who cannot afford customized mega prostheses, or in centres which do not have the facilities. As Dr. Mayilvahanan Natarajan, the world's leading expert on orthopaedic oncology, has repeatedly stated: *There is no place for amputation in bone tumours, so long as they are diagnosed early*. Where the resection gap cannot be replaced by a customized megaprosthesis, Ilizarov offers the only hope.

In my opinion, there are four situations where an Ilizarov construct can be used: In lower femur, upper tibia, distal radius and mid shaft humerus. Otherwise, it is better that tumours be managed by existing established methods.

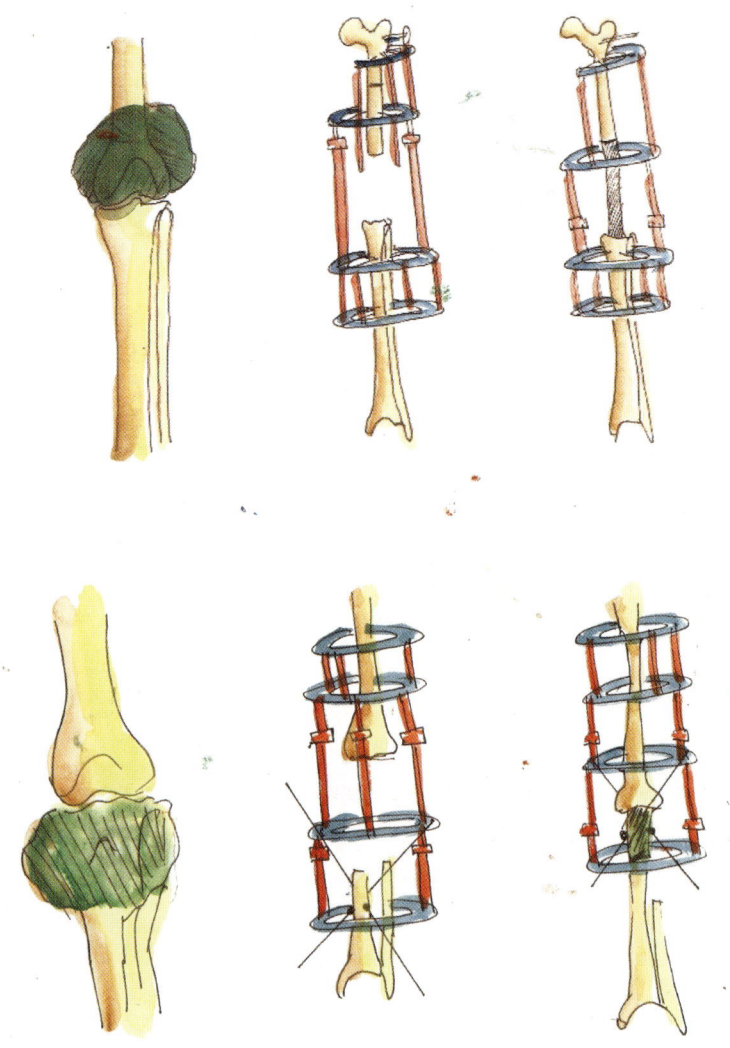

Picture 251: Frame constructs for tumors of upper tibia and lower femur.

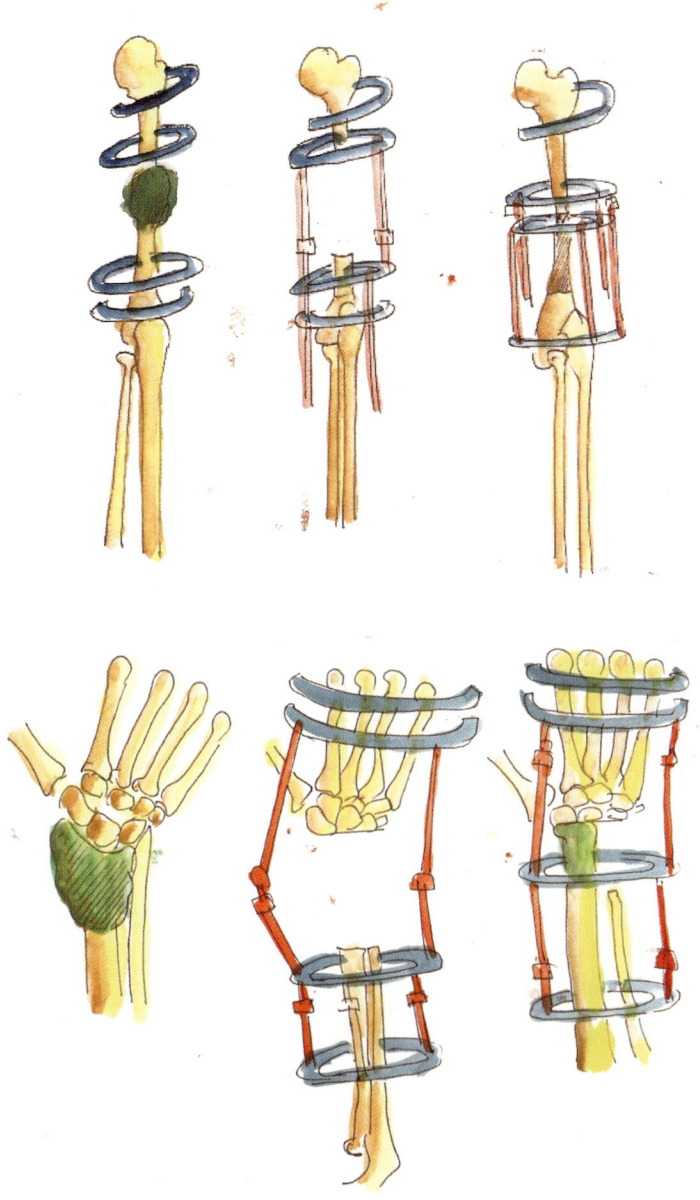

Picture 252: Frame constructs for tumours of diaphyseal femur and distal radius.

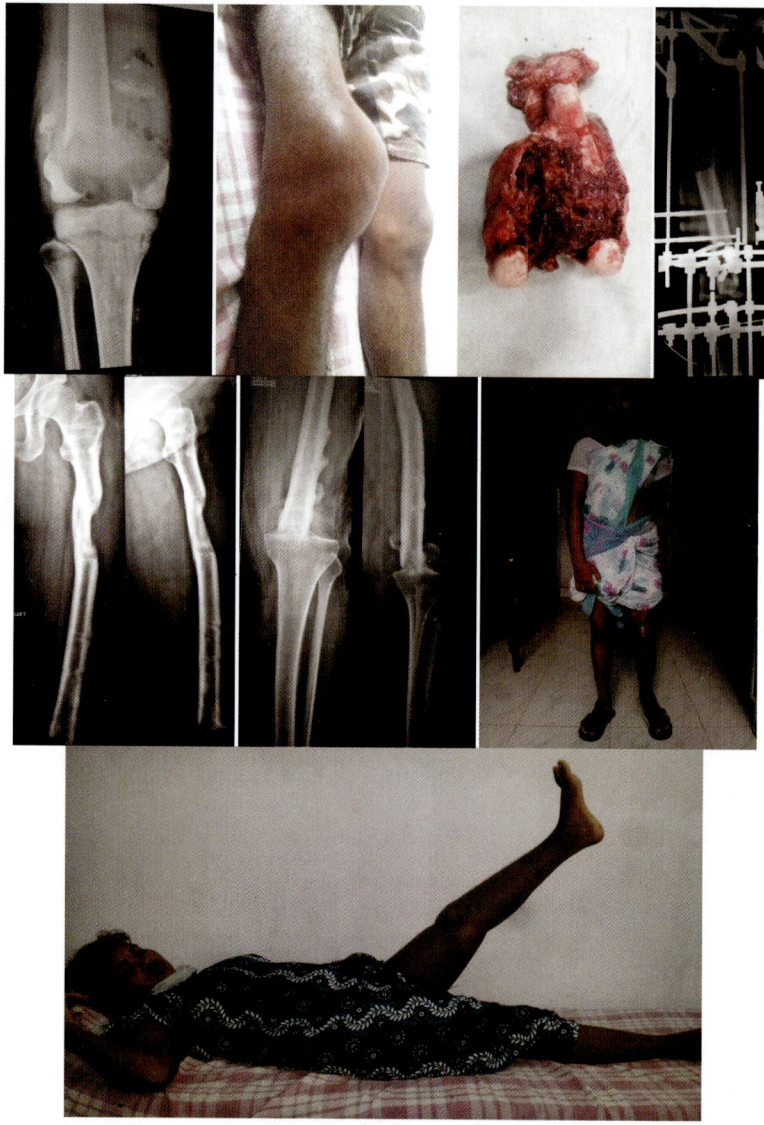

Picture 253: Clinical example of an aggressive giant cell tumour, successfully treated by Ilizarov method

Ilizarov for soft tissue problems

Ilizarov often stated that the term *Transosseus Osteosynthesis* was a misnomer, because sustained continuous traction stretches not only the bone, but all the soft tissues around it: nerves, vessels, muscles, tendons, subcutaneous tissue and even the skin. Thus the Ilizarov system can also be used for pathologies other than skeletal problems. We must appreciate that a cortical bone is non-stretchable, and thus needs a cortical breach to elongate. The soft tissues on the other hand stretch, except in case of really tight tendons or scarred tissue where small percutaneous tenotomies may be needed. This principle can thus be successfully applied to non healing ulcers, skin defects, and other similar situations.

Not much has been written in literature about the *gardening* aspect of Ilizarov, as all books only stress on the *carpentry* part. Thus no established procedures or standard protocols for soft tissue surgery with Ilizarov have been explained or documented. The surgeons who do this procedure do it by their own individual techniques, all mirroring the original Ilizarov principles. The basic concepts are simple.

1. K-wires are inserted into soft tissues, leaving enough margins to avoid tear through.
2. Occasionally, one has to use twisted wires or even flexible wires.
3. A judicious use of olive wires helps in applying and dissipating forces uniformly across the area of interest.
4. Tight, scarred and fibrosed tissues are percutaneously slit, to ease the stretching.

5. The usual rate of stretch is 1 mm per day. Anatomy teaching tells us that nerves regenerate at this rate. This is true of all tissues stretched properly and immobilized biologically.

6. Once the soft tissue defect has been reasonably corrected, plastic surgery procedures can be used as a final step. However, this becomes unnecessary in many cases.

7. The following clinical examples illustrate the magic of Ilizarov.

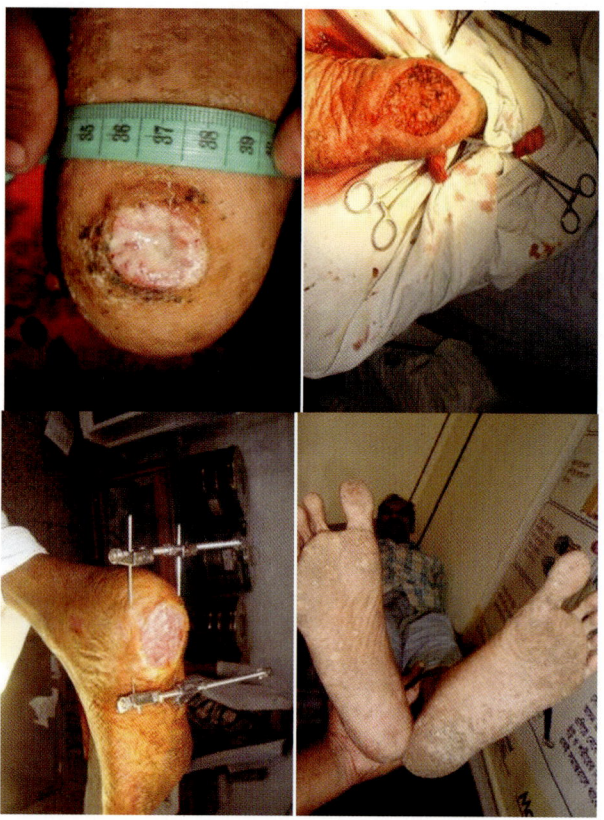

Picture 254: Arsenic induced squamous cell carcinomatous ulcer treated by Ilizarov method

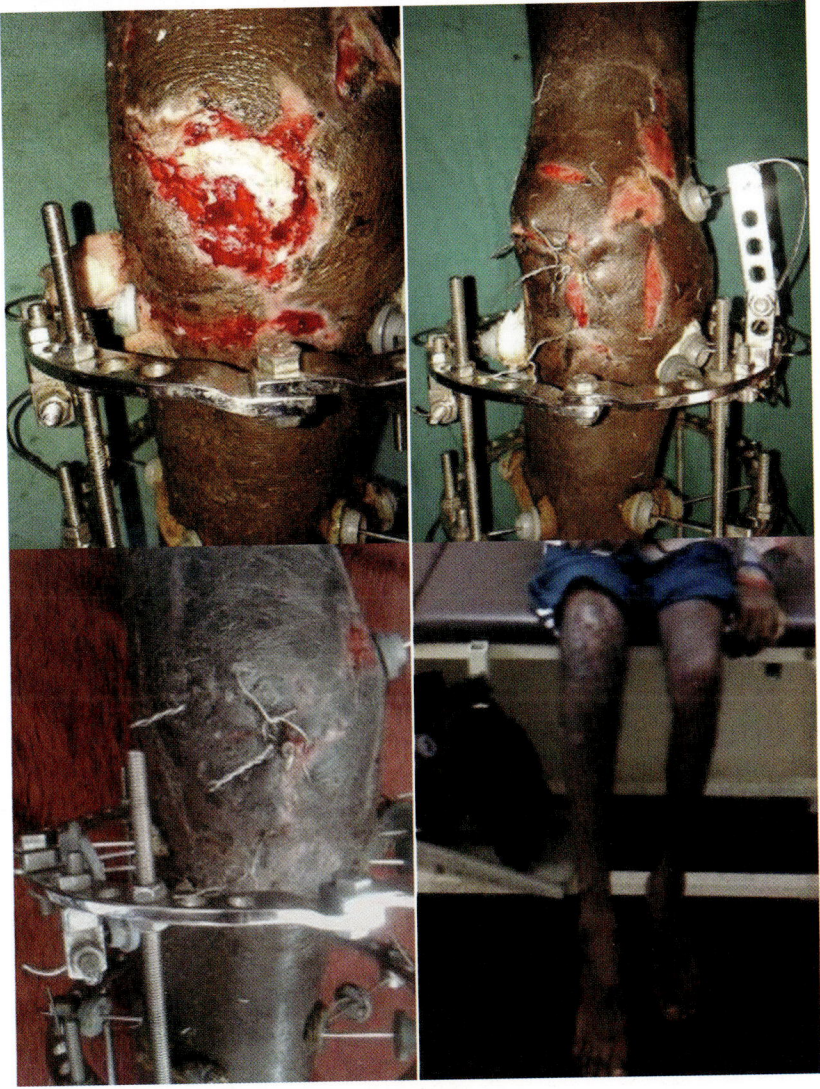

Picture 255: Compound tibial fracture with skin loss managed without skin or bone grafts

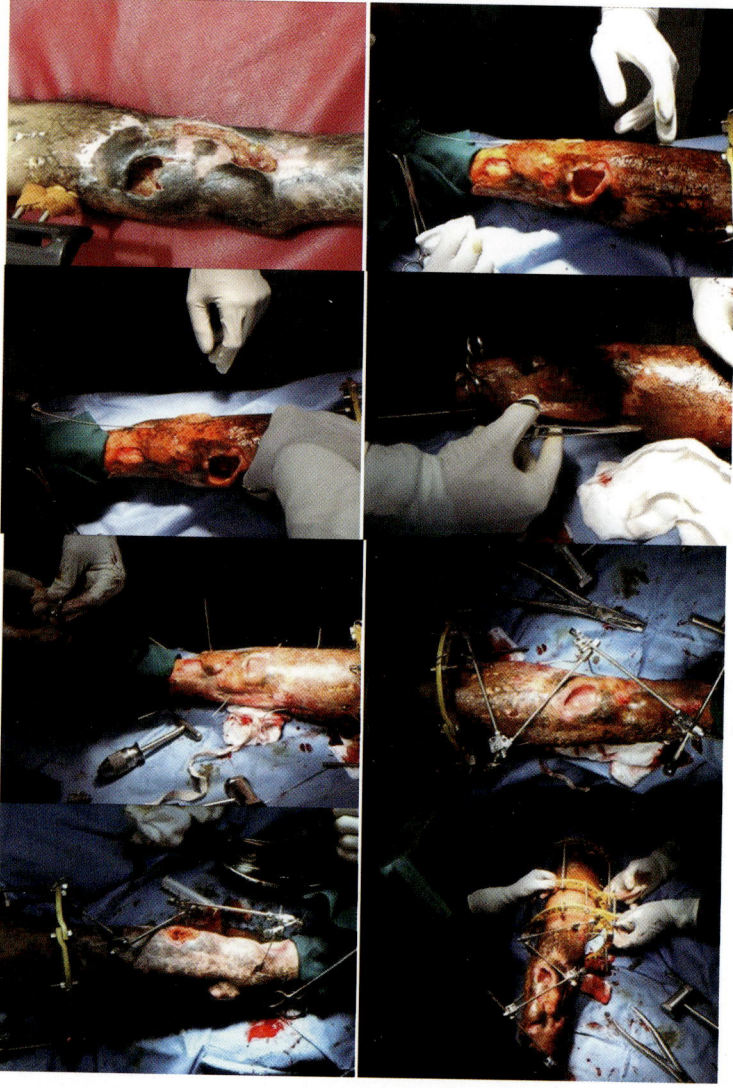

Picture 256: Ilizarov system can replace or facilitate plastic surgery procedures

Ilizarov in Arthrodesis

The ring fixation system can be used in performing most arthrodesis procedures. However, it is commonly used in the arthrodesis of knee and ankle joints. Use of ring fixators is too cumbersome for other joints like shoulder and hip; joints like elbow and wrist can be fused using much simpler methods.

ARTHRODESIS OF THE KNEE JOINT:

The following are the steps of the procedure:

1. Resection of the joint surfaces is done in the standard manner.
2. Two rings are placed in the distal femur and two in the proximal tibia.
3. The wires are tensioned and the rings are joined together by telescopic rods.
4. Compression is exerted between these pairs of rings at the arthrodesis surface.

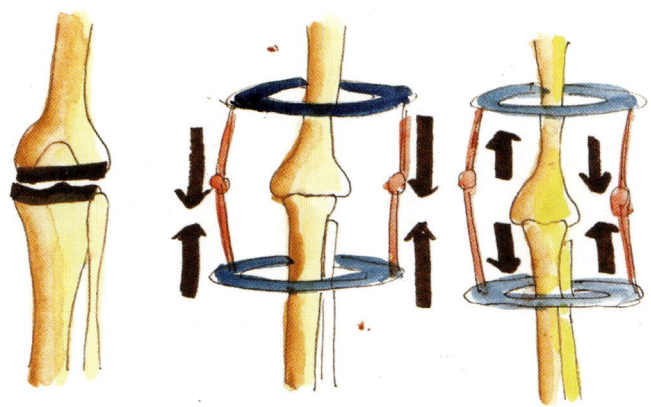

Picture 257: Schematics for arthrodesis of the knee joint

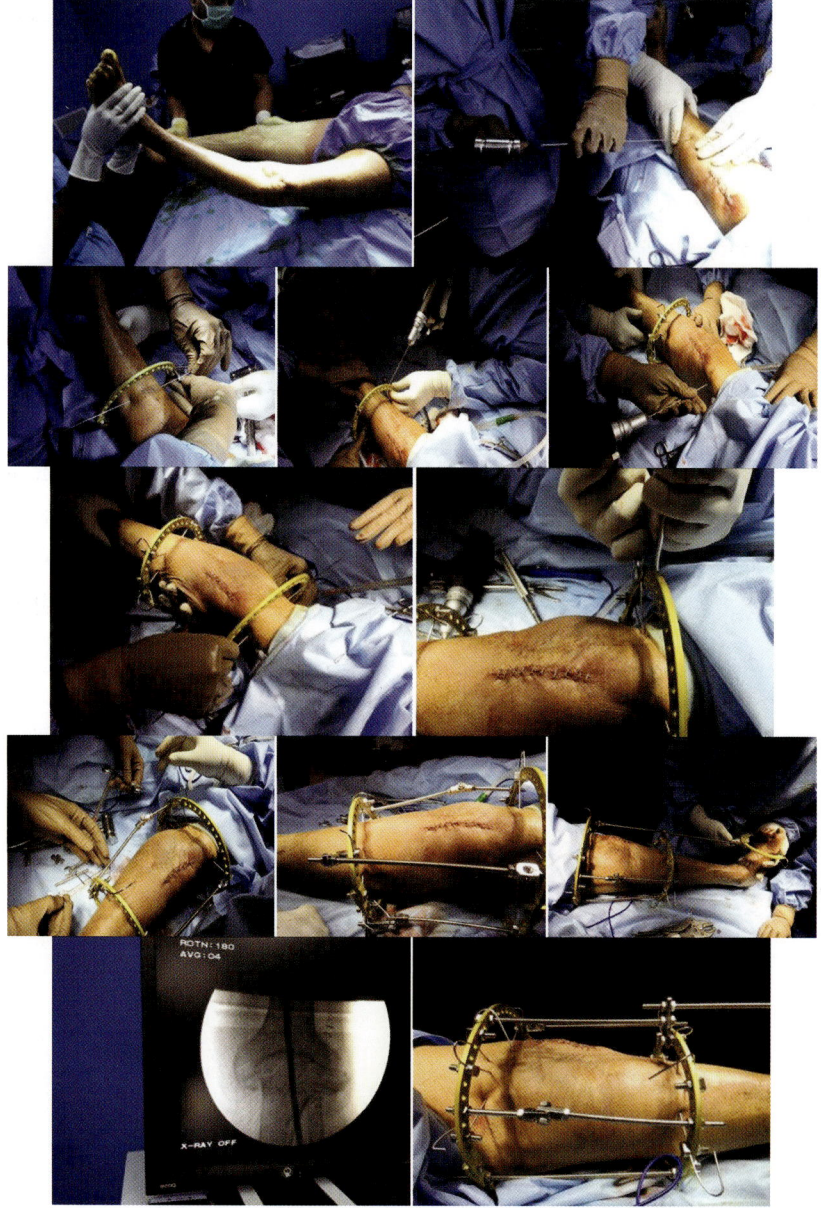

Picture 258: Steps and construct for knee arthrodesis

5. The linear micromotion provided by the system due to the inherent resilience of the tensioned pins is sufficient to achieve rapid fusion.

6. Hinges in the correct axis will retain a 5 degrees valgus and 15 degrees flexion, which is desired.

7. The patient is encouraged to walk from day one, and union is achieved in about 6 to 8 weeks.

ARTHRODESIS OF THE ANKLE JOINT:

1. In foot deformities in an adult, one may elect to arthrodesis the ankle and simultaneously correct the other existing foot deformities.

2. The joint exposure and the resection of the joint surfaces are done in the standard manner. The frame construction is similar to that described for the correction of foot deformities.

3. An additional wire might be passed through talus and connected to the calcaneal ring with posts.

4. Threaded rods exert compression at the talo-calcaneal junction.

5. Simultaneous correction of other existing deformities can now be done.

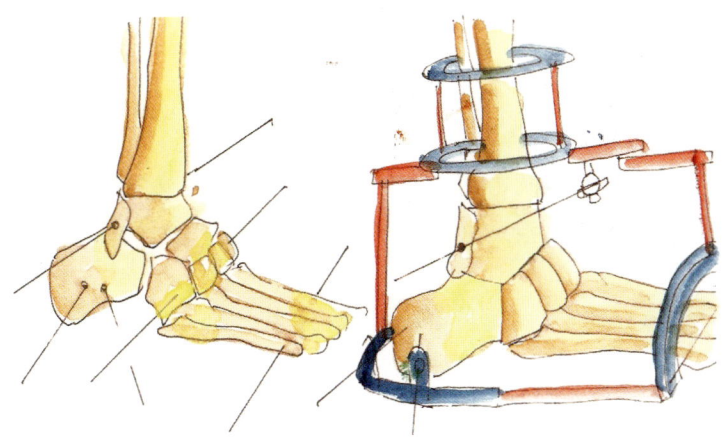

Picture 259: Schematics for ankle arthrodesis by Ilizarov methods

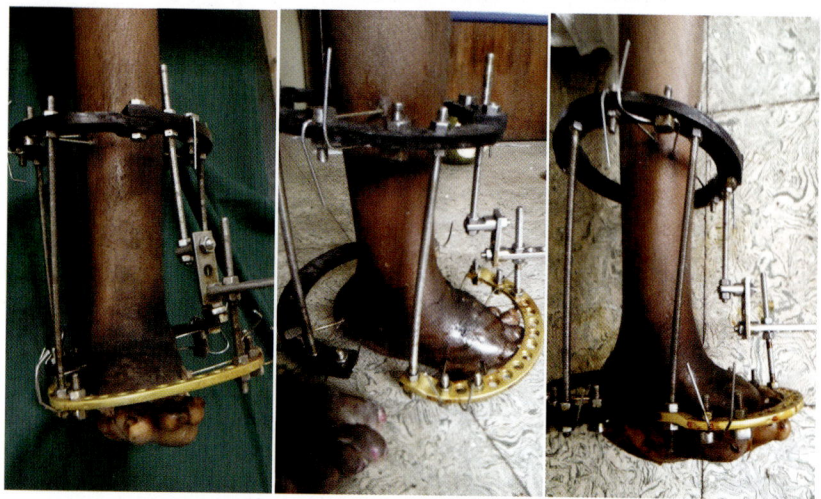

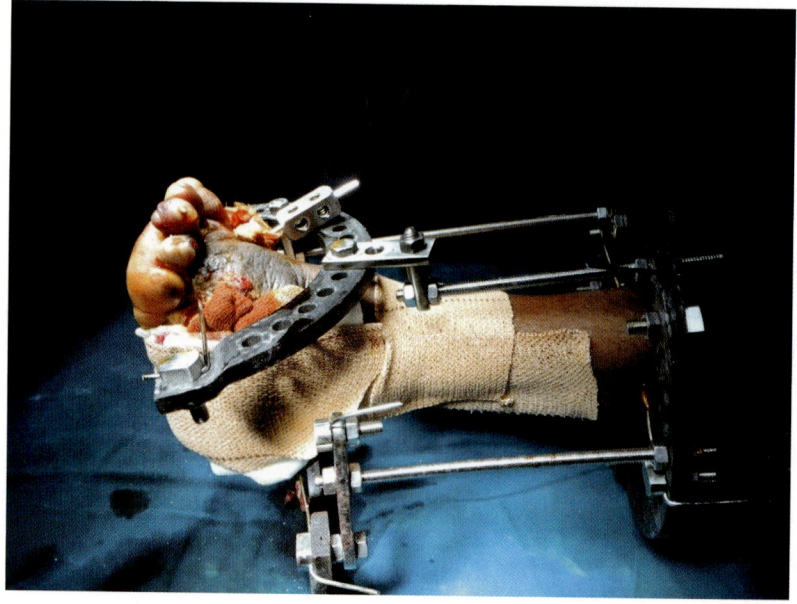

Picture 260: Clinical examples of frames for ankle Arthrodesis.

Conclusion

There is doubt that the advent of transosseous osteosynthesis has been one of the revolutions of orthopaedic surgery. Yet the method is not without inherent risks and disadvantages. Massive research evidence accumulating from Russia, Italy, France, Canada and America provides us with newer and more exciting applications of this system. Based on the current literature and personal experience, the following are the salient advantages and disadvantages of the Ilizarov method.

ADVANTAGES:

1. UNIVERSAL SYSTEM WITH MULTIPLE APPLICATIONS:

The system has a wide range of applications. As described in previous chapters, it can be used for diverse applications like fractures, non-unions, deformities, pseudoarthrosis, congenital deformities, poliomyelitis, arthrodesis, tumours, etc.

2. SIMPLICITY OF METHODS:

Once the basics of frame assembly and wire passage are mastered, the application of the apparatus becomes relatively simple.

3. MINIMALLY INVASIVE SURGERY:

As most modalities in transosseous osteosynthesis do not involve long incisions, soft tissue, bone damage or tissue destruction, complications like blood loss and post operative care are minimized.

4. ACCEPTANCE OF THIN WIRES

Thin transosseous wires of 1.6 to 1.8 mm diameter are far better tolerated (than pins and nails of larger diameter) and cause much less damage to muscles, tendons, skin and bone. The magic of the original Ilizarov system is the pins. We exchange them for thicker Shanz screws only for surgical convenience.

5. THREE DIMENSIONAL CORRECTION:

Axial compression, distraction, medial lateral angulation, rotational corrections or a combination of these is possible with the comprehensive apparatus.

6. EASE OF REMOVAL:

The removal of the frames and wires can be done simply and easily as an out-patient procedure without any problems.

7. BONE GRAFTING IS NOT NEEDED:

The possibility of supplementing an internal regeneration process for bone formation without the use of grafts is in itself a revolutionary concept and should be heralded as one of the greatest achievements of orthopaedic surgery.

DISADVANTAGES OF THE ILIZAROV SYSTEM

1. LONG LEARNING CURVE:

As the assembly of the apparatus is much more complex and time consuming than the uniaxial frame, it takes some time to master the various aspects of the meccano set like constructions of the system.

2. CAREFUL MONITORING AND PATIENT CO-OPERATION:

A patient has to clean at least 10 to 20 pin sites and has to turn nuts over a dozen time each day. The surgeon has to closely monitor the frame and the patient. Unlike the *fit and forget* approach of internal fixations, Ilizarov is a high maintenance surgery.

3. PAIN:

Stretching process to bone and soft tissue is not well tolerated by all patients.

4. POSSIBLE NEUROVASCULAR INJURY:

Because a large number of pins are passed in various axes, the possibility of causing damage to blood vessels and nerves leading to aneurysms or neuroma is present. A thorough knowledge of the topographic anatomy is necessary to minimize this risk.

5. REGULAR OUT-PATIENT MONITORING:

Patients need to be regularly monitored during the period of treatment, which requires a larger number of time-consuming post-operative visits.

6. PSYCHOLOGICAL ACCEPTANCE:

To retain the frame on the body and carry on with one's normal social activities requires a lot of psychological courage. There is a good percentage of patients who are not able to bear the psychological trauma of the assembly. In a few cases, psychological factors combined with severe pain have necessitated a premature removal of the implant.

In closing, I would like to emphasize that it is not as simple as procuring the apparatus and starting to operate. First time users are strongly advised to study the literature thoroughly and familiarize themselves with all aspects of the apparatus. They must also view videos of surgical procedures to acquaint themselves with the various modalities. If opportunities exist, one can spend some time learning the procedure first-hand in an institution where it is being regularly performed in large numbers.

In the beginning of one's learning curve, it is best to start with simple applications, then to progress to more difficult and complicated problems. One must not be reluctant to refer difficult cases to senior colleagues or a senior surgeon who is more experienced than oneself.

With these words of caution, I would like to thank you, dear reader. You have not only paid for this book, but have also spent time and effort reading it right till the end! I am confident you will put this knowledge to good use. I will be very grateful to receive all your comments and criticisms.

References

Ali A. M., Burton M., Hashmi M., Saleh M.: **Outcome of complex fractures of the tibial plateau treated with a beam-loading ring fixation system.** *J Bone Joint Surg Br* 2003, **85**–5:691–9.

Ali A. M., El-Shafie M., Willet K. M.: **Failure of fixation of tibial fractures.** *J Orthop Trauma* 2002, **16**–5:323–9.

Aronson J., Harrison B. H., Stewart C. L., Harp J. H. Jr.: **The histology of distraction osteogenesis using different external fixators.** Clin Orthop Relat Res 1989 Apr(241):106-16.

Aronson J.: **Experimental and clinical experience with distraction osteogenesis.** Cleft Palate Craniofac J. 1994;31:473–81.

Aroson J.: **Biological and clinical evaluation of distraction osteogenesis.** Clin Orthop 1994;3012-3.

Aroson J.: **Biology of distraction osteogenesis In:** Bianchi-Maiocchi A., Aronson J., editors. Operative principles of Ilizarov. Baltimore: Williams & Wilkins 1991pp.27-32.

Baratz M., Watson A. D., Imbriglia J. E.: ***Orthopaedic surgery: the essentials.*** New York: Thieme Medical Publishers; 1999:517.

Bianchi Maiocchi A., Aronson, editors: **Operative principles of Ilizarov.** Baltimore, MD: Williams and Wilkins 1991pp.63-4.

Boszotta H., Helperstorfer W., Kölndorfer G., Prunner K.: **Long-term results of surgical management of displaced tibial head fractures.***Aktuelle Traumatol* 1993, **23**–4:178–82.

Boyd H. B.: **Congenital pseudoarthrosis treatment by dual bone grafts.** J. Bone Joint Surg 1941 Jul;23(3):497-515.

Boyd H. B., Lipinski S. W., Wiley J. H.: **Observations on non-union of the shafts of the long bones, with a statistical analysis of 842 patients.** J Bone Joint Surg 1961 Mar;43(2):159-68.

Boyd H. B., Lipinski S. W.: **Nonunion of trochanteric and subtrochanteric fractures.** Surg Gynecol Obstet 1957 Apr;104(4):463-70.

Calhoun J. H., Li F., Bauford W. L.: **Rigidity of half pins for the Ilizarov external fixator**. Bull Hosp J Dis.1992;52:21–6.

Campbell's *Operative orthopaedics*. 11th edition. Philadelphia: Mosby Elsevier; 2007.

Catagni M., Ottaviani G., Maggioni M.: **Treatment strategies for complex fractures of the tibial plateau with external circular fixation and limited internal fixation.** *J Trauma* 2007, **63–5:**1043–53.

Checketts R. G., Otterburn M., Mac Eachern A. G.: **Pin track infection; definition, incidence and prevention.** *Int J OrthopTrauma*1993,3(Suppl 3):16–18.

Cierny G. 3rd, Zorn K. E.. **Segmental tibial defects. Comparing conventional and Ilizarov methodologies.** Clin Orthop Relat Res 1994 Apr(301):118-23.

Codivilla A.: **On the means of lengthening, in the lower limbs, the muscles and tissues which are shortened through deformity.** Clin Orthop Relat Res 1994 Apr;3014-9.

Codivilla A.: **On the means of lengthening in the lower limbs, the muscles and tissues which are shortened through deformity.** Am J Orthop Surg. 1905;2:353–69.

Coglianese D. B., Herzenberg J. E., Goulet J. A.: **Physical therapy management of patients undergoing limb lengthening by distraction osteogenesis.** J Orthop Sports Phys Ther. 1993;17:124–32.

Colletti P., Greenberg H., Terk M. R.: **MR findings in patients with acute tibial plateau fractures.** *Comput Med Imaging Graph* 1996, **20–5:**389–394.

Corrales L. A., Morshed S., Bhandari M., Miclau T. 3rd: **Variability in the assessment of fracture-healing in orthopaedic trauma studies.** *J Bone Joint Surg Am* 2008, **90–9:**1862–8.

Cross A. R., Lewis D. D., Murphy S. T.: **Effects of ring diameter and wire tension on the axial biomechanics of four ring circular external fixator constructs.** Am J Vet Res. 2001;62:1025–30.

Davies R., Holt N., Nayagam S.: **The care of pin sites with external fixation.** *J Bone Joint Surg Br* 2005, **87–5:**716–719.

Davis B. J., Roberts P. J., Moorcroft C. I., Brown M. F., Thomas P. B., Wade R. H.: **Reliability of radiographs in defining union of internal fixed fractures.** *Injury* 2004, **35–6:**557–61.

Dendrinos G. K., Kontos S., Katsenis D., Dalas A.: **Treatment of high-energy tibial plateau fractures by the Ilizarov circular fixator.** *J Bone Joint Surg Br* 1996, **78–5:**710–7.

Dirschl D. R.., Del Gaizo D.: **Staged management of tibial plateau fractures.** *Am J Orthop* 2007, **36–4**:12–7.

Dujardyn J., Lammens J.: Treatment **of delayed non-union ro non-union of tibial shaft with partial fibulectomy and Ilizarov frame:** Acta Orthop Belg 2007 Oct;73(5):630-4.

Eggli S., Hartel M. J., Kohl S., Haupt U., Exadaktylos A. K., Röder C.: **Unstable bicondylar tibial plateau fractures: a clinical investigation.** *J Orthop Trauma* 2008, **22–10**:673–9.

Egol K. A., Tejwani N. C., Capla EL, Wolinsky P. L., Koval K. J.: **Staged management of high-energy proximal tibia fractures (OTA types 41): the results of a prospective, standardized protocol.** *J Orthop Trauma* 2005, **19–7**:448–55.

Farmanullah Khan M. S., Awais S. M.: **Evaluation of management of Tibial non-union defect with Ilizarnv fixator.** J Ayub Med Coll Abbottabad 2007 Jul–Sep;19(3):34-6.

Fitch R. D., Thompson J. G., Rizk W. S., Seaber A. V., Garrett W. E. Jr.: **The effects of the Ilizarov distraction technique on bone and muscle in a canine model.** Iowa Orthop J 1996;1610-19.

Fleming B., Paley D., Kristiansen T., Pope M.: **A biomechanical analysis of the Ilizarov external fixator.** *Clin Orthop Relat Res* 1989,241:95–105.

Fowler B. L., Dall B. E., Rowe D. E.: **Complications associated with harvesting autogenous iliac bone graft.** *Am J Orthop* 1995, **24**:895–903.

Frierson M., Ibrahim K., Boles M., Bote H., Ganey T.: **Distraction osteogenesis. A comparison of corticotomy techniques.** Clin Orthop. 1994;301:19–24.

Galardi G., Comi G., Lozza L., Marchettini P., Novarina M., et al.: **Peripheral nerve damage during limb lengthening. Neurophysiology in five cases of bilateral tibial lengthening.** J Bone Joint Surg Br.1990;72:121–4.

Gasser B., Boman B., Wyder D.: **Stiffness characteristics of the circular Ilizarov device as opposed to conventional external fixators.** J Biomech Eng. 1990;112:15–21.

Gaston P, Will EM, Keating JF: **Recovery of knee function following fracture of the tibial plateau.** *J Bone Joint Surg Br* 2005, **87–9**:1233–6.

Gausewitz S., Hohl M.: **The significance of early motion in treatment of tibial plateau fractures.** *Clin Orthop Relat Res* 1986, **202**:135–8.

Gershuni D. H., Pinsker R.: **Bone grafting for nonunion of fractures of the tibia: a critical review.** J Trauma 1982 Jan;22(1):43-9.

Gustilo R. B.: **Fractures of the tibial plateau.** In *Fractures and dislocations.* St. Louis: CV Mosby; 1993:945.

Ilizarov G. A.: **Clinical application of the tension-stress effect for limb lengthening.** Clin Orthop Relat Res 1990 Jan(250):8-26.

Ilizarov G. A.: **The tension-stress effect on the genesis and growth of tissues. Part I. The influence of stability of fixation and soft-tissue preservation.** Clin Orthop Relat Res 1989 Jan(238):249-81.

Ilizarov G. A., Emilyanova H. S., Lebedev B. E.: **Perosseus compression and distraction osteosynthesis. Traumatology and Orthopaedics.** Kurgan: 1972. Some experimental studies. Mechanical characteristics of Kirschner wires; pp. 34–47. l.

Ilizarov G. A., Ledyasev V. I., Shitin V. P.: **Experimental studies of bone lengthening.** Eksp Khir Anesteziol.1969;14:3.

Ilizarov G. A., Shevistov V. I.: **Compression, distraction-osteosynthesis apparatus of G.A Ilizarov for the treatment of pseudoarthrosis and bony defects of humerus.** In: Transosseous osteosynthesis in traumatology and orthopaedics. Vol. 1. Kurgan, USSR 1972p.144.

Ilizarov GA. **Clinical application of the tension-stress effect for limb lengthening.** Clin Orthop.1990;250:8–26.

Ilizarov G. A.: **The tension-stress effect on the genesis and growth of tissues**: Part I. The influence of stability of fixation and sort tissue preservation. Clin Orthop. 1989;238:249–81.

Ilizarov GA. The **tension-stress effect on the genesis and growth of tissues: Part II**. The influence of the rate and frequency of distraction. Clin Orthop. 1989;239:263–85.

Ilizarov G. A.: **A New Principle of Osteosynthesis with the Use of Crossing Pins and Rings.** In *Collected Scientific Works of the Kurgan Regional Scientific Medical Society.* Edited by: Ilizarov G. A. Kurgan: Union of Soviet Socialists Republic; 1954:145–160.

Ilizarov G. A.: *Transosseous osteosynthesis.* 1st edition. Berlin Heidelberger New York: Springer Verlag; 1992.

Ippolito E., Peretti G., Bellocci M., Farsetti P., Tudisco C., et al.: **Histology and ultrastructure of arteries, veins and peripheral nerves during limb lengthening.** Clin Orthop. 1994;308:54–62.

Kemefuna O., Saqib H., Cary B., Chapman M. D.: **Ilizarov external fixator for stump salvage in infected non-unions.** Orthopaedics 2013 Aug;36(8):e.99094.

Lee D. Y., Choi I. H., Chung C. Y., Chung P. H., Chi J. G., Suh Y. L.: **Effect of tibial length ening on the gastrocnemius muscle. A histopathologic and morphometric study in rabbits.** Acta Orthop Scand.1993;64:688–92.

Lee D. Y., Chung C. Y., Choi I. H.: **Longitudinal growth of the rabbit tibia after callotasis.** J Bone Joint Surg Br. 1993;75:898–903.

Lee J. A., Papadakis S. A., Moon C., Zalavras C. G.: **Tibial plateau fractures treated with less invasive stabilisation system.** *Int Orthop* 2007,31–3:415–418.

Lucht U., Pilgaard S.: **Fractures of the tibial condyles.** *Acta Orthop Scand* 1971, **42**:366–76.

Ma C. H., Wu C. H., Yu S. W., Yen C. Y., Tu Y. K.: **Staged external and internal less-invasive stabilization system plating for open proximal tibia fractures.** *Injury* 2010, 41–2:190–196.

Maripuri S. N., Rao P., Manoj-Thomas A., Mohanthy K.: **The classification systems for tibial plateau fractures: how reliable are they?** *Injury* 2008, 39–10:1216–1221.

Marsh J. L., Buckwalter J., Gelberman R., Dirschl D., Olson S., Brown T., Llinias A.: **Articular fractures: Does an anatomical reduction really change the result?** *J Bone Joint Surg Am* 2002, **84A**–7:1259–71.

McKee M. D., Wild L. M., Schemitsch E. H., Waddell J. P.: **The use of antibiotic-impregnated, osteoconductive, bioabsorbable bone substitute in the treatment of infected long bone defects: Early results of a prospective trial.** J Orthop Trauma. 2002;16:622–7.

McKee M. D., Yoo D., Schemetisch E. H.: **Health status after Ilizarov reconstruction of post-traumatic lower-limb deformity.** *J Bone Joint Surg Br* 1998, **80**–2:360–4.

Mehtab A., Pirvwani M., Aslam Siddiqui, Yunis H.: **Management of infected nonunion tibia by intercalary bone transport.** Pak J Surg 2008;24(1):26-30.

Mikulak S. A., Gold S. M., Zinar D. M.: **Small wire external fixation of high energy tibial plateau fractures.** *Clin Orthop Relat Res* 1998,**356**:230–8.

Milch H.: **Tibiofibularsynostosis for non-union of the tibia.** Surgery 1950 May;27(5):770-9.

Moore T. M., Patzakis M. J., Harvey J. P.: **Tibial fractures: definition, demographics, treatment rationale, and long-term results of closed traction management or operative reduction.** *J Orthop Trauma* 1987, **1**–2:97–119.

Müller M. E., Nazarian S., Koch P., Schatzker J.: *The comprehensive classification of fractures of long bones.* New York: Springer; 1990.

Paley D.: **Problems, obstacles and complications of limb lengthening by Ilizarov technique.** Clin Orthop Relat Res 1990 Jan;25081-104.

Paley D., Catagni M. A., Argnani F., Villa A., Benedetti G. B., Cattaneo R.: **Ilizarov treatment of tibial nonunions with bone loss.** Clin Orthop Relat Res 1989 Apr;241146-65.

Paley D., Testworth K.: **Percutaneous osteotomies with osteotome and gigli saw technique.** Oethop Clin North Am 1991 Oct;22(4):613-24.

Paley D., Testworth K. D.: **Deformity correction by the Ilizarov technique.** In: Chapman MW, Editors: Green S. A., Aronson J., Paley D., Tetsworth D., Taylor J. C. **Operative Orthopeadics** 3rd ed 2001:Lippincott Williams publicationp.883-948.

Paley D.: **Principles of Deformity Correction.** Berlin: Springer; 2001.

Papagelopoulos P. J., Partisinevelos A. A., Themitocleous G. S., Mvrogenis A. F., Korres D. S., Soucacos P. N.: **Complications after tibial plateau fracture surgery.** *Injury* 2006, **6:**475–484.

Parameswaran A. D., Roberts C. S., Seligson D., Voor M.: **Pin tract infection with contemporary external fixation: How much of a problem?** *J Orthop Trauma* 2003, 17–7:503–7.

Park S., Ahn J., Gee A. O., Kuntz A. F., Esterhai J. L.: **Compartment syndrome in tibial fractures.** *J Orthop Trauma* 2009, **23**–7:514–8.

Piza G., Caja V. L., Gonzalez-Viejo M. A.: **Hydroxyapatite-coated external-fixation pins. The effect on pin loosening and pin-tract infection in lengthening for short stature.** J Bone Joint Surg Br. 2004;86:892–7.

Podolsky A., Chao E. Y.: **Mechanical performance of Ilizarov circular frame exter nal fixators in comparison with other external fixators.** Clin Orthop. 1993;293:61–70.

Pommer A., Muhr G., David A.: **Hydroxyapatite-coated Schantz pins in external fixators for distraction osteogenesis: a randomised, controlled trial.** J Bone Joint Surg Am. 2002;84:1162–6.

Rasmussen P. S.: *A functional approach to evaluation and treatment of tibial condylar fractures. Ph.D. thesis.* Gothenburg: Gothenburg University Elanders Boktryckeri Aktiebolag; 1971.

Rockwood and Green's *Fractures in adults*. 6th edition. Philadelphia: Lippincott Williams & Wilkins; 2006.

Rodriguez-Merchan E. C., Forriol F.: **Nonunion: general principles and experimental data**. Clin Orthop Relat Res 2004 Feb(419):4-12.

Rosen H.: **The treatment of nonunions and pseudarthroses of the humeral shaft**. Orthop Clin North Am 1990 Oct;21(4):725-42.

Rozbruch S. R., Ilizarov S.: **Limb Lengthening and Reconstruction Surgery**. New York: Informa Healthcare; 2007.

Russel T. A., Leighton R. K.: **Comparison of autogenous bone graft and endothermic calcium phosphate cement for defect augmentation in tibial plateau fractures. A multicentre, prospective, randomized study.** *J Bone Surg Am* 2008, **90–10**:2057–61.

Sahu R. L., Sikdar J.: **Fracture union in closed interlocking nail in femoral fracture.** JNMA J Nepal Med Assoc 2010 Jul–Sep;49(179):228-31.

Saleh Al-Harby W.: **Ilizarov technique in correcting limb deformities**. Bahrain Med Bull 1995 Jun;17(2):-00.

Schatzker J., McBroom R., Bruce D.: **The tibial plateau fracture. The Toronto experience 1968–1975.** *Clin Orthop Relat Res* 1979, **138**:94–104.

Schatzker J.: **Tibial plateau fractures**. In *Skeletal trauma*. Edited by: Browner B. D., Jupiter B. B., Levine A. M., Philadelphia WB Saunders; 1993:1745.

Segal D., Mallik A. R., Wetzler M. J., Franchi A. V., Whitelaw G. P.: **Early weight-bearing of lateral tibial plateau fractures.** *Clin Orthop Relat Res*1993, **294**:232–7.

Seiler J. G. 3rd, Johnson J.: **Iliac crest autogenous bone grafting: donor site complications.** *J South Orthop Assoc* 2000, **9**:91–7.

Sen C., Eralp L., Genus T.: **An alternative method for the treatment of nonunion of tibia with bone loss.** J Bone Joint Surg Br 2006 Jun;88(6):783-9.

Tejwani N. C., Achan: **Staged management of high-energy proximal tibia fractures.** *Bull Hosp Jt Dis* 2004, **62**:62–66.

The Canadian Orthopaedic Trauma Society: **Open reduction and internal fixation compared with the circular fixator application for bicondylar tibial plateau fractures. Results of a multicentre, prospective, randomised clinical trial.** *J Bone Joint Surg Am* 2006, **88–12**:2613–2623.

Tscherne H., Lobenhoffer P.: **Tibial plateau fractures: management and expected results.** *Clin Orthop* 1993, **292:**87–100.

Vauhkonen M., Peltonen J., Karaharju E., Aalto K., Alitalo I.: **Collagen synthesis and mineralization in the early phase of distraction bone healing.** Bone Miner. 1990;10:171–81.

Velazquez R. J., Bell D. F., Armstrong P. F., Babyn P., Tibshirani R.: **Complications of use of the Ilizarov technique in the correction of limb deformities in children.** J Bone Joint Surg Am. 1993;75:1148–56.

Wagner H.: **Operative lengthening of the femur.** Clin Orthop. 1978;136:125–42.

Watson J. T., Coufal C.: **Treatment of complex lateral plateau fractures using Ilizarov techniques.** *Clin Orthop Relat Res* 1998, **353:**97–106.

Ylmaz E., Belhan O., Karakurt L., Arslan N., Serin E.: **Mechanical performance of hybrid Ilizarov external fixator in comparison with the Ilizarov circular external fixator.** *Clin Biomech* 2003, **18–6:**518–522.

Young M. J., Barrack R. L.: **Complications of internal fixation of tibial plateau fractures.** *Orthop*

ZumBrunnen J. L., Brindley H. H.: **Nonunion of the shafts of the long bones. A review and analysis of 140 cases.** JAMA 1968 Feb;203(9):637-40.